Mental Health and Care Homes

Mental Health and Care Homes

Edited by

Tom Dening
Consultant Psychiatrist and Medical Director,
Cambridgeshire and Peterborough NHS Foundation Trust,
Cambridge, UK

Alisoun Milne
Reader in Social Gerontology,
School of Social Policy, Sociology and Social Research
University of Kent, UK

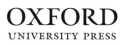

OXFORD
UNIVERSITY PRESS

OXFORD
UNIVERSITY PRESS

Great Clarendon Street, Oxford OX2 6DP

Oxford University Press is a department of the University of Oxford.
It furthers the University's objective of excellence in research, scholarship,
and education by publishing worldwide in

Oxford New York

Athens Auckland Bangkok Bogotá Buenos Aires Cape Town
Chennai Dar es Salaam Delhi Florence Hong Kong Istanbul Karachi
Kolkata Kuala Lumpur Madrid Melbourne Mexico City Mumbai Nairobi
Paris São Paulo Shanghai Singapore Taipei Tokyo Toronto Warsaw

with associated companies in Berlin Ibadan

Oxford is a registered trade mark of Oxford University Press
in the UK and in certain other countries

Published in the United States
by Oxford University Press Inc., New York

British Library Cataloguing in Publication Data
Data available

Library of Congress Cataloguing in Publication Data
Library of Congress Control Number: 2011923159

Typeset in Minion by Glyph International, Bangalore, India
Printed in Great Britain on acid-free paper
by CPI Antony Rowe, Chippenham, Wiltshire

ISBN 978–0–19–959363–7

10 9 8 7 6 5 4 3 2 1

Whilst every effort has been made to ensure that the contents of this book are as complete,
accurate and up-to-date as possible at the date of writing, Oxford University Press is not able to give
any guarantee or assurance that such is the case. Readers are urged to take appropriately qualified
medical advice in all cases. The information in this book is intended to be useful to the general
reader, but should not be used as a means of self-diagnosis or for the prescription of medication.

Dedication

This book is dedicated to our families and to older people in care homes, wherever they may be.

Foreword

Dame Philippa Russell

Mental health and care homes: promoting quality care and good practice

The publication of *Mental Health and Care Homes* could not be more timely, as we debate the future of care services in the context of an ageing population. It is particularly encouraging to see that the two related issues of care homes and the mental health of care home residents are starting to attract much greater attention, both in terms of public policy and good practice. As the launch of the National Dementia Strategy and the creation of the Care Quality Commission in 2009 demonstrate, there is national commitment to raising and monitoring high standards of care. But we are all well aware of a challenging agenda ahead in achieving these objectives.

Although prevalence of mental health problems in care home residents is high, it is relatively under-researched. The sector is large, with over 400,000 residents in the United Kingdom. Similar numbers of staff are employed and residential care is therefore an area of considerable social and economic significance. It is also a growth area. The past decade has seen major changes in policy, practice, and expectations around the care and support of older people. The personalization agenda has seen a philosophical shift towards greater independence, choice, and control for service users of all ages, with social care to both younger and older disabled people being increasingly provided in the community. But support in a family home is not necessarily the best option when the person concerned is very frail and has dementia or related mental health problems. Care home residents are often very old; many have multiple physical and mental health problems. Their admission to a home often follows a crisis such as hospital admission and their care poses particular challenges. Sadly, this population tends to be profoundly marginalized and is often invisible in the wider debates about quality of care. But residential care should matter to all of us, although it is too often seen as a 'last resort' and the result of a failure to care by family and friends. Yet good group care can, and should, be seen as integral to any high quality national care system and the elderly residents valued as equal citizens with the right to a good life in a *care home* that is very definitely their *own home*.

As the UK's population ages, so the challenge of how best to achieve a good quality of life in later life will affect us all. Many residential care homes have closed and there have been several high profile cases about institutional abuse. But improved life expectancy has also brought more complex health needs and in some cases much greater dependency in old age. Dementia is one of our greatest challenges for the future and, with greater dependency, recognition that residential care may actually be a positive choice rather than a last resort.

Communal living has always been the preferred option for some older people and self-funders in particular have made conscious choices to move into a residential home. My own mother-in-law, anxious about remaining in her own house with multiple health problems and failing sight, declined to move in with either of her two sons. She (and we) chose a small care home and she was very happy. Her only anger at the big changes in her life was when a grandson talked about '*Granny lives in a home now*'. 'I do NOT live in a home', she retorted, '*this is MY home and I chose to come here*'.

In recent years, there has been increasing research interest into various aspects of mental health in care homes, for example depression, prescribing of psychotropic drugs, but there is no single account that synthesises this work into a single text. This book importantly addresses this deficit and provides a coherent, clinically informed, and evidence-based review of the key issues that are in, and round, the delivery of good quality care in care homes around mental health. One of the book's key strengths is that it successfully fuses expertise and research from both the health and social care fields as well as offering perspectives from inside and outside the care home sector. Very positively, it presents complex issues in an accessible manner for a potentially wide readership. This will not only include professionals but also care workers, researchers, those advising or representing the interests of older people, and families of those in care homes or considering admission.

The contributors to *Mental Health and Care Homes* bring a fresh, rich, and illuminating perspective to an area of policy and practice that is often viewed negatively. Most importantly, the book reminds us that entering residential care need not be seen as a 'last resort' but rather one of the range of options available to all of us when we need additional support in later life. As the author Diana Athill commented in a BBC interview with Alan Yentob,

> I dreaded going into a "home". I thought all the other residents would be asleep all the time, no interest, nothing to do. But actually I found the other residents to be really interesting people with a richness of experience that more than compensated for physical fragility. We have found plenty of shared interests. The most important thing is to see yourself "at home" and not "in a home". And it is comforting to know that there is always someone to look out for you when you are ill.

Not everyone entering a care home can have Diana Athill's intellectual energy and positive outcomes. But this book should help to ensure that many more older people and their families do have good experiences when they move into a care home and find their mental, emotional and physical well-being enhanced rather than diminished by the experience.

Dame Philippa Russell,
Chair,
Standing Commission on Carers
July 2010

Acknowledgements

The editors would like to thank all our authors for their enthusiastic support of this enterprise, and Charlotte Green and Martin Baum at Oxford University Press for their encouragement. You have all been a great pleasure to work with. TD thanks Cambridgeshire and Peterborough NHS Foundation Trust for allowing time spent on this book. TD is a member of the Cambridgeshire and Peterborough NIHR-CLAHRC (National Institute for Health Research-Collaboration for Leadership in Applied Health Research and Care). AM is a Trustee of the Alzheimer's and Dementia Support Services in Kent and a member of the NIHR Mental Health Research Network on Personalisation in Dementia and the Standing Commission on Carers.

Contents

List of contributors *xiii*

Introduction *1*
Alisoun Milne and Tom Dening

Part 1 **The inside view—living in a care home**

1 A resident's view *9*
Pat Singer

2 A carer's account *13*
Eric Berger

3 A care home manager's view *21*
Marsha Tuffin

4 Creative work with residents *29*
John Killick and Lynda Martin

5 Hearing the voice of older people with dementia *41*
Dorothy Runnicles

6 Living with dementia in a care home: a review of
research evidence *53*
Alisoun Milne

Part 2 **The outside view**

7 Regulation and quality *69*
Rekha Elaswarapu

8 Funding: paying for residential care for older people *89*
Theresia Bäumker and Ann Netten

9 Legal aspects *101*
Amanda Keeling

10 Abuse in care homes for older people: the case for safeguards *113*
Hilary Brown

11 Long-term care: an international perspective *131*
Ricardo Rodrigues and Frédérique Hoffmann

Part 3 **Mental health and care**

12 Meeting mental health needs *149*
Tom Dening

13 Dementia in care homes *161*
Janya Freer and Vellingiri Raja Badrakalimuthu

14 Depression in care homes *179*
Briony Dow, Xiaoping Lin, Jean Tinney, Betty Haralambous,
and David Ames

15 Functional mental illness *191*
Catherine Hatfield and Tom Dening

16 Psychosocial interventions in care homes *205*
Graham Stokes

17 Support to care homes *221*
Amanda Thompsell

18 Working with minorities in care homes *237*
Jill Manthorpe and Jo Moriarty

19 Physical health issues *251*
Clive Bowman

20 Palliative care and end-of-life care *265*
Elizabeth L. Sampson and Karen Harrison Dening

Part 4 **Promoting health and well-being**

21 Promoting health and well-being: good practice
inside the care homes *279*
Dawn Brooker

22 Good practice outside the care homes *297*
Claire Goodman and Sue L. Davies

23 Risk and choice *313*
Sheila Furness

24 Dementia training in care homes *327*
Buz Loveday

25 *My* home life: exploring the evidence base for best practice *345*
Julienne Meyer and Tom Owen

26 Conclusion: key themes and future directions *365*
Tom Dening and Alisoun Milne

Index *373*

List of contributors

David Ames
Professor of Ageing and Health,
University of Melbourne and Director,
National Ageing Research Institute,
Victoria, Australia

Vellingiri Raja Badrakalimuthu
Specialist Registrar in Old Age
Psychiatry, Cambridgeshire and
Peterborough NHS Foundation Trust
Cambridge, UK

Theresia Bäumker
Research Officer, Personal Social
Services Research Unit, University of
Kent, Canterbury, UK

Eric Berger
Was the main carer for his wife Daisy,
who had dementia.
Cambridge, UK

Clive Bowman
Medical Director, Bupa Care Services,
UK

Dawn Brooker
Professor and Director of the
University of Worcester Association
for Dementia Studies,
University of Worcester,
Worcester, UK

Hilary Brown
Professor of Social Care at Canterbury
Christ Church University
Tunbridge Wells, UK

Sue L. Davies
Research Fellow, Centre for
Research in Primary and Community
Care Older People's Health,
University of Hertfordshire,
Hatfield, UK

Karen Harrison Dening
National Practice Development Lead for
Admiral Nursing, Dementia UK and
seconded to National Council for
Palliative Care and Marie Curie
Palliative Care Research Unit, UCL,
London, UK

Tom Dening
Consultant Psychiatrist and Medical
Director, Cambridgeshire and
Peterborough NHS Foundation Trust
Cambridge, UK

Briony Dow
Director of the Preventive and Public
Health Division, National Ageing
Research Institute,
Victoria, Australia

Rekha Elaswarapu
Strategy Development Manager
(older people), Care Quality
Commission and Honorary Senior
Visiting Fellow, City University,
London, UK

Janya Freer
Consultant in Old Age Psychiatry,
Cambridgeshire and Peterborough NHS
Foundation Trust, UK

Sheila Furness
Senior Lecturer, Division of Social
Work and Social Care,
University of Bradford, UK

Claire Goodman
Professor of Health Care Research,
Centre for Research in Primary and
Community Care, University of
Hertfordshire,
Hatfield, UK

Betty Haralambous
Research Fellow, National Ageing
Research Institute,
Victoria, Australia

Catherine Hatfield
Specialist Registrar in Old Age
Psychiatry, Cambridgeshire
and Peterborough NHS
Foundation Trust, UK

Frédérique Hoffmann
Researcher and International Relations
Attachée, European Centre for
Social Welfare Policy and Research,
Vienna, Austria

Amanda Keeling
Research Assistant, Cambridge
Intellectual and Developmental
Disabilities Research Group,
Department of Psychiatry,
University of Cambridge
Cambridge, UK

John Killick
Poet and writer and one of the partners
of Dementia Positive

Xiaoping Lin
PhD student at the National Ageing
Research Institute,
Victoria, Australia

Buz Loveday
Lead Trainer, DementiaTrainers
(Buz Loveday and Associates),
London, UK

Jill Manthorpe
Professor of Social Work,
King's College London and
Director of the Social Care
Workforce Research Unit
London, UK

Lynda Martin
Partnership and Development Manager,
Cambridgeshire Libraries,
Cambridgeshire, UK

Julienne Meyer
Professor of Nursing, Care for Older
People, and Executive Director,
My Home Life Programme,
City University London, UK

Alisoun Milne
Reader in Social Gerontology,
School of Social Policy,
Sociology and Social Research
University of Kent, UK

Jo Moriarty
Research Fellow, Social Care Workforce
Research Unit, King's College London,
London, UK

Ann Netten
Professor of Social Welfare and Director,
Personal Social Services Research Unit,
University of Kent,
Canterbury, UK

Tom Owen
Director, My Home Life Programme,
City University London,
London, UK

Greg Prior (cover design)
Lives in Cambridge, UK

Ricardo Rodrigues
Researcher, European Centre for Social
Welfare Policy and Research,
Vienna, Austria

Dorothy Runnicles
Older person advisor, researcher, and
advocate

Dame Philippa Russell
Chair, Standing Commission on Carers,
c/o National Children's Bureau,
London, UK

Elizabeth L. Sampson
Senior Lecturer in Psychiatric and
Supportive Care of the Elderly,
Department of Mental
Health Sciences, UCL,
London, UK

Pat Singer
Lives in an Abbeyfield Society Care
Home in Cambridge, UK

Graham Stokes
Director of Dementia Care,
Bupa Care Services, UK

Amanda Thompsell
Consultant in Old Age Psychiatry,
South London and Maudsley NHS
Foundation Trust
London, UK

Jean Tinney
Research Fellow, National Ageing
Research Institute,
Victoria, Australia

Marsha Tuffin
Registered Manager of Brown's
Field House, an Abbeyfield Society Care
Home in Cambridge, UK

Introduction

Alisoun Milne and Tom Dening

First of all, what is a care home? Throughout this book, the term 'care home' is used to refer to two previously distinct groups of long-term care facilities: nursing homes and residential homes, or alternatively, care homes with and without nursing. Care homes can be provided by either the independent or voluntary sector, or public agencies (local authorities or the National Health Service [NHS]). Approximately three-quarters of all homes are run by private providers, a sixth by not-for-profit organizations, and just over a tenth are operating within the public sector (Laing and Buisson, 2009).

In the United Kingdom, 5% of those aged 65 years and over live in a care home. The proportion increases with age; while this is the case for only 0.8% of the 65- to 74-year-old cohort, the figure rises to16.2% for those aged 85 years and over (Laing and Buisson, 2009). About one person in five will eventually move into residential or nursing care; 150,000 people are admitted every year. Approximately two-thirds of care home residents are women aged 75 years or over. Older people from ethnic minorities are underrepresented. Overall, there are approximately 500,000 places in about 18,500 homes in the United Kingdom (Laing and Buisson, 2009; Office of Fair Trading, 2005). Care homes constitute a substantial sector of the economy, employing some 450,000 staff and representing a total value of over £13 billion (Laing and Buisson, 2009).

Most care home residents have multiple health problems, particularly in relationship to mobility, mental health, and continence (Dening and Milne, 2009). It has been estimated that at least two-thirds of residents have dementia irrespective of whether the care home provides 'specialist care' for this population or not (Alzheimer's Society, 2007a; Matthews and Dening, 2002). In fact, dementia—in combination with difficulties in performing activities of daily living—is the strongest health-related determinant for care home admission (Department of Health, 2009a,b). In addition, an estimated half of all care home residents have depressive disorders that would warrant intervention and other mental health problems such as anxiety are not uncommon (Dening and Milne, 2008). Certainly the care home population is older and frailer than it was 10 years ago and significantly more dependent (Commission for Social Care Inspection, 2008a). Care homes constitute the second most common location for death after acute hospitals.

It is important to recognize that care homes operate within a complex context of user need, funding, providers, and policy initiatives (Froggatt et al., 2009; Wanless, 2006). The policy agenda has increasingly moved towards offering service users more personalized care and choice, the promotion of independence, and joined-up care. Several recent policies aimed at improving the quality and nature of care include: *Shaping the Future of Care Together* (HM Government, 2009), the *National Dementia Strategy* (Department of Health, 2009a), and the recent *Building a National Care Service* (HM Government, 2010).

These policies, particularly the National Dementia Strategy, highlight the need to improve the quality of care and support in care homes (Department of Health, 2009a). In order to achieve this, care homes need a well-trained specialist workforce; consistent and coherent access to NHS primary care and specialist mental health services; and to be supported by an inspection regime that is committed to driving up quality (Care Quality Commission, 2010; Department of Health, 2008). They also place considerable emphasis on user involvement (HM Government, 2007). For example, there is an expectation that residents' experiences will be captured in inspection activities, including those with advanced dementia (Commission for Social Care Inspection, 2008b). Initial funding of £150 million over the next 2 years has been committed to fund the implementation of the strategy, a portion of which will be invested in workforce development including care home staff (Department of Health, 2009b).

There is limited consensus in the available literature about what factors affect quality of care in care homes but it is likely to be influenced by a mix of internal and external issues (Warner et al., 2010). Factors outside the control of individual homes include the regulatory and competitive environment. It has been suggested that staff attitudes, behaviours, and interaction with residents are mediating factors between features of the care home environment (facilities, management, workforce) and outcomes in the form of residents' well-being and quality of life (Gage et al., 2009). We have to bear in mind that these establishments are places where older people live, so there is an important balance to be struck between regulation and homeliness, as well as the inevitable compromises of taste involved in communal living. Not everything that happens in a care home is necessarily viewed as 'care': much of it is activity. Residents are participants as well as recipients. We hope that the contents of this book will shed new and additional light onto these complex intersecting issues.

There is certainly a gap in our knowledge of the experiences of people living in care homes and for various reasons there has been very limited investment in research to capture their needs and wishes (Milne, 2010). Residents of care homes form an almost invisible population since they are often physically frail and do not venture far beyond the walls of the home, or perhaps because many of them have dementia and lack the capacity to do (some) things for themselves. They also tend to exist outside the boundaries of 'ordinary society' and community and are 'off the radar' of the majority of initiatives that aim to engage citizens or address marginalization. If a yardstick of active citizenship is having a front door opening onto the street, then care home residents live a long way back from this point. If social inclusion is about being able to access the things that most of us take for granted, then older people in care homes are excluded in the most fundamental way. There are a number of serious difficulties in being able to engage freely in dialogue with people who may have dementia and/or communication problems and/or sensory difficulties. However, if we are serious about improving the quality of care in care homes it is pivotal that we find ways to engage with care home residents across these practical barriers, and across the social barriers of prejudice and ageism. Some approaches to meeting these challenges are described in the book (Alzheimer's Society, 2007b).

In view of the accumulating evidence, it is perfectly reasonable to argue that mental health has become the core business of care homes. Even for those without a formal diagnosis, quality of life *and* care are inextricably entwined with residents' mental health. We confidently expect that this issue will become more, rather than less, important in the future as a consequence of the projected increase in the number of very old (over 85) people and the likely growth in demand for care home places, especially for people with dementia.

We believe that there is a distinct need for a book that highlights mental health issues in care home settings and brings together recent research findings and experience of good practice. However, it needs to be more than just a textbook of old psychiatry aimed at care home staff and to have a focus that is broader than dementia, important though this is. Existing work can be divided into two camps: relatively general accounts of care homes, written from social care or general medical perspectives and texts which offer summaries of mental health problems among care home populations. The strength of our approach is that we cover both aspects. Not only do we discuss mental health issues *within* the care home itself, but we also consider what constitutes 'good quality care' and have used a wide lens of analysis of the issues that can influence the experience of living in a care home.

We also think our orientation is quite different. It's the mental *health* of care home residents this book is focusing on, not just their mental health *problems*; even among those people with advanced dementia there is still potential to enhance or promote mental health rather than just treating or managing the symptoms of mental illness (Livingstone et al., 2008; Milne, 2009). The book also faces in two directions: it seeks ways to promote good practice and enhance residents' quality of life internally—towards the home itself including staff, resources, and practice—and externally—towards health services, inspection regimes, and training initiatives.

This book offers a coherent and evidence-based overview of the issues around mental health in care homes for older people. It opens with first-hand accounts of care home life, from a resident, a carer, a manager, and people who work directly with listening to and/or capturing the voices of people with dementia. The second section moves on to discuss the regulatory, funding, and legislative context in which care homes operate including drawing on international experiences. In the third section, we explore the mental health and other needs of care home residents in detail and the last section brings together a range of expert chapters—providing key examples—on good practice in delivering high quality care and supporting care home residents and staff. We conclude the book by summarizing key themes and looking to the future.

Inevitably there are some boundaries in our subject matter. We have largely concentrated on the United Kingdom, and some of the detail about policy and regulation may be more applicable to England than anywhere else. However, the broader principles are applicable across many countries, and the ageing population and increasing prevalence of dementia are global phenomena that should interest an international audience. The book is about older people in care homes, so it does not deal with children or with people who spend their whole lives in residential care, such as some people with complex needs and learning disabilities. We do discuss older people with learning disabilities but only in relation to their long-term care needs as they age, and how this intersects with the general provision of residential care for older people.

The book is intended to be a source text accessible to a wide readership and is targeted at a broad professional and vocational audience. Readers will include: staff managing and working in care homes, health and social work students and professionals, and researchers. We also hope that it will attract readers among third sector organizations, carers and relatives, and older people themselves. Contributors are experts in their fields and are from a mixture of health and social care backgrounds; some authors are experts by experience. This not only ensures that all the key perspectives are represented but also situates the book, quite rightly, inside both the health and social care arenas and discourses. Our main aim is to stimulate discussion, capture good practice, and advance work to improve the quality of care of elderly residents in care homes. After all, they are our future selves, and even if we never need the services of residential care directly, almost all of us will have our lives touched by care homes in some way at some point.

References

Alzheimer's Society (2007a). *Dementia UK*. London: Alzheimer's Society.

Alzheimer's Society (2007b). *Home from Home*. London: Alzheimer's Society.

Care Quality Commission (2010). *The State of Health Care and Adult Social Care in England*. London: Stationary Office.

Commission for Social Care Inspection (2008a). *The State of Social Care in England 2006/07*. London: Commission for Social Care Inspection.

Commission for Social Care Inspection (2008b). *See Me, Not Just My Dementia: Understanding People's Experience of Living in a Care Home*. London: Commission for Social Care Inspection.

Dening, T. & Milne, A. (2008). *Mental Health in Care Homes for Older People*. In: R. Jacoby, C. Oppenheimer, T. Dening, & A. Thomas (Eds.), *The Oxford Textbook of Old Age Psychiatry* (pp. 355–370). Oxford: Oxford University Press.

Dening, T. & Milne, A. (2009). Depression and mental health in care homes. *Quality in Ageing Special Issue: Depression, Suicide and Self-harm in Older Adults, 10*(2), 40–46.

Department of Health (2008). *High Quality Care for All: NHS Next Stage Review*. London: Department of Health.

Department of Health (2009a). *Living Well with Dementia: A National Dementia Strategy*. London: Department of Health.

Department of Health (2009b). *Living Well with Dementia in a Care Home: A Guide to Implementing the National Dementia Strategy*. London: Department of Health.

Froggatt, K., Davies, S., & Meyer, J. (2009). Research and development in care homes: setting the scene. In: K. Froggatt, S. Davies, & J. Meyer (Eds.), *Understanding Care Homes, a Research and Development Perspective* (pp. 9–22). London: Jessica Kingsley Publishers.

Gage, H., Knibb, W., Evans, J., Williams, P., Rickman, N., & Bryan, K. (2009). Why are some care homes better than others? An empirical study of the factors associated with quality of care for older people in residential homes in Surrey, England. *Health and Social Care in the Community, 17*(6), 599–609.

HM Government (2007). *Putting People First*. London: Stationery Office.

HM Government (2009). *Shaping the Future of Care Together*. London: Stationery Office.

HM Government (2010). *Building the National Care Service*. London: Stationery Office.

Laing & Buisson (2009). *Care of Elderly People: UK Market Survey 2008*. London: Laing & Buisson.

Livingstone, G., Cooper, C., Woods, J., Milne, A., & Katona, C. (2008). Successful ageing in adversity—the LASER longitudinal study. *Journal of Neurology, Neurosurgery and Psychiatry*, *79*, 641–645.

Matthews, F.E. & Dening, T.R. (2002). Prevalence of dementia in institutional care. *Lancet*, *360*, 225–226.

Milne, A. (2009). Addressing the challenges to mental health and well being in later life. In: T. Williamson (Ed.), *Older People's Mental Health Today: A Handbook* (pp. 31–42). Brighton: Mental Health Foundation and Pavilion Publishing.

Milne, A. (2010). The care home experience. In: M. Abou-Saleh, C. Katona, & A. Kumar (Eds.), *Principles and Practice of Geriatric Psychiatry*, 3rd Edition (pp. 205–209) London: Wiley-Blackwell.

Office of Fair Trading (2005). *Care Homes for Older People in the UK, a Market Study*. London: Office of Fair Trading.

Wanless, D. (2006). *Securing Good Care for Older People: Taking a Long Term View*. London: The Kings Fund.

Warner, J., Milne, A., & Peet, J. (2010). *'My Name is Not Dementia': Literature Review*. London: Alzheimer's Society.

Part 1

The inside view—living in a care home

Chapter 1

A resident's view

Pat Singer

Abstract

This is an account by a resident in a care home, who tells her story of how she came to move into residential care and her experience over several years of living there. She describes the ambience of the home and the care she receives, as well as other matters such as food and the activities that are on offer.

A resident's view

I have lived here for over 5 years now. Before that I had a flat in London. I was living alone since I was widowed at the age of 59 back in 1974. So I lived on my own for quite a long time, about 30 years altogether. In the end, I couldn't go on living alone. I got very lonely and depressed. I didn't feel safe in the flat. I had intruders on one occasion. I wanted company. Although I had thought about moving into a home for some time, in the end it was the depression that sealed my decision to move.

My son asked me if I wanted to stay in London near my friends or move to Cambridge where he lived at the time. I said I wanted to be near family so we started to look here. He had a big list of homes and we got down to a shortlist of three, which I visited. I can't remember the names of the other two homes I looked at but they were awful—smelly with poor bedrooms and lacking a good atmosphere. So coming here wasn't a difficult choice for me to make.

I certainly have no regrets about moving here. I have been very content and I have not hankered after living independently again. When I moved in, I was still very depressed. It didn't take much adjusting to as I was so lonely at that time. I don't remember feeling especially relieved to be here, maybe because I was still feeling so low. However, I settled in fine and things have turned out much as I might have expected. There weren't any things that really surprised me. I continued to have spasms of depression for a while but with medication this has settled down and I have been fine recently.

At the time I moved, I hadn't got any plans for my flat. In the event, my son had to move to London within a couple of months so he has lived there ever since. I would have left it to him anyway so it was fine for him to have it a bit earlier than planned. He also has my car too. I am pleased he was able to make use of it as it meant there wouldn't be any problems with squatters or the like. Because the flat has stayed in the family, I haven't had the issues that many other people must have with having to dispose of most of their possessions. I came here with very little, just clothes and personal effects really, so all the furniture has remained back in London. So, although it is a bit ironic that we moved in opposite directions at about the same time, it seems to have worked out quite well.

What I like about this place is that it has a good atmosphere. It is homely and living here is really no strain at all. I feel safe and very comfortable here. It is always clean and tidy, and I appreciate that. The manager is excellent and the carers are very patient especially as some of the residents can be unreasonable at times. They are willing to do little extras, for example, special lunches for Valentine's Day, or for St. David's and St. Andrew's days. For example, they would have some Scottish food and suitable music for St. Andrew's day. Obviously, it's not perfect but I only have minor gripes, such as the horrible thick teacups they use. But that's nothing really.

On a typical day, I get my newspaper and read it right through. I go down for meals at lunch and teatime and I watch TV in the evening. I'm not very steady on my feet so I don't walk far outside, but I do enjoy walking in the garden. There are some animals, a couple of chickens, and some guinea pigs as well as some goldfish. We quite often have outings. There is a programme covering the whole year, with about three scheduled events a month, plus there are always some extra outings. We have been to places like Anglesey Abbey (a local National Trust garden) and the Norfolk coast. We recently had a Caribbean evening with a steel band. They were a bit deafening but quite enjoyable. We also get taken out for pub lunches sometimes.

The other residents are mainly pleasant, and we make an effort to make new residents feel welcome. Most of them seem reasonably content. Some people have dementia, though by no means all, and perhaps they are sometimes less happy. Maybe that would be so wherever they were though. I've made some good friends here, I tend to sit with the same people at mealtimes. I'm friendly to some of the people with dementia but there's a limit to how much you can talk about. Most of the other residents seem to have visitors but they are not intrusive. I have no difficulty in being private and undisturbed in my room if I want to be on my own.

My son visits every fortnight, and my granddaughter comes up from London as often as she can. He takes me out for meals, including at Christmas, but I haven't been back to London. For some reason, I have no wish to see my flat again. I have managed to keep in touch with some old friends from London. I do see them sometimes but they aren't very keen on driving up the motorway. I am able to go out and into town. I take a taxi. If I need clothes, I tend to get them in Cambridge. There is somebody who comes here from time to time to sell clothes. They aren't exactly great. I might buy the odd thing, something like a cardigan maybe.

There isn't a visiting hairdresser but one of the staff does hairdressing in her own time. She's OK, certainly keeps things clean and tidy for me. Some residents go out to hairdressers, though I don't do so myself. There is a chiropodist, in fact they were here this morning. The district nurses quite often come to do dressings and so on. Most of the residents are with the local general practitioner (GP) surgery, which is a few hundred yards away, but I'm with a different GP. When I came to Cambridge, I registered with the practice my son was with and I've stayed with them. They've been fine. I have been visited here by the doctor but I have also been to the surgery, for example to visit the nurse to have this thing on my cheek frozen every now and again. I used to go to church regularly but, in later life, I've rather lost interest. Besides, I can't kneel to take Communion. I make sure that I vote in general elections. Last time we got a lift to the polling station. I'm less bothered about the local elections.

I think the home is able to cope with a wide range of people, so far as I know. They would put themselves out to try and make people feel at home. The staff group is quite stable, a lot of them seem to be related to each other and most of them live locally. They are a very good team. They work well together and you can see that they rally round, for example if somebody is off. The manager doesn't like to have temporary staff—you can understand why not, you don't know who you are getting. There are sometimes temporary staff in the kitchen but not usually among the care staff. They have started to wear uniforms but I don't mind whether they do or not. It's up to them.

Everyone has a care plan and they review mine with me each month before I sign it off. I'm quite happy with what's in it and I'm sure they would change it if I wasn't happy.

The food has improved tremendously. When I first came here, it was pretty grotty. The present cook is very good and there is a reasonable choice of food. There is always yogurt available, which I like. That's useful if I don't care for the dessert on the menu. Of course, there are sometimes moans about the food, but not entirely reasonable. There's one old fellow who thinks he should have two roast dinners every day! Another was complaining there weren't any dates in his date pudding the other day. For people's birthdays, they make quite a fuss and we have birthday cakes with candles and all that sort of thing.

As I have said, I'm pretty content and I think most of the others are too. There is a complaints box but I've never used it. Not sure if anyone else has either. There is a residents' meeting every month. The staff aren't allowed and it's chaired either by the manager or by a volunteer who was on the management committee in the past. Various things get discussed, but it's mainly just the usual nonsense, moaning about food and such like. Occasionally, I have seen people from head office about the home. They come to see the manager from time to time. I haven't spoken to them myself. That doesn't concern me. I suppose it would do if things were bad. But if things did get bad, there would probably be a revolution! Like not getting dates in your pudding, maybe. But more seriously, I'm not sure what I would do if things were difficult. I wouldn't want to move anywhere else. Seeing that the other homes I looked at here weren't any good, I'd probably look for somewhere in London, I suppose. I don't think it's going to come to that though. I know that the home is inspected every now and again. I have talked to a young man who came on one of these visits. I don't think the home makes any special effort in advance of a visit, as it is always kept very tidy anyway. Some of the visits may be unannounced so there's nothing you can do to prepare for that.

My son looks after my affairs for me. He has a power of attorney and he pays the fees and other bills on my behalf. I still have my own bank account, with a debit card so I can make cash withdrawals and use it to buy things when I go to town. It all seems to work fine and I don't have any worries about money. I also have a living will. I drew it up several years ago, well before I came here. I think it is in the manager's office. I don't know exactly what it says. I haven't looked at it for some time. I haven't revised it since it was drawn up. So far as I can remember, it says mainly that I don't want to be resuscitated unnecessarily. I don't know whether other residents have living wills or not.

Obviously, from time to time, some of the residents move away or they die. Sometimes, with the people who have dementia, the managers decide with their families that they may need to be elsewhere, somewhere that is more in keeping with their condition. And then they move, but actually that doesn't happen very often. We don't usually have many problems with people who have dementia behaving oddly, so we aren't too worried by their behaviour. When someone dies, we do get told. Usually, the carer just tells you quietly in the morning, 'So-and-so has died'. After that it's dropped. What else would there be to say? The manager and her deputy go to most of the funerals.

By now, I think I'm the longest established resident here. If anything, that is cause for some satisfaction. I've had three different rooms in this time. The present one is good because of the en suite bathroom and the lovely view over the garden. Since I've been here, not a great deal has changed so far as I can tell. We've still got the same manager who was here when I moved in. I can't think of much else that's different apart from the improvement in the food. Maybe if anything, it's got generally better all round.

Chapter 2

A carer's account

Eric Berger

Abstract

This chapter discusses the problems confronting the author after his wife, who had been diagnosed with Alzheimer's disease, could no longer be cared for in her own home. In this journey without maps, he was faced with the timing of the move, the choice of a care home, the frequency of visits, the relationships with the home manager and staff, the relationships with the other residents and their families, and the need to establish some form of communication with a wife who had undergone profound personality changes and lost the ability to speak. The author considers the adaptations, both emotional and practical, that he found necessary to maintain his inner strength in a world where the abnormal had become the norm.

Living in a care home: a carer's account

Many matters the gods bring to surprising ends.
The things we thought would happen do not happen.

Medea, Euripides

Don't think too hard about the future. The future has its own script. A retirement that had once held out the promise of freedom to spend more time together with my wife, listening to music and looking at paintings and travelling, became something else. Uninvited, a thief in the night, Alzheimer's arrived.

As dementia set about establishing its dominion, the earlier hopes were discarded. Horizons shrank and life slowly became reduced to the house and to walks, interminable walks, walks with no seeming aim, walks propelled by a mission with no goal, certainly no goal I could fathom. My own earlier multiplicity of goals now narrowed down to one: to ensure that my wife could continue to live in her own home for as long as possible.

In the world of Alzheimer's, a world utterly new, embarked on a journey without maps, the carer adapts. The progression of dementia can be slow, painfully slow. Each day seems like the day before, the decline almost invisible except when seen retrospectively in a longer time frame. The carer adapts almost without realizing that he is adapting. The abnormal slowly, gradually, becomes the norm: the hot water bottle in the refrigerator; the umbrella on the breakfast table; the cornflakes wrapped in a sweater in a wardrobe. The slow changes in the sufferer march hand in hand with the slow adaptations of the carer. The carer, almost unconsciously, lapses into a mode of alienation. This is not really happening to me, the carer tells himself. It is happening to someone resembling the carer, just as the carer's wife, husband, parent, resembles the person who was once wife, husband, or parent. Sufferer and carer; they both change. There is an unspoken agreement. This is now it.

And so we lived at home. I had read all the books, knew what could lie in store, convinced myself, or tried to convince myself, that not everyone suffering dementia became incontinent, and at my monthly support group meetings I took guilty heart when I heard of situations worse than my own. My situation, our situation, was bad, terrible, but it could be worse, even more terrible. And trying to look ahead into a fog that mirrored the fog that had descended on my wife, I told myself that I must carry on in surroundings my wife knew, sort of knew, and with me, whom she knew, sort of knew, knew emotionally, although she had long forgotten my name as she had long forgotten our children's names. We managed.

We managed, and then we sort of managed, and finally we did not manage. There can only be one result. Alzheimer's always wins. And so the day arrived when it became clear, as clear as anything can become clear, that even my one single goal was no longer attainable. The day arrived when home became a Home.

For many weeks, months, years, I had been steeling myself for this day, confronted by the mounting evidence that there was no way back. I had had some training for this day. Some months before the move to the care home, my wife had entered a hospital assessment unit. The assessment, I knew, could have only one outcome. My wife could not come home. How could I disagree with this outcome? It had to happen. I could not be faulted. I had made the correct decision, correct for her and correct for me. Everyone was eager to tell me that I had made the right decision in agreeing to her admission to hospital and then to a care home. The professionals, family, and friends all told me that this was what had to be. I could not have done otherwise. I could not be faulted. My decision was universally validated. And, naturally, I was consumed with guilt.

A couple of years earlier, in an attempt to think ahead, the one piece of planning I could envisage, the one aspect of our future over which I could exert some control, I had visited a large care home close to where we were living. Although I had read all the books, I found myself quite unprepared to see people in the late stages of dementia, sufferers lying in the fetal position and unable to feed themselves. I had thought I was prepared, but no one is ever prepared. The reality is sharper than anything on the printed page. I gave up thinking about care homes, allowing myself a period of denial, before learning from a neighbour of a small home where her mother had been given exceptional nursing care. I visited, and finding an atmosphere that seemed calmer and less institutional, and meeting a home manager who gained my confidence, I made a decision. I put down my wife's name. Here, I decided, was where she would spend her final days. Here was where she would live and here was where she would die.

After some weeks in the hospital assessment unit, my wife appeared to have 'settled', Alzheimer's requiring us to put a new twist on vocabulary. She smiled at the nurses and hugged the carers. She had a new family. The settling was a good thing but this good thing was also a bad thing. She could not remain here. Others were waiting to take her place. The hospital, understandably from its perspective, wanted the bed. But I, equally understandably from my perspective, was not prepared to agree to a move to the first home which had a place available. I was now waiting for the home I had selected. But to be admitted to the home of my choice, someone else had to die. I waited but no places became available. I heard that things would get 'better' in winter. In winter residents were more likely to succumb. How strange to be hoping, eagerly I might add, that some stranger would die. I would just have to wait. I waited, not prepared to compromise. I was standing up for my wife, someone who had long ceased to be able to stand up for herself. But I could not hold out indefinitely and as the days and weeks passed I was pressured to be more flexible, to look elsewhere.

How does one choose a home? There are the Care Quality Commission reports, readily available online. But after putting to one side those homes criticized for severe failings, how does one go about evaluating the others? I was advised to take these reports with a pinch of salt. How can a short visit provide a real feel for what a home is providing, something above the paperwork and the drugs trolley and the number of fire extinguishers?

Some homes ask you to make an appointment before visiting, others do not. Instinctively, one feels more confidence in a home prepared for you to wander in at any time. But in any short visit you can only obtain a snapshot. Your visit may coincide with some of the residents exhibiting what is euphemistically called 'challenging behaviour'. Are you aware of a discomforting smell? Nothing can appear more off-putting than smell. How typical are these experiences? How can you tell? But you have to decide.

Unable to wait indefinitely for a bed to become available in my first and only choice, I looked again and finally came upon a home I thought could be suitable. It was also small and the setting as homely as one could expect in the context of this dreadful illness. The home manager again impressed. She was straight-talking, had a sense of humour, and put me at my ease. She would undoubtedly now become a key figure in my life. I was handing my wife over into her care. There are times in life when one has to act on instinct, when the time is not available for a detailed analysis. I requested a place and, my luck now in—it was winter and how my concept of 'luck' had changed—one soon became available.

On the day of the move, I arrived early, so early that I spent an hour walking round the block, trying to convince myself that I had chosen well. How I hated my God-like powers after all those years of sharing decisions. I entered the home and waited for her arrival. The ambulance from the hospital finally came into view and my wife was helped out and ushered in through the door from which she would never exit. She was pleased to see me, more than pleased, excited. This was not in doubt. For a moment I felt cheerful. But she soon left me to wander the corridors, trying the doors that were locked to the outside. How did you get out of this place?

As evening approached, I had to leave. This was now her home, not mine. I slipped out when she was not looking, a furtive skill I had developed during her stay in hospital. I phoned the home manager on how to handle the next days and weeks. Would it help my wife to settle, as some had advised, to stay away for a few days? No, I was told. Come the next day.

The first few days were difficult. The attempts to find a way out continued. Resistance to help in personal care was as expected. ('How would you feel', the home manager asked me, 'if you were changed by three Martians?') Slowly she settled into her new home, slowly the Martians became family. How often should I now visit? An outreach worker for the Alzheimer's Society had advised me not to look at what other carers were doing. This was not a competition, she told me. I decided to visit every other day. This somehow felt 'right', if 'right' still meant anything. I could have visited once a week, once a fortnight, once a month. If I visited infrequently would my wife be aware? Did she have any concept of time, or what I knew as time? I was well aware that if a problem occurred, I could be contacted by phone and could be there within the hour. But the decision to visit three or four times a week was an emotional rather than a practical decision, a decision not accessible to simple analysis. Whatever my wife understood, using the term understood in as broad a manner as possible, I felt comfortable visiting every other day. It gave me the feeling that I had some control over an uncontrollable situation. And the days I did not visit, I tried to persuade myself, would constitute a parallel life, days I could do something else, days I could go to concerts or visit friends or do nothing. Doing nothing seemed particularly attractive, after the years of caring at home when every minute had been accounted for. How long had it been since I had done nothing? And I knew, I knew—how could I not know?—that I was already preparing for those days in the future when there would be no one to visit.

Over time the care home became 'home from home'. A pattern developed. I would arrive mid-morning, ring the bell, and wait for someone to let me in. After the door was unlocked there would be some cheery badinage with the home manager or her administrative assistant and then with the nurses and care staff. They were now key figures in my life. They had taken over the care of my wife. They had become, in an important way, more important than family or friends. They had taken my place. The cheery badinage was there to lighten a situation that had to be somehow lightened so that the visitors and the care staff could get on with things. We whistled in the wind. In the weeks and months that followed, I felt a compulsion, if not to normalize a situation that defied normalization, to lighten the darkness. Humour was essential, often black humour, but without humour one risked going under. This light-hearted repartee with the busy staff would take place against a background of someone somewhere shouting 'No! No!' and someone hanging around the door hoping to slip out and someone endlessly navigating the corridors in one of Dante's circles. The carer must take this in his stride. The abnormal has become the norm. And the carer, who is no longer the 24/7 carer, still has to care for himself. The tragedy that has overwhelmed their lives will not defeat him. He must keep whole because he is the carer. He has a duty to care for himself. And always, the sneaking suspicion: if he never visited, disappeared under a bus, would she notice? She now has a new family, nurses and carers from the Philippines, Kerala, Thailand, Brazil, and Poland. Did I now have a function? Had I written myself out of the script? But I continued to visit every other day and I still got my smiles, as the nurses and the carers still got their smiles. I received some uplift from those smiles. Perhaps my wife was finally finding some peace after the years of turmoil. It took me time to acknowledge this calm in the storm. I told myself to loosen up.

And always the same question, the question that refused to go away, a question without an answer: who was I visiting when I visited? I was visiting someone who resembled my wife. And what was this person who resembled my wife thinking? The inability of the carer to understand what the other is thinking, whatever is now meant by thinking, permeates everything.

The abnormal becomes the norm. The carer holds the hand of his silent partner. We cannot solve the thinking conundrum but it is clear that something is communicated by touch. At times his hand is gripped tightly. He likes it when his hand is gripped tightly. He persuades himself that even with her new family he is still the special one. There is a need for physical contact. The carer holds a hand, kisses a brow, a brow not the lips, as if acknowledging that the normal intimacy of husband and wife has become another intimacy, perhaps deeper, but one that cannot be put into words.

The need for physical contact, as a passing nurse or carer strokes a face or hugs a shoulder, spreads over into contact between residents, a contact that on occasions seems painful as a man wanders unsteadily but determinedly over to a woman in an armchair and attempts to sit on her lap. At times this leads to screams and fights, but it can also herald some form of bonding. A good thing, the carer tells himself, but at times painful for those carers who now find that their partner is now showing a greater affection for another resident.

The carer is on his treadmill. He turns up every other day, greets his wife who is always seated in the same armchair in a public room. She has lost the power of speech but he holds her hand and watches television. He watches people at auctions buying run-down properties to refurbish and sell. He becomes interested. What a strange way of spending a morning. But what else is there to do? For the carer, his job now handed over to the professionals, watching a programme, any programme, provides some respite from watching the man in the corner armchair, head slumped, nose endlessly dripping, or staring at the woman endlessly drumming her knuckles on a tray until her cup is knocked over. Would he really want to listen to the woman down the corridor calling out for a mother long dead? No, he will watch house auctions. Should the people on the screen sell or rent? The carer becomes involved. He has to get through his visits. He has to make the best of it. He goes with the flow. There are no longer any choices to be made. What will be, will be. Will his wife, gripping his hand, watching but not watching the television, live another month, another year, longer? He needs to stop thinking about a future over which he has no control. And yet, when on leaving he catches a glimpse through a half-open bedroom door of a bed-ridden resident in a grotesque posture, the carer knows what he wants.

Making the best of it. The carer tries hard not to analyse his situation, put it in a wider perspective. He must not ask 'why me?' How can he ask 'why me?' in a world where the evening news endlessly relays human tragedies in floods and earthquakes and wars, and babies are born with crippling defects and friends succumb to cancer and heart attacks. As the saying goes, stuff happens. No use howling at the moon. A visiting chaplain, all pep and fizz, assures the residents that we live in a wonderful world. I look round the room and silently beg to demur. But then, he has belief. How comfortable to have belief. I look at my wife and try not to go over the same thoughts again and again. But under the radar the thoughts creep in. How could this person who had been so intelligent, so vivacious, so bursting with life, be reduced to this?

One observes other visitors. Some attempt to jolly up a husband or a mother by talking loudly and slowly. The visitors' nervous tension finds some release in an attempt to ginger up the situation when perhaps what is 'wanted' is simply a silent holding of hands. The touch means something. Perhaps everything. Everything that is now possible, that is. When a person with dementia finally loses the ability to speak, what else is available but touch?

And then there are the people who appear to have no visitors. Perhaps they have visitors at a time of day when I'm not there. I occasionally alternate morning and afternoon visits and the suspicion mounts that some people never have visitors. Or maybe they have just once-a-year Christmas visitors. Some may have no remaining family. Some may have family living far away. Some, one cannot help thinking, may have been shunted here, never to be seen again. One feels the need to say something, anything, to the people with no visitors, to stroke a shoulder and offer a smile. We keep on smiling, particularly now that there is so little to smile about.

In time, the carer swaps stories with those visitors who seem eager to talk, visitors who also need to fill in their time. Gradually, a picture of the other residents begins to take shape. These broken people were once whole. The lady who wanders endlessly from room to room closing the curtains and shutting doors, busy busy, always busy, was once a primary school head. Perhaps closing curtains and shutting doors was once, in that former life, that predementia life, a daily practice. The man muttering and endlessly rubbing his knee was once a university professor, an esteemed physicist. The big, thick-set man, who argues fiercely and hurls his daily bowl of cornflakes on the floor, was once a farmer and a bachelor. The blind lady, addressing an invisible audience in overrefined tones—'Mr Jenkins is in a meeting but will answer your call this afternoon'—was, one discovers, a telephonist.

The staff remain, on the whole, cheery. Watching the carers and nurses taking people to bathe, taking people to the lavatory, residents who sometimes do not wish to be bathed or taken to the lavatory, residents who can sometimes scream and scratch and punch as they resist help, watching the nurses and carers keeping their cool, showing endless patience, attempting to calm the situation, I feel better about the human race.

Holding a hand, stroking a brow, the carer watches television. In the evening, in his own home, he will watch another documentary on care homes. Care homes, he will be told, do many things wrong. After bathing, dressing, and feeding, residents are simply dumped in armchairs in front of the television. No doubt that some homes restrict themselves to this basic formula. But my home, our home, tries to do more. If the resident can arrange flowers, let her arrange flowers. If he can help to chop an onion, an onion will be chopped. But for the resident who cannot arrange flowers or chop an onion, what is there left? Ah, cry the pundits, the media psychiatrists, and authors of books with titles like Contented Dementia (golly gosh! Alzheimer's! almost as good as winning the lottery), those experts who have never had to care for someone with dementia, the answer is to listen and observe what the sufferer wants, go along with their illusions, enter their world. They have an answer. The sufferers do not have to suffer.

There is a paradox here. The television that screens documentaries that shun the full horrors of Alzheimer's, the physical abuse and anger that many carers experience as their loved ones descend into the uncomprehending fog, too often portrays care homes as heartless institutions drugging their residents. The balance is all wrong. Dementia is, for much of the time, a nightmare for the sufferer and the carer. And in many care homes there are poorly paid nurses and care staff doing a splendid job, a job most people would not do for 10 times the salary.

We would all want there to be one member of staff who when we leave would constantly be at the side of our loved one, sensitive to his or her needs. But beds need to be changed, carpets hoovered, meals cooked. There is simply not the staff available to run a parallel service to give unreserved one-to-one care. Care homes are already costly enough. The economics cannot be ignored. And where are the trained carers ready to fill these roles?

In recent times, there has been great publicity regarding the use of atypical antipsychotic drugs. Newspapers and television and the Alzheimer's Society have all waded in, condemning 'the chemical cosh'. I do not doubt that these drugs have been dispensed too readily, but when I hear how 'challenging behaviour' can be handled more effectively, more safely, by listening carefully to the disturbed person, bringing sensitive psychological intervention techniques into play, techniques that will do away with the need for medication, I can only wonder yet again how many of these professional dispensers of wisdom have ever had to cope with care. Future generations will doubtless see antipsychotic drugs as crude. But one can only use what is available at the time. Mental health problems are real problems.

My wife had a room, a pleasant room, a room overlooking a garden. Entering this room, this pleasant room with its floral curtains, brought it all home. I did not like coming into this room, searching in the small wardrobe for a sweater, a small wardrobe that now holds all her clothes, all she needs. She once had many clothes and had a job and cared for a family. She had a life. She now spends her days in an armchair. Spending days in an armchair requires little in the way of clothing. The room, the wardrobe, the bathroom I did not like to enter, the safety sides on the bed . . . I did not like this room, this pleasant room with its floral curtains, this pleasant room overlooking a garden. She once had a house. She once had a life.

I become aware that I have not seen one of the residents, normally a familiar face, for some time. I wonder. I do not wish to pry. Perhaps he is now too ill to be brought into the communal rooms. And then I hear that he has 'passed away' some weeks earlier. I look again at my wife. Do I really want her to go on like this day after day? Do I want her to travel the full stretch of this disease? Feeding by tube, fetal position. I know what I want. I know what I want but I want it to happen painlessly, almost painlessly. I do not want it to be drawn out.

One day pneumonia arrives. It all seems to happen very quickly. She struggles for breath as I hold on to her hand. She is fighting, fighting, fighting for breath, fighting for life. And then, suddenly, it is all over. She has ceased to struggle.

A nurse comes into the room and closes the curtains.

Finis.

Chapter 3

A care home manager's view

Marsha Tuffin

Abstract

The author manages a residential care home with 27 beds. Over her time working at the home, the major change has been that the proportion of people with dementia has greatly increased. The chapter describes how the home operates. The staff team is relatively stable, with obvious benefits for getting to know the residents and maintaining good standards of care. There is a considerable emphasis on staff training. This account outlines how care is provided, describes the home environment, and the varied activities provided. Relationships with outside agencies, including primary care and mental health services is important, as is the contribution made by volunteers. Care practices have had to adapt to the needs of individuals, with imaginative care planning that takes into account people's identities both past and present in order to understand their feelings and behaviours.

A care home manager's view

Only too often in life we say, 'Where has the time gone?' Just how true this statement is!

Welcome to my account, giving a staff perspective on working in a residential home.

I have been employed in the same residential care setting for 14 years and the time has flown by without any opportunity to look back until now. Writing this chapter is a wonderful chance to reflect and evaluate this time of achievement, change, and collaboration within a team.

I commenced employment in January 1997 at Brown's Field House in Cambridge, a residential care home run by the Abbeyfield Society, a national charitable organization. At that time, it provided 24-hour care for 23 older people, mainly physically frail with old age, and rarely seeing people diagnosed with dementia. It is striking to see just how the provision of care has changed during these 14 years. The mixture of residents has changed, along with changes in systems and structures within the home itself, and also new national frameworks within a regulatory system ensuring quality and safety of all vulnerable people within residential care homes.

I started working as a care assistant in another home when I was 18 and I soon realized that this was what I wanted to do. I was concerned with some of the poor practice that I saw, for example staff not showing proper respect for the residents they were looking after. I moved away to obtain more experience and to train for a National Vocational Qualification (NVQ), which I completed when I got to Brown's Field House. More or less straightaway I became an assistant manager and for the last 7 years I am now the Registered Care Manager.

The biggest change has been that our main work is now looking after people with dementia. Originally, Brown's Field House was registered for only three people with dementia but this has been increased so that the entire 27 registered places can provide this service now. A staggering 85% of residents within my care have either been diagnosed with a form of dementia or have a mental health problem. When I first entered the caring field it was very rare to come across people diagnosed with dementia in residential care, so Brown's Field House has had to change its ways of caring and training to keep up with the demand for this particular client group. Regulators such as the Care Quality Commission (CQC) have also recognized the demand for more provision for dementia care.

The staff team

My care team is amazing. They are highly committed, very loyal, dedicated to the home and indeed to each other, especially working in such a challenging and demanding role. Many of my care team have been employed since the opening of the Abbeyfield Society in Cambridge, over 20 years; in total the carers have delivered a staggering amount of 280 years of commitment within the home. My staff are very diverse in terms of characters, skills, and qualifications, but they all have one vision for residents at Brown's Field House and that is to promote their well-being in every aspect of their lives. We are very fortunate that we have been able to retain our staff, as high turnover is often a problem for other homes. We try to look after each other. For example, we have a short debrief session at the end of each shift, where we discuss how the shift was for each of us. This is very helpful as there are times when residents may appear to be picking on certain members of staff. This is of course more likely if the resident has dementia as he or she may misinterpret what is going on. Sometimes male carers can have a hard time from female residents, who may be flirtatious or else start accusing them of misconduct.

Another feature is that we do not employ agency staff but cover shifts from our own resources. This requires flexible working patterns sometimes but it maintains quality care provided by familiar staff. There is an on-call rota for senior staff. Fortunately, these days, I don't get called very often whereas, in the past, I would get phoned about trivial things. That must indicate that we are all on the same wavelength.

I was thinking that I would write something about a typical day in the life of the home but, in fact, it isn't like that at all. There really isn't a typical day. The day starts to take shape from the moment I come in through the door, depending on how the residents are and what they seem to want to do.

So for these reasons therefore I feel Brown's Field House is a very special and experienced care home in meeting the needs of all residents especially around dementia care.

There is no real hierarchy around the place and everyone is willing to do any of the tasks that may be required. Obviously, there is a fair bit of paperwork and record keeping, which mainly is shared between me and my deputy. Each member of staff is encouraged to develop their skills, especially around real person-centred care and not just in theory or in practice exercises. Having a consistent group of staff has enabled me to provide specialist training on a regular basis, training which is accredited and meaningful. Our next project is to obtain training in dementia care mapping.

My Deputy Manager shares my passion for all older people and especially mental health. It is a privilege to work with her. We share common goals, values, opinions, honesty, and mutual respect, which give a strong management and leadership team. We both place a strong emphasis on training. For example, we have been able to introduce some really good training packages, such as courses provided by the Open University, especially the units covering life history work. All staff, including the housekeepers and catering department, have had training through the Yesterday, Today, Tomorrow package from the Alzheimer's Society. My inspiration is for the staffs to achieve their maximum potential, to equip them with sets of knowledge and skills which will enable them to care for all our residents, and to enable them to grow within themselves as carers. We have a robust supervision and annual appraisal system and in these discussions, we have identified that sometimes courses outside the usual run of mandatory or academic courses can benefit both residents and carers. For example, some carers felt that linking up to the local college to undertake courses in the beauty department would be very rewarding and therapeutic, as well as massage which is an excellent way of relaxing people. Not only does it relieve people when experiencing anxiety, it is also a way to alleviate loneliness and lack of affection, common feelings that are often experienced by older people who have a mental health problem.

I feel strongly that training is at the heart of a successful home. I have a personal commitment, for example having done an Open University degree in Social Care in my own time, and senior members of the team often pay to attend courses from their own money. In an ideal world, I would choose to invest more money in training, though of course it has to be borne in mind that ultimately this money would come from the residents' fees.

Providing care

We have a robust, holistic pre-admission procedure, which is as person-centred as possible. This ensures a positive approach and promotes well-being from the beginning while maintaining positive outcomes for the person entering a care setting for the first time. Some pre-assessments can be too hurried due to time pressures imposed by hospitals. However, it is imperative for people with dementia that their needs and behaviours are understood prior to admission so a smooth transition can take place. This admission process provides an excellent framework for positive person work, especially within the field of dementia care. The move into residential care is a major upheaval, often involving personal losses such as ill health or bereavement, as well as some loss of independence, so getting this right from the outset is very important and it can be extremely rewarding.

Life history work is vital to this process. We start this before a person enters the home and it is continued through reminiscence work. By constructing the person's life story, we can recognize their past life and achievements as well as help them to maintain their identity, something that can be lost in the advanced stages of dementia. Furthermore, there is good evidence that this can help to relieve anxiety and open up avenues of conversation and social interaction. Knowing the past experiences of residents has helped us to understand when a person is caught up in the past and is displaying what is described as challenging behaviour. The more we know about someone, the more meaningful these apparently unpredictable behaviours seem to be. This can also help us to understand the feelings being experienced so that the carers can help to validate those feelings. In general, we manage behaviour problems quite well. We try to understand what is going on and to prevent things from escalating. In recent years, people wandering out of the building and being at risk of getting lost has become more of a problem. We want to strike a balance between liberty and safety and we don't want to make the front door so impassable that none of the residents can come in and out. We are looking at different types of door catches at present.

One interesting change in practice is that, in my early years of being educated in dementia care, we would work hard at trying to re-orientate people at all times, bringing them back to reality as we see it. This may have involved trying to tell someone who believed they needed to collect their children, as they once did in their past, that this could not possibly be the case due to their age and situation. This more often than not led to increased agitation, anxiety, and ultimately what is described as challenging behaviour. By contrast, today's approach is to try and enter that person's reality and validate feelings of abandonment or possible loss. This has reaped rewards as it seems that people become less anxious and agitated, and display fewer behaviour problems, due to these feelings being addressed and validated. Family members often find this difficult to come to terms with at first, but once they have seen the results—fewer behavioural problems requiring less medical intervention and almost never prescribing antipsychotic drugs—they appreciate our approach.

We provide a lot of end-of-life care. Most of our residents eventually die here rather than in hospital. We encourage residents to draw up advance directives, as we have found that simply writing in the care plan that someone does not wish to be sent to hospital is not enough to stop this happening if the events are happening out of hours with unfamiliar general practitioners (GPs) involved. We have been participating in locally organized research on end-of-life care and we also have a good relationship with staff at the local hospice. We quite often keep in touch with the relatives of deceased residents, several of whom have become enthusiastic volunteers.

The environment

Having a consistent staff base helps to maximize the feelings of familiarity, and a feeling of home and belonging has made Brown's Field House a true home for many of our residents with mental health problems. People are encouraged to make their rooms their own by making them as personalized as possible. Having familiar furniture and belongings around emphasize the sense of home. This is vital for people with memory problems as it is not uncommon for people to question why they are here or indeed where they are. Having visual reminders, in the form of personal belongings, help enormously with these confused and at times frightening feelings of displacement.

The whole care environment has to be considered, not just personal rooms, but outside areas need to be made available for residents to make it their own. Although perfectly landscaped gardens look wonderful in some care settings, I wonder exactly how much actual input residents have had and whether they get the opportunity to maintain these themselves? Many of our residents have been, and still are, avid gardeners and this helps to make our gardens very much resident owned. People are encouraged to contribute in whatever way they can. As well as being a meaningful activity, sharing our garden demonstrates true ownership and again proves to be very therapeutic.

Animals also have led the way to making a homely environment both in and outside the house. Naturally, animals have in the past played a large part in many people's home lives and we have developed a small menagerie, much to the pleasure of many residents and visitors. Animals that can be petted offer a therapeutic opportunity to display and receive affection by stroking them. Having egg-laying chickens in the garden has given a focus for residents to go outside for a definite purpose and with the tangible result of collecting the eggs.

Some residents need and benefit from having routines in their daily living and this has enabled them to preserve certain daily living skills that can slowly be lost with dementia. Other residents have very different expectations and their days vary enormously to keep them occupied and stimulated and therefore content within the setting of the home. Again it proves that no one box fits all and care delivery needs to be very individually planned so that good outcomes can be achieved.

Activities

I'm very excited and proud of the daily activities which are carried out at the home. Some have a structure with a finished product and other activities are less formal and are simply ongoing from day to day. Daily activities have changed and have evolved over the years all depending on the individual and their personal history and lifestyle. Some residents take great pride in growing home grown salads and vegetables in the raised beds of our garden and proudly demonstrating their achievements with the produce at mealtimes at the dining table. Others enjoy the lovely aspect of joining in and helping out around their home, assisting with carers and housekeepers in laying the tables for the daily meal or folding the napkins and towels for the next day. These pleasant and worthwhile tasks give the individual a sense of running their own home, recognizing that they still have a vital, important role within Brown's Field House to fulfil.

On the other hand, some activities have taken a much less expected direction, as follows. One lady came to England from France 50 years before, and she had worked in the past as a French teacher in Cambridge. Although she was diagnosed with dementia, she inspired other residents at the home to learn French. Provided with some learning materials that we purchased, and supported by two carers who could speak this language from school days, she taught basic French to four residents for about a year, until sadly she became too frail and died. The wonderful aspect of personhood here was how she—the client—would revert to her native language, and the carers and some of the residents could engage with her by speaking French, reassuring her that in this transition of her life she was safe and cared for.

Another important aspect of our activities is the art therapy sessions that we provide, particularly for those residents with quite advanced levels of dementia. Art can be especially helpful for people whose verbal communication is very impaired. Art therapy can help to alleviate one's anxieties and express oneself through an activity which does not have a structured finished product. The outcome is a valid reflection of what that individual encounters at that given time and how they have encountered their feelings within such an activity session. Many residents still have their artwork displayed around the home, given to their families, or proudly on show in their bedroom, a positive non-frustrated activity but also an interesting focal point for discussion with any resident, a meaningful activity but with a different outcome.

We do not of course have organized activities at night but there is a certain amount of coming and going during this time. If people want to be up and if they want to do certain things, then of course they can, as it is their home. We are certainly not going to give out sleeping tablets for our own convenience.

Support from outside

We currently use three GP surgeries to serve the healthcare needs of the residents who are given the opportunity to be reviewed by their own GP regularly. Those who have advanced dementia or other mental health problems need the support of me and my team to communicate any problems on their behalf. I am lucky enough to have a good working partnership with these surgeries. They understand that when they are called concerning a mental health issue, it has arisen after we have applied our own skills to try to understand the cause of the problem, excluded any obvious physical problems, and tried to manage it ourselves. With the increased number of residents with dementia, we are passionate as a team about supporting mental health problems of whatever kind. The team monitor and document any concerns so at the review stage a full picture can be presented and an informed decision can be made. Sometimes, this can involve referrals to the mental health team. Once the referral has been established, everyone collaborates for the best possible outcome for the resident. Community psychiatric nurses with the back up of a psychiatrist and at times a social worker assist in giving a holistic approach to managing the various issues identified. We are keen that, where appropriate, residents do receive a diagnosis of dementia. This is not to do with funding but we need the diagnosis so that we can understand their needs better.

Some mental health issues are very complex, for example if someone has dementia together with a lifelong history of chronic depression. Caring for such individuals has required sensitive and innovative ways of thinking. It can be a challenge to keep the staff motivated in caring for someone if they are persistently negative about everything, but it is our responsibility to keep going and provide people with respect and dignity even if they don't give much warmth back in return. Being a small home compared with others is an advantage, as it gives our care team the bonus of really being able to get to know individuals and therefore be able to recognize when intervention is required. Having this consistent team who offer the security of a familiar face is one of the most important aspects of the care service, this is not only true for residents but also for the whole multidisciplinary team. When professionals visit, they need to be given an up-to-date concise breakdown of what has transpired and a close team can deliver this.

Another really useful part of my team is the Friends of the Abbeyfield Society, volunteers who kindly give up their valuable time along with staff at Brown's Field House to raise the profile of the Society. They help with fund raising, which provides items for the home, but also other activities such as excursions. Such trips are a meaningful and interesting way of reminding residents of the community we live in, such as river boat cruises, trips to the seaside, or to formal gardens like Sandringham House. However, a luncheon at the local pub is always appreciated by all residents. The staff and volunteers will always make the extra effort to ensure that even a trip to the local food or chemist shops, polling station, or even to post one's own letter into the street post box is meaningful and connects to the person's past life.

Where next?

The carers fulfil an amazing role in enhancing the lives of all our residents. No matter how diverse their personal care plan is, it is implemented, reviewed, and updated throughout monthly care plan reviews, with the resident, relative, or sponsor. Everyone is treated with dignity, choice, and respect and our emphasis is to deliver truly person-centred care. By working together as a home team and within a multidisciplinary team, everyone has created a true home from home for the older people within our care, while maintaining an excellent rating under CQC. For these reasons Brown's Field House was the runner up in the National Care Awards in 2008–2009 in the Care Team category and proudly, in May 2010 we won the East of England award for best 'Care Home Team' hosted by the Great British Care Awards.

None of these awards would have been achieved without the whole team working together and having one goal—achieving the best possible person-centred practices and care for all vulnerable people at our home. This makes me both very proud and very grateful for the support from our staff and our organization. The Abbeyfield Society's mission is 'to enhance the quality of life of older people', and the Society has certainly responded positively to the challenges of our changing group of residents.

What keeps me going is lots of personal passion and enthusiasm for the here and now, as well as looking ahead to develop our learning and skills within dementia care. We are all lifelong learners!

Chapter 4

Creative work with residents

John Killick and Lynda Martin

Abstract

This chapter describes a creative writing project run jointly by the
authors as resident poet and on behalf of Cambridgeshire Libraries.
The project worked with people with dementia in various settings,
including inpatient wards and care homes. The poems arise from
conversations between the poet and the persons with dementia,
using their words to bring out the main threads of the story. The
poems are read back to the persons with dementia to ensure that
they are content with the end product. Altogether almost 70 poems
were written in 6 months and many of these appeared in a
published volume. The project received much positive feedback and
provides a viable model for creative work with even the most
disabled of individuals.

Introduction

'Home' is a concept which means many things to many people, and is a most significant one: think of the many song titles with the word 'home' in them. But for many
older people with mental health problems it takes on a new significance: 'A Home' is
where one ends one's days.

Can 'A Home' ever be 'home'? One suspects, rarely. In many instances people have
not chosen to be there—the decision has been made by others on their behalf. The
move to 'A Home' has probably been accompanied by other changes in the person's
circumstances, which can be classified as 'losses': independence, mobility, and partner
are some of these, not the least significant, of course, being the loss of 'home' itself.

'Homes' often make a real effort to be 'home-like', encouraging the move to be
accompanied by the transfer of limited amounts of furniture and familiar objects for
the person's room. The rest of the décor, the shared facilities, the menus, in general are
imposed rather than the result of choice or even a modicum of consultation. The loss
of decision-making in these areas is often keenly felt. And, of course, an individual has
had no say in who their fellow residents are, or the staff who are there to respond
to their needs. It is hardly surprising, therefore, that many who are faced with these

profound changes towards the end of their lives contrast unfavourably their new 'Home' with the 'home' they have left behind.

Those experiencing confusion, for instance those with dementia, can find the whole business of living in an institution a whole further layer of distress to their condition. Peter Hollingsworth, a man with dementia in a care home in Cambridgeshire, reflects this state of mind cogently in his poem 'Statement':

Statement

. . . And this can happen, I have found, so easily:
it's happening to many in here—
they can't understand what's happening to them;
they can't understand why they can't go out;
they can't understand why they have a room number.

It was said to me today
'When you've nothing to do
and all day to do it in.....'
I'm still perplexed by it, to some extent.
But it's true: I return to my room
and bang my brains about. (Killick, 2009)

The first verse here makes the point about failure to understand the new situation people are in. The second makes a new point about lack of stimulation. This is a criticism that is often voiced: that people in care homes are left very much to their own devices, and lacking stimulus, deteriorate rapidly into groups to whom things are done rather than doing things by and for themselves. Debbie Everett, a hospital chaplain in Canada, sums up the situation in the following words:

> The condition of dementia abounds in waiting, thus, when people with dementia are unable to control their lives or do purposeful activity, they often feel useless. (Everett, 1996)

We would agree with those who would put activity high on the agenda for change for care homes. Both the quality and quantity of what is offered need to be improved, and much can be achieved by self-help initiatives. Tessa Perrin has identified where the groundswell of this cultural change is to be found:

> The prime movers are not professionals at all. They are those untrained unqualified members of the care team who either redeploy to the roles of activities organiser or who leave and set up in the activity business on their own. What we are seeing is the coming together of a body of people who have an intuitive understanding of the critical need for occupation in elder care settings and a whole-hearted commitment to meeting that need. (Perrin, 2001)

Although this is undoubtedly a correct assessment of where we must look for development, it does not seem to us to tell the whole story of what is required to accelerate innovation. Many of those who have identified the need lack knowledge of the possibilities and what procedures to adopt to ensure a successful outcome in enhancing the lives of residents. For this to occur we maintain that professional example and advice must play an essential role, and while money to employ such people is in short supply (and indeed the numbers of persons prepared to give time and effort in this area is also limited), nevertheless by the cascade principle approaches and techniques can be spread relatively quickly.

In the rest of this chapter, we propose to give an account of a project in which we were both involved, which, we hope, will illustrate some of the strengths and rewards of this approach, and the outline of which may give a kind of template for work elsewhere involving different individuals and organizations and different creative approaches. We do not claim perfection for this project, but we do believe that we got the balance right here between a variety of opposing claims—the individual and the group, the personal and the public, the organized and the spontaneous—which helped it to reach something approaching its maximal potential. We begin with a factual description of what occurred. This is followed by John's personal evaluation of the residency. Lynda then gives her own reactions to the piece of work. We will end with some comments from some of the participants.

General account

The inception of the project came when Lynda heard a series of broadcasts by John on BBC Radio Four in January 2009. She contacted him through his website and we agreed to put together a joint bid to Eastern Region of the NHS for a small pot of money (£15,000) that was being made available to the most innovative project under the national 'Dignity in Care' initiative. The project would also link with Cambridgeshire Libraries' older person's post funded jointly by the County Council Library Service and Adult Support Services.

We saw our proposal as aiming to address some of the needs of a group in the community marginalized both through their communication difficulties and the stigma surrounding their condition, which makes them doubly disadvantaged. People with dementia are also a group which the library service has tended to ignore. Yet they are just the kind of minority (and an increasing one!) which the library service needs to be catering for.

In the following list, we have listed the aims of the Dignity in Care campaign, and below each we have set out how we would design the project to respond to them:

1 Support people with the same respect you would want for yourself or a member of your family.
   ◆ Respect and recognition of each person's unique experience would form the basis of the project.

2 Engage with family members and carers as care partners.
   ◆ Care workers, relatives, and friends would be enriched by the results of the work and involved in the opportunity to continue understanding the power of creativity in this context.

3 Treat each person as an individual by offering a personalized service.
   ◆ The poet would work on a 1:1 basis with the people taking part.
   ◆ The finished piece of work would be the personal creation of the individual.

4 Assist people to maintain confidence and a positive self-esteem.

- ◆ Confidence and self-esteem would be enhanced in all those taking part by seeing their work published and performed, and by the opportunity to take part in shaping the project.

5 Act to alleviate people's loneliness and isolation.

- ◆ The project would promote inclusion and understanding of people with dementia.
- ◆ The project would seek to dispel loneliness and isolation by giving time and attention to those taking part.
- ◆ The project would seek opportunities to equip care workers with the knowledge and enthusiasm to continue with creative activities.
- ◆ The project would encourage those taking part to visit libraries for poetry performances.
- ◆ The project would encourage home carers and those they look after to participate in existing library activities together, such as 'Engage' Clubs for older people.
- ◆ The project would also encourage supportive dialogue among carers and promote the library 'Carers Café Clubs'.

We were successful in receiving the sum of money and set about drawing up plans for the residency. Among the factors that weighed with us were:

1 It was to be suitably celebratory, so it would begin and end with special events.
2 It would involve as many institutions and persons with dementia in the county as possible.
3 It would have a training component with special sessions and also a mentoring element.
4 It would have a strong public relations slant with talks, readings, and broadcasts, with the object of countering stigma.
5 There would be tangible products such as publications.
6 An advisory group would be convened, to include a person with dementia, which would steer and monitor the project.

Lynda approached all day centres, nursing homes, and hospitals by means of an attractive leaflet explaining the project and offering John's services. Eventually, he worked in 6 day centres, 9 nursing homes, and 1 hospital ward; these facilities were spread across the county. Over the span of 25 working days, he saw 77 people in one-to-ones, producing 67 poems and 10 pieces of prose. He gave readings and workshops to 127 people with dementia in groups, saw 294 home carers and professional staff in training sessions or through mentoring, and 232 members of the public came to talks and readings. The special events of the project consisted of a launch on 30th April, and a celebratory reading and launch of the materials at the Central Library on 29th October. He gave 6 other readings in libraries, made 3 broadcasts on local radio, a training video was shot, and a book and calendar were published. The representative advisory group, including a person with dementia and her home carer, met regularly. John was given supervision by a senior member of the County Council's Adult Support Services staff on a number of occasions; this high-level professional support was important for advice on issues raised during John's conversations with participants.

John's account

I should explain, first of all, what the one-to-one work, which was the major component of the residency, consisted of. I began by establishing rapport with persons with dementia, and then invited them to talk about anything that interested them. At some stage I would, with their permission, begin writing down or tape-recording their words. Later I would edit the texts in such a way as to bring out what I perceived to be the main thread of the person's story. The unbreakable rule was to add nothing to the person's words, but only select from the material given to me. The draft poem would then be taken back to the person for his or her approval. All those which I subsequently read in public and/or appeared in the book or calendar had been released for sharing in this way.

I was gratified by the eagerness with which I was received by residents in the nursing homes where I worked. There were usually more people who wished to see me than I could accommodate in the schedule. Sometimes they had already chosen what they wanted to say to me (and even proposed a title!). Almost without exception the finished poems were enthusiastically received, and permission to share granted without hesitation. When readings were given in their presence they responded with pride. I have no doubt that writing down the words of someone, and then their publication in some form, is confirmatory of their personhood. It makes one speculate as to what extent in their daily lives in the homes they are genuinely listened to and their preferences acted upon.

Many of the poems which came from residents did not refer to where they were currently living or their mental health problems but concentrated upon retelling memorable events from their past. A sizeable proportion referred to occupations or hobbies, such as teaching, cleaning, kite flying, skating, cake-making, and crocheting. It was not lost on me that these were reflections on keeping active in mind and body. But here, as an example, is one that did encompass the present situation. It is by Sally Jane Pettit:

Miffed
I'm a bit miffed
that I've got this horrible thing.
I know there's nothing I can do about it
and that there's nothing you can do about it.
It takes me a long time to say things.
This is what happens:
as soon as I want to say something
this happens...... and then I can't do it.
We used to look after children.
We had some fun

with the children that came:
there was one girl that came
and she was so naughty we loved her.
I knew exactly what I would do
when I retired—it was fostering.
And then I couldn't go down that road,
and that was such a shame.
'Why?' you wonder,
'What makes things like this happen?'
I say to myself
'Ok, you've got it.'
And I go to church
and they're wonderful to me,
they look after me
and do things for me—
people are very kind, so kind.
I try not to look at the future.
I want to try to keep going
just as long as I can. (Killick, 2009)

This poem is obviously valuable for the self-awareness and courage that it shows, but it is important not to overemphasize the end product here. I am convinced that the process is even more significant to the person: that is what goes straight into the emotional memory of the individual and stays there, while other aspects of remembering deteriorate.

The effect of these interventions on staff was more difficult to measure. Some seemed enthused by my visits, and asked for more; others appeared to attach little importance to them. In some instances a member of staff was lent to me (as had been planned) and some mentoring could occur; in others I was left alone and no-one observed the process that was occurring. One person from outside any of the homes volunteered to take part, worked alongside me on a number of occasions, and is carrying on the project in her own way in one of the homes singlehanded.

Lynda's account

In the current climate we all need to be creative in accessing any funding opportunities for development work. It was very timely that, having heard the inspirational broadcast from John, the opportunity arose to bid for the Dignity in Care award. The campaign was drawn to my attention by a health colleague on the Cambridgeshire Celebrates Age Steering Group, and shows the value of developing local cross-department networks in an area.

1 Learning point: look outside your immediate area of work and join appropriate local networking groups.
    ◆ We all learned a great deal by working with John on this project, and by meeting residents and staff in homes. Also by making useful links to the Alzheimer's Society Group meetings and county day centres, and working with, and learning from, the Steering Group for the project.

2 Learning point: find appropriate partners in your local care, health, learning, creative, library, arts, and voluntary organizations and invite them to work on joint projects and funding bids.

- ◆ The highlight of John's residency in Cambridgeshire has to be the legacy of the poems themselves. These words of our local people with dementia are precious for their insight and honesty, and for the fact that without this project they would have been lost. Sadly, some of the participants are no longer with us, but their poems have been read at their funerals, and have been a great source of amazement and comfort to their relatives. The celebration event in the Cambridge Central Library was a truly memorable and moving experience, with some participants reading their own poems to an audience of people from health, libraries, adult social care, voluntary sector, carers, and relatives.

3 Learning point: we should value and celebrate the creative work of people with dementia and bring it to a wider audience.

- ◆ I am very proud of this project: it has been a privilege for us to work with John. Four members of library staff were involved directly in the project, and all libraries in the county had the calendars and the 'Elephant in the Room' book of poems that we produced for sale. The project generated good publicity and promotion for the Library Service and I believe has helped sustain the funding we receive from Adult Social Care for our joint post focusing on developing library services for older people. The joint regional training events with library, nursing, and care staff were especially valuable for all who took part—John imparted a great deal of experience and knowledge and practical exercises in a short dynamic session.

4 Learning point: share training and learning opportunities with other agencies, and promote and publicize achievements.

- ◆ Libraries are all about words, making sure we have access to words that can inform, enlighten, amaze, and inspire. Here the poem from our contributor Peter Van Spyk shows exactly this:

It can be done
This is heaven
because for a lot of people it helps them.
You do it on a one-to-one
and that's right.
I feel I'm very lucky
because I've got something like poetry.
I've lots of memories, good and bad.
Most of my friends, they never say a thing—
I think they're frightened:
I've got a friend in London
and he's only phoned once in three years
We've just come back from Madeira.
My wife noticed it and told me.
I said "I've got Alzheimer's."

I could see the same signs.
He was there with his wife.
She had it. On the last three days
we stayed together,
we found a rapport.
I'm pretty healthy.
You're not in it, are you?
I was trying to look at your badge
just to make sure!
Some people can't handle it.
They think, how can I carry on?
But I don't think I want these things round my neck—
I want to live!
I'm not looking to get rid of myself,
I've never even thought of it.
I really mean it:
if you take your courage in both hands
it can be done! (Killick, 2009)

Learning points for libraries

I'm not aware of any public libraries in the United Kingdom with a designated service for people with dementia; the only research available is from Denmark (Mortensen and Nielsen, 2007). If we are to genuinely seek to deliver a comprehensive and inclusive service to the community, we need an urgent rethink of how to reach this group of people and assist care homes in providing an innovative, stimulating, creative, and learning environment.

Libraries are good at providing information. Most library authorities will have a Books on Prescription or health information service with information on dementia and memory loss for health and care professionals, carers, and people with dementia.

But libraries can do so much more. I am convinced library services can make difference by using all the wealth of their resources such as:

- ensuring robust links with Adult Social Care colleagues, relevant organizations such as the Alzheimer's Society, Older People's Partnership Boards, and by becoming a Dignity Champion;

- creating and using special collections of books, such as Pictures to Share (see ref), music, films, local history collections, and family history;

- promoting libraries as an inclusive venue for events—poetry readings, creative writing, talks, and visits from the mobile library. Using Friends Groups and library volunteers to provide a network of help such as buddying for computer use or to help to attend a reading group in a library;

- building links to other agencies such as museums for hands-on loans of artefacts and schools for intergenerational activities;

- building confidence in library staff with opportunities such as our project to see experts at work and to meet people with dementia;

COMMENTS FROM PARTICIPANTS | 37

- joint training and discussion with staff in homes and libraries to build links and apply for joint funding for new initiatives;
- seeking and applying for funding for more creative work with people with dementia; and
- involving and listening to people with dementia and memory loss.

5 Last learning point for care staff: use your local library and work together with library staff to build better resources and creative opportunities for people in care homes, and especially for people with dementia who are too often forgotten.

Comments from participants

I find it absolutely overwhelming that I've got all this bubbling up inside and then someone comes along who actually wants me to give him all the specific details of what Alzheimer's is like, rather than having their eyes glaze over when I rabbit on about myself all the time.

Molly Brown

You've made me try and use my brain in a way no-one else here has, and I thank you.

Bryan Kingman

It's not often you get somebody to talk to like this who listens! You talk about things that ordinary people don't. A lot of conversation is just casual.

Connie Nevill

Writing is important. We want to be recording what has gone on, and what is still going on.

Iris Snow

This book you're writing in—it's just the right size and the right shape for everything. The only time I shall ever know is when it suddenly decides to be writing there for me.

Daisy Miller

When I was at school I didn't have any interest in poetry at all and I've ignored it most of my life. John has made me interested in poetry for the first time in my life and I've found it very inspiring.

Bryan Kingman

To these should be added the first verse of Peter Van Spyk's poem previously quoted.

Jim Downes is the husband and carer of Karen, who participated in the project. He commented as follows:

Karen was very pleased to take part in the project, and doing the poem and the prose enabled her to bring closure to a part of her illness that had been preying on her mind for some time.

I was pleased that she was able to open up to a non-family member and this took some pressure away from me.

As for John, we both felt that we had met someone that we now think of as a friend, who can turn listening to a person with dementia and translate their words into a poem or prose—a great skill.

The person who was mentored by John and is now replicating the process in a care home on her own is Kate Durrant. These are her words:

> The Celebration Event was the ultimate for me. Some of the people attending were those who had contributed to the poems. John holds the hand of a lady who bravely shares her story of her family's response to her illness. Another sits in the audience mouthing the words as John reads out a poem confirming her existence.

Jacqueline Wieczorek was one of the librarians involved in the project:

> Learning and inspiration from John has helped me understand more about the users of libraries who have dementia, the importance that the library plays in their lives, that they still come and visit, try to take a book or two, even though they can't remember where they live or even their name at times. Some have come on their own; others with their carer, and it means a lot to that carer to be able to choose their own reading at the same time as having their loved one in a safe place.
>
> It has also helped me to be more patient with my own mother-in-law who at 85 may or may not have dementia—she can't speak or communicate very much since she had a stroke 24 years ago, it is difficult to know. John's help on communication is very much appreciated. I found it hard to convince her care home staff of the importance of spending quality time with their residents, just listening to them, and wish that John, or others that he has trained, could work in Surrey.

Richard O'Driscoll, Head of Older People's Commissioning in Cambridgeshire offered the following comments:

> This project was truly wonderful in so many ways. What really impressed me was how it managed to transcend the usual service boundaries, and genuinely put the service user at the centre. In so doing, it achieved outcomes which for many were just a distant dream. Reaching the often forgotten residents and recognising their creative potential was a fantastic achievement. As for the celebration event, it was so moving it brought a seasoned manager to tears.

Conclusion

To return to the theme with which we started: can projects such as this make a home seem more 'homely' and make a difference to the mental health of residents? We think it can, and in the following ways:

- By confirming the person in their personhood, reinforcing their essential identity to themselves—a very important service to perform for those coming to terms with a communal experience.
- By giving the person a creative achievement to take pride in.
- By showing other residents and the staff that they are interacting with an individual, with their own unique personality, whose views and tastes must be catered for.
- By refreshing the ethos of the place in countless small ways just by introducing novelty to environments that can so easily grow stale.
- By giving the staff ideas, techniques, and approaches which they can maintain and develop long after the formal project has been completed.

References

Everett, D. (1996). *Forget Me Not: The Spiritual Care of People with Alzheimer's*. Edmonton, Alberta: Inkwell Press.

Killick, J., Ed. (2009). *The Elephant in the Room: Poems by People in Cambridgeshire with Memory Loss*. Cambridgeshire: Cambridgeshire Libraries.

Mortensen, H.A. & Nielsen, G.S. (2007). *Guidelines for Library Services to Persons with Dementia*. IFLA Professional Report No. 104. The Hague: International Federation of Library Associations and Institutions.

Perrin, T. (2001). Don't despise the fluffy bunny: a reflection from practice. *British Journal of Occupational Therapy*, *64*, 129–134.

Pictures to Share Community Interest Company create and supply high quality illustrated books, specifically designed for people with dementia. Available at: www.picturestoshare.co.uk (accessed 13 February 2011).

Chapter 5

Hearing the voice of older people with dementia

Dorothy Runnicles

Abstract

Dementia is probably the condition that people nowadays fear the most. However, there is increasing attention paid to the subject, for example in the media and in the form of first person accounts. This chapter gives several examples of how people with dementia can make their voices heard and how they can be helped to express themselves. The author emphasizes the importance of understanding the person with dementia through knowing his/her life history and encouraging family members to maintain their close and supportive relationships, even when the person with dementia has moved into residential care. Hearing the person's voice enables us to understand many of the apparently unpredictable behaviours of people with dementia, and this can help in the provision of better care.

Introduction

This chapter focuses on the need for better services and social inclusion for those going through the dementia pathway in their last stage of life. In order to improve things we need to understand better what people with dementia want and to do this we have to listen to them more attentively. So this chapter explores the contribution of care homes and how they can support other housing by providing day care and respite care as well as permanent residential care. However, most people living with dementia are not living in residential care homes. They may be living at home with or without carers, in sheltered housing units, or in extra care housing, so this chapter takes a somewhat broader perspective than other chapters in this book.

The main evidence in this chapter is drawn from my own experiences during the last 20 years. Part of this experience derives from my role as a daughter and carer, sharing in my mother's life as her dementia increased in the last decade of her life. I have also learnt of other people's difficulties in adjusting to and living through this end-of-life pathway; through friendship networks and work as an advocate and older person researcher.

'The voices of older people who need a lot of support are largely absent; other people (professionals, families) speak for them' (Bowers et al., 2009).

About dementia: fear of dementia and safeguarding

One in three people over 65 will die with dementia. Despite the prevalence of dementia being close to that of cancer, it is still frequently misunderstood, misdiagnosed, or written off as a natural symptom of old age when it is actually far more complex. Usually, the first feature of dementia is short-term memory loss and during the first years of dementia life can be relatively tolerable and people can continue to undertake normal roles. Throughout the progress of dementia, people can be given choices in their lives and treated with dignity and respect. As dementia progresses, the focus turns more to the care and support that is provided for people with dementia while still maximizing their opportunities to exercise choice. At all stages of the dementia pathway, people respond positively to the experience of feeling secure and experiencing continuity of care in familiar surroundings. This can reduce the mood swings, anger, fear, and subsequent challenging behaviour that are sometimes seen in moderate to severe dementia. Staff and family members need to try to trace the frequent environmental causes of anxiety which may create a change of mood.

Without support, dementia can be a crippling fearful journey to the end of life. Dementia seems to be the most feared condition of all, ahead of fear of cancer, heart disease, stroke, and diabetes (Alzheimer's Society, 2009). The diagnosis of dementia or related condition carries with it stigma, fear, and apprehension because of the progressive nature of this illness for which there is currently no cure.

Recent media attention including people with dementia speaking up for themselves has been a powerful lever for promoting change, tackling people's fear, and the stigma attached to those who have this diagnosis. Films such as *Iris* and novels like *Still Alice* (Genova, 2009) have also helped to promote public awareness of dementia. The advocates for change include people who have personal or family experiences of living with dementia and seek to maximize positive life experiences, enjoyment, and social inclusion. People with this diagnosis are now publicly asking to be given more understanding, equal respect and dignity as others on different end-of-life journeys. For example, Sir Terry Pratchett, the well-known English novelist, has spoken on several occasions about the experience of being diagnosed with dementia. He has emphasized the difficulties faced by partners of patients and also drawn attention to the meagre spending on dementia research, a mere 3% of which goes to find cancer cures.

Dr Daphne Wallace, a retired consultant psychiatrist, found herself needing support after being diagnosed with vascular dementia (Pitt, 2010): 'I didn't have any specialist follow-up and for the next three and half years I had an increasing sense of abandonment. There is a sense of bereavement and loss and a total change in how you look at your life ahead of you'. She says poor care is at the root of people's fear of the disease. This fear leads to people being scared to report that they are having problems, potentially delaying diagnosis of the disease. Also, she comments that the education and understanding of primary care professionals is still lacking and this can lead to patients being turned away. She points to hospitals as an ongoing area of concern and refers to her own experience in practice: 'I've had patients on my books who have terrible problems when they fall ill and go into hospital—a higher proportion end up in care homes'. Dr Wallace is optimistic about the government target for reducing antipsychotic drugs for dementia patients. She affirms that delivering more understanding care will bring other benefits and, as a result, she believes people's whole quality of life will improve.

In considering care for people with dementia, it is important to think about how the nature of the condition can render older people with dementia vulnerable and at risk of abuse or exploitation. In relation to this, various recent legal and policy developments are to be welcomed. The Mental Capacity Act 2005 encourages the involvement of people in taking their own decisions where appropriate, and introduces lasting powers so that people have a say in the future arrangements for their property and for their care and welfare. It also introduces a criminal offence of mistreating a person who lacks capacity. The National Dementia Strategy advocates that people with dementia should be involved as much as possible in their own care and in making decisions about their future. Recognition is also given to the fundamental role played by family carers and the need to ensure that their support needs are identified and met.

It is important that local people should make use of the influence that they can bring to bear in improving standards of care, whether through the Care Quality Commission or by other means. In one recent case, a community group of advocates, ex-staff, and family witnesses collected evidence about the abuse and ill treatment of people with dementia after a change of ownership of a residential care home. After 8 years of presenting the evidence to various regulatory bodies, action was taken by the Fitness to Practice Committee of the Nursing and Midwifery Council which 'found that the facts which it has found amounted to misconduct'. The Registrant was a clinical manager in charge of residential care home (NMC, 2009).

Moving through the dementia pathway towards the end of life

There is now much literature, media, and material available to illustrate this journey. One example from my personal experience follows.

Case study

The experience of my mother's death in her 100th year occurred when I was 74. In keeping with the East London tradition, she had come to live near to me when she retired aged 70. She was by then already a widow. She wanted to share parts of her daily life with her grandchildren and family. This arrangement was mutually useful as she helped with the care of her grandchildren while I worked. From the age of 85 she gradually suffered memory loss and developed symptoms of dementia. However, she was still an active volunteer in her early 90s in a club for older people who were blind. Her memory loss began to be more severe in her mid-90s but with adaptations to keep her safe remained in her home until her 99th year. As her symptoms became more severe, she was willing to enter a residential care home of her choice.

Although still at home she valued her freedom to go out and used the bus from outside the front door. 'Yes I've had a lovely outing on the bus to its terminus but I don't know where I've been, I came back on the same bus and everybody chatted to me. It was much more fun than the day centre'. While living alone in her flat she had a daily 'social programme' continuing with her hobbies, friends, and interests with appropriate support. Her weekly support included a nurse, a home help, a shower attendant and friends, and lunch delivery 3 days a week. She also had a daily contact from me, her 'care manager'.

Her move into a care home of her choice in her 99th year became necessary when her dementia began to affect the neighbours in her block of flats. By the time of her admission to a care home, she had lost much more than her short-term memory but she was still enjoying walks and outings, stimulating events, and a choice of food. Caring staff provided a continuity of personnel and there was a trained activities organiser who provided a range of choices each day, enabling people to choose and participate as they wished. She played an active role in the life of the care home by being allowed to lay the table.

Gradually over her last 18 months, she lost her ability to speak, walk, understand concepts, recognise most friends and relatives, read, watch television, feed herself, or stand alone. But, even when she was totally silent, she was still able to communicate by lifting her arm on my arrival in readiness for the massage that she knew that I would provide. Regular visits and outings were continued to ensure her feeling of security and belonging. Throughout this period of deterioration she managed to retain key words which expressed her emotions.

It was important for my mother to remain active to maintain her maximum mental and physical capacity. This involved continuing engagement and stimulation, which maintained her self-esteem and prevented boredom. Staying active gave her a purpose and a role. By maintaining contact with friends, others in a similar position, and the outside world, she was able to maintain a sense of identity linked to her past. From the earliest years of her dementia it appeared that her well-being was helped by providing the continuity of a familiar environment in which she felt safe and supported. Being recognized by others and treated with dignity and respect maintained her high morale most of the time. However, she also suffered with low and volatile moods when she became aware of her deteriorating memory or was made fearful by her environment. Usually it was possible to help her, by taking time to establish the causes of her fear and providing reassurances where possible. Doing so helped to encourage more positive moods. On one occasion, in her advanced stage of dementia, my mother became angry and aggressive towards the person sitting next to her in the care home. In response staff removed her stick and investigated what had caused this unusual outburst of challenging behaviour. It apparently started from anxiety relating to a change in seating arrangements which had occurred and which had disturbed her sense of security.

Housing: care homes and extra care settings

Although only a third of people with diagnosed dementia currently live in care homes, nearly two-thirds of care home residents have a form of dementia.

Care homes can play a wider role than simply providing long-term residential care. There are often opportunities for them to diversify by acting as hosts for day centres or by providing short-term respite care. Such different activities help to place the home as a focal point for the community it serves. There is also potential for homes in the same locality or run by the same provider to share skills and expertise, or to offer training and work experience for people working elsewhere. This model, which places the home at the centre of its community, can help to overcome the prevailing fear of dementia and improve carers' (paid and family) understanding and practice. This can be a useful route for some people with dementia living in local housing, in sheltered housing, or in 'extra care housing'. The trained staff in residential establishments can be a resource and a model for others working with people with dementia in local services. These care homes can become centres of expertise in their own right.

A care home operating as a centre of expertise excellence in dementia care offers a range of activities and activation for all its residents. This includes, among other things:

- A designated activities coordinator
- Training to staff involved with activities
- Variety of equipment and resources
- Monthly calendar of activities
- Tailored care plans, personalized for each resident

The philosophy of this care home is described by a staff member:

> For residents with dementia it is even more important that each resident pursues their hobbies and recreational interests. Activities and activation can have a huge impact on the quality of life for residents, helping to reduce depression, loneliness and boredom.

One of the most significant constraints on developing outstanding care for residents with dementia is, of course, money. The dominance of economic and market factors, and their implications for residents in care homes, cannot be ignored. 'They are regarded as and treated like commodities, not consumers with rights, entitlements, or purchasing power . . . funding and market factors dominate discussions of long-term care (rather than focus on older people's lives). "I had to sell my flat to pay for X care home so no I haven't got a choice—this is my home because it is all I've got left"' (Bowers et al., 2009).

Arising from concerns about both the cost and quality of residential care homes is a growing interest and investment in models of 'housing with care' for older people. These reflect high hopes for possible improvement in the promotion of independence, reduction of social isolation, improvement of quality of life, and provision of a viable alternative to residential or institutional care. The Joseph Rowntree Foundation report entitled 'Social well-being in extra care housing' (Evans and Vallelly, 2007), concluded that 'a person-centred approach to care provision can contribute towards social well-being. This should be based on comprehensive personal profiles developed in collaboration with tenants, their relatives and referrers'.

Case study

The extra care housing unit in the Cambridgeshire village of Burwell offers a range of different facilities which support and enhance the life of people with high support needs, arising from both physical and mental ill health. The managers of this facility work in collaboration with other local providers. For example, liaison with the local day centre enables residents including those with early stage dementia to go once or twice a week to attend enjoyable activities, exercises, recreational events, and lunch. Voluntary and statutory service providers meet together at networking lunches in this facility to discuss local issues, and find solutions where possible to areas of concern including referrals and integrated responses to areas of concern.

Developing communication skills to stimulate discussion and participation

People with dementia living in care homes often demonstrate great interest in topics from their past lives. People with dementia are often not talking about time and place in the same way as others. This means that the listener/hearer needs to try to understand clues from their accessible memory. Several examples of good practice are discussed below.

When two residents were asked what they liked to do, they were able to say:

> My garden . . . I did . . . I could help (an 82-year-old man with dementia in a care home). I like folding towels . . . I do a lot of that (an 84-year-old lady who had worked in a care home before her diagnosis of dementia).

Opportunities to help were not being offered to these residents at that time which might have helped to maintain identity and a sense of belonging.

Training programmes are increasingly using a life history approach to enable staff and family to relate with and connect to interests of the person's past. The life history approach provides a written document with photos and memorabilia including information on hobbies and skills, aspects of identity and roles, obtained from family and friends. This document is open for all to view in order to help people with dementia to connect to aspects of their earlier life. The benefits of this approach are illustrated in the following case study.

Case study

I met John, an 86-year-old man, during his weekly visit to a day centre which gave his wife respite from her role as carer. This day centre is part of a residential care home. John has advanced dementia.

The day centre manager introduced me to all the members attending that day saying that I had come to see how they were managing. The manager provided a little 'life history' about all the people to whom I was introduced.

After a few conversations with people with varying degrees of dementia I encountered John, who appeared to be low in mood and sat next to him to encourage conversation. I asked John about his well-being and then moved to his previous life as a local headmaster. His reaction was to apologize saying 'I cannot help you; I cannot remember my work as headmaster'.

My approach then was to go further back in his history by asking about his life as a pilot in the Royal Air Force (RAF). When I asked a question about flying in Spitfires, his face came to life. He was suddenly animated as he said 'Only for 10 hours'. We discussed in detail different planes used in the latter part of the war about which we shared information. We had found common ground (I had also been involved with these planes at that time) in which we could hold an interesting and detailed conversation. It appeared that this conversation transformed his day as he followed me around during the rest of my visit.

This encounter highlighted the possibility of improving quality of life and communication by finding and triggering past memory which is still accessible to the person with dementia.

It also demonstrated the importance of staff knowledge of people's backgrounds including their previous occupation, hobbies, and interests.

This life history approach, via a brief introduction by the well-informed day centre manager enabled me to trigger a profitable and informative conversation. She had said in her introduction that John had been a pilot during the Second World War and a local head teacher.

Another approach has been led by research conducted at Glasgow Caledonian University. Working in partnership with the Scottish Football Museum, Alzheimer Scotland, and member clubs of the Scottish Football Heritage Network, Schofield and Tolson (2010) demonstrated that showing football memorabilia to men with dementia stimulates their memories with quite remarkable results. The project used match photographs and programmes as the subject of one-to-one or group discussions over a period of 12 months and found that the men responded positively to the memorabilia and were able to chat with others about their memories of players and events. The wife of one of the men involved in the study, said: 'I drive here with this sad person with dementia and I take home my husband'. Thus, there appears to be more scope for the use of football in stimulating the mind, along with the possibility of extending this work to other popular sports in other countries, for example using ice hockey memorabilia in Canada. One of the researchers commented: 'This was a fascinating study that revealed impressive results. The men's life-long interest in football connected them to their former selves and shared memories. There is very little provided specifically for men with dementia and this is a welcome and positive innovation'.

Another tool to trigger memories, 'Many Happy Returns 1940s' has been developed by Sarah Reed. This is a set of cards to share and enjoy with anyone who can remember the decade and includes stories, questions, and conversational prompts, for example events, what people did at the time, etc. (www.manyhappyreturns.org). The box of 26 cards is designed to be used by younger people (anyone under 65 years old) with those over 70 years old. The card subjects—researched among more than 120 people between the ages of 70 and 99 years old—are those that can lead to insight and fascinating conversations about people's life experiences during the 1940s (e.g. getting to school, washday, rationing, and romance). The decade means a great deal to this group because for most, however young they were, it is the one that will carry some of their most vibrant and enduring memories.

The use of 'Talking Mats' as an interview tool has enabled frail older people with communication. Talking Mats is a low-tech communication framework involving sets of symbols. It was originally developed by the AAC (Alternative and Augmentative Communication) Research Unit to support people with communication impairment. Since its original conception, additional research has taken place and now it is an established communication tool, which uses a mat with pictures symbols attached as the basis for communication. It is designed to help people with communication difficulties to think about issues discussed with them, and provide them with a way to effectively express their opinions. A recent study found that people with dementia thought that the mats helped them clarify their thoughts and enabled them to express themselves, while family carers felt more 'listened to' by the people with dementia (Murphy et al., 2010).

Social inclusion: involving community resources to improve the quality of life for people with mental health needs

There are numerous examples of where community support and social inclusion can enhance the quality of life for people with dementia, their carers at home, or in care homes. The Joseph Rowntree Foundation report quoted above (Evans and Vallelly, 2007) refers to the risk of social exclusion for 'some tenants including those who have recently moved in, people who don't receive regular contact from family or friends, and people who have impaired mobility and/or reduced cognitive function'.

Cambridgeshire Celebrates Age provides an annual programme of community events held around the International Day of Older People. This community-bred movement promotes social inclusion, intergenerational integration, and offers an opportunity for anyone or any organization during the month of October to organize community activity/events, publicize them widely, and encourage participation in activities promoting inclusion and well-being.

A well-known leader, who promotes singing, offered to provide a church-based event. The chairs were cleared to allow people arriving (no tickets required) in wheel-chairs and baby buggies access to space, as well as mobile people of all ages who wandered around or sat down curious about what was to come. Starting with chants, the inspiring leader led the group step by step towards the awareness that they could enjoy singing together. Their widespread sense of uncertainty gradually evaporated as people relaxed and voices got stronger and a sense of common support prevailed. The breast-feeding mother and the older man with dementia joined in. The initial anxiety and restlessness of the man with dementia was well handled by his carer who also enjoyed the event. This example provides some evidence of how community events can include all people with disabilities including people with dementia. It is based on a value held by a community that social inclusion is the responsibility of everyone. This allows for different behaviours at community events to be tolerated with compassion.

Case study: an integrated community approach

In Burwell, a Cambridgeshire village, there is a broad community access to a range of facilities, which maximize available space and expertise, benefiting the mental health and well-being of all village residents who attend. The day centre works as a community 'hub', providing other services including hearing aid services, a shop, vaccinations from the health service, chiropody, and massage. It can also be used by people not needing or eligible to attend the day centre for the main daily functions. Social service assessments also take place there.

Another facility used by people needing support is a 'drop in' centre in the middle of Burwell, run by the local church and staffed entirely by volunteers. It is used by a number of people including those with mental health problems and family carers. It provides coffee, information, and relaxation at an informal level. Books and cards are sold there and the Parish nurse is available to give advice and support to the volunteers.

There is also an active self-help carers group run by family carers which offers support, regular meetings, information, and relaxation for family carers in the village. Another community group in the village provides a home visiting service for people who are hard to reach. The way in which public and voluntary services work collaboratively and maximize available resources and expertise depend on their willingness to be partners. They have shared values and are prepared to share power in the interests of the changing needs of the village. The village community has an inclusive ethos which accepts people living in residential care, sheltered housing, or in their own homes with support needs.

Not all villages offer this range of support and services. In this village facilities and resources of all kinds are maximized, including the expertise of the staff team of the housing with care home who take a positive approach to include people with dementia. The care home is closely linked to other village services and facilities. It is an integral part of village life and operates an open access policy. Burwell demonstrates that an integrated approach is possible and can benefit not only those with dementia but also the whole community (Cambridge Older People's Reference Group, 2009).

Personalization: maintaining freedom in spite of advancing dementia

Most dementia sufferers live in their own homes. According to the National Dementia Strategy, only one-third of patients receive a formal diagnosis and those who do often receive it too late to take effective action. There is considerable variation between the lives of people with dementia in the community and those admitted to care homes and medical units.

Case study

Harry had his diagnosis of Alzheimer's when he was 82. He had the advantage of a caring daughter-in-law with whom he shared his home. She managed to arrange a memory clinic appointment for him without undue delay and therefore he benefited from treatment with the drug donepezil (Aricept), which delayed progress.

A year later he announced, 'I am better, I don't have Alzheimer's'. The problem of denial and difficulty accepting this one way deteriorating journey is common and becomes a way of coping with an unacceptable diagnosis. He was still able to freely travel around on his bicycle. As his condition developed and if he got lost, he had access to family links, a mobile telephone, and an address card in his hat. His routine included walking, enjoying cinema, and eating out thus encountering a network of people who grew to understand his condition and were willing to help him return safely home. His personal integrity and dignity were maintained even with his gradual memory loss.

Community and family support meant that this man was not subjected to the confinement of institutional care for several years despite his advancing dementia. His early, reliable family support illustrated the significance and importance of an understanding attitude and a stable home background. His community links and networks learned about his needs and helped to maintain his non-institutional life.

Despite the risks involved with this freedom he survived for 3 years until he lost his key family support member, his daughter-in-law. Following this, there were three house moves which further confused him and his freedom became more of a risk and problematic leading to the consideration of his entering a residential home. Like many other people with dementia, he had not been of major interest to the health services. However, recently Harry has been admitted to a care home with the loss of his family carer. He now misses his freedom.

Over the past 10 years, there have been various policy developments to encourage personalization. Pilot schemes relating to 'personal health budgets' are now (in 2010) under way. The social model of promoting the well-being of people with physical and mental disabilities is beginning to gain ground. Personalization aims to tailor support to meet individual's needs. It is a wide ranging concept that is attempting to transform attitudes and practice towards people. It can help the frontline workers and carers to be more effective. It moves away from the traditional service-led provision so that all systems, processes, staff, and services are more geared to put people first. It aims to provide more choices and enrich lives. It is also aimed at supporting family carers more appropriately with help that enables them to give the loving care that many provide to their family members with mental disabilities including dementia. It means having access to the right information, advice, and advocacy to make good decisions about the support people need. Personalization can apply wherever people live, for example if they live at home, in sheltered housing, in a care home, or in hospital. It starts with the assumption that people with disability have arrived at the later stage of life having lived a range of different earlier lifestyles, in which they had hobbies, interests, jobs, and skills which could give added value to their older lives. It requires a life history approach in preparing a personal plan in which their present identity is recognized by having knowledge of their earlier lives.

Case study

Michael sat silently alone after lunch in the respite care unit to which he had been coming intermittently for some years. Michael was not communicating verbally. I sat close to him. I knew nothing about Michael but was able to engage with him while he responded to my words with nods, touches, gestures, and body language. A visitor arrived and uncovered a keyboard hidden in the corner of the room. When Michael saw the keyboard his face lit up, he stood up, opened it, and played fluently. He was at this point able to communicate using a skill which nobody knew that he had. His demeanour was transformed with joy. Staff were very surprised at this episode as Michael came to life. They had no knowledge of his past life, interests, and hobbies despite the fact that he stayed regularly in the care home for short respite periods. After discussion, their interest in creating life histories was increased by this unexpected incident.

To summarize, in my experience the following factors can be important in improving the quality of life for people with dementia and their carers:

◆ The importance of understanding and knowing life histories, that is, skills, hobbies, interests, activities, work, pleasures, etc. These are more likely to be known by loving carers than by paid carers in a care home. However, there are ways in which promoting a life history approach in all situations could influence the experience in the setting.

◆ Caring and loving make a difference. Keeping family members involved and overcoming their fears, building on life experiences, and understanding what 'works well', providing support and respite can all help to retain their central role in the life of the person with dementia. The quality of relationships before dementia hits can be an important variable factor for the person with dementia and the carer. In the longer term, what is better for the person with dementia is better for the carer as well.

◆ Investigating causes of and factors giving rise to challenging behaviour and taking action to alleviate environmental triggers is a key to improving quality of life.

In conclusion, this chapter has included a range of issues that affect people living with dementia and their carers. Hearing their voices, and remaining in touch with them, is the way forward to improving their quality of life and understanding this end-of-life pathway. The final imperative is a cure to be more actively pursued.

References

Alzheimer's Society (2009). *Public Awareness of Dementia: What Every Commissioner Needs to Know*. London: Alzheimer's Society.

Bowers, H., Clark, A., Crosby, G., et al. (2009). *Older People's Vision for Long-term Care*. York: Joseph Rowntree Foundation.

Cambridge Older People's Reference Group (2009). *Unsung Heroes in a Changing Climate: A Cambridgeshire Community Study of Older People's Involvement in Community Groups*. *COPRG*. Available at: http://www.rowans-scientific.co.uk/books.html (accessed 13 February 2011).

Evans, S. & Vallelly, S. (2007). *Promoting Social Well-being in Extra Care Housing*. York: Joseph Rowntree Foundation.

Genova, L. (2009). *Still Alice*. London: Simon & Schuster.

Nursing and Midwifery Council (2009). Available at: http://www.nmc-uk.org/Documents/FTPOutcomes/Reasons%20CCCSH%20Mitchell_Whiteford%2020100217.pdf (accessed 24 June 2010).

Murphy, J., Oliver, T.M., & Cox, S. (2010). *Talking Mats Help Involve People with Dementia and their Carers in Decision Making*. York: Joseph Rowntree Foundation.

Pitt, V. (2010). *Dr. Daphne Wallace: Determined to Play Her Part in Improving Dementia Care*. *Community Care*. Available at: http://www.communitycare.co.uk/Articles/2010/03/29/114163/the-25-former-old-age-psychiatrist-who-now-has-vascular-dementia.htm (accessed 13 February 2011).

Schofield, I. & Tolson, D. (2010). *Scottish Football Museum Reminiscence Pilot Project for People with Dementia: A Realistic Evaluation*. Glasgow: Glasgow Caledonian University. Available at: http://www.gcu.ac.uk/newsevents/news/bydate/2010/1 /name,8774,en.html (accessed 13 February 2011).

Chapter 6

Living with dementia in a care home: a review of research evidence

Alisoun Milne

Abstract

Living in a care home with dementia is an enormous challenge: in addition to their declining cognitive powers, residents often have to cope with physical frailty, communication problems, and dependency on others. These combined difficulties routinely result in their perspectives being ignored. Research instruments, interviews, and observational methods have made a significant contribution to our appreciation of what is important to residents with dementia. More recent research that is attempting to capture the lived experiences of residents is adding further to our understanding of both quality of life and care. Specifically, residents prioritize non-disease-related domains of quality of life which is somewhat different to those identified by relatives, care home staff, and 'objective' measures. Not only is it evident that residents are able to describe aspects of their situation but they also appear to retain a sense of self and identity. There is a distinctive need for assessment of quality of life among residents with dementia to place their subjective view at its core.

Introduction

Despite the extent of recent policy and practice attention paid to care homes in the United Kingdom, surprisingly little is known about residents' lived experience (Department of Health, 2008; Social Care Institute for Excellence, 2009). In part, this reflects the liminal status of people with dementia inside and outside the health and social care system, as well as the genuine complexity of collecting data from people whose cognitive capacity is impaired and whose communications skills are limited (Dening and Milne, 2009). It is notable that an accumulating body of evidence offers valuable insights into the subjective experience of living with early stage dementia in community settings (Milne and Peet, 2008). It is also increasingly accepted that people in the middle to late stages of dementia retain the capacity for emotional expression and many can reliably express preferences or report aspects of their own experience, such as mood (Phinney, 2008). Research is only now beginning to take account of the perspective of people with dementia living in care homes and is embarking on the not inconsiderable task of developing methodologies that can meaningfully capture their perspectives (Brooker, 2008a).

The care home experience

Currently, there are four sources of evidence about 'the care home experience'. The first relies on research tools or measures to evaluate—in a relatively objective way—the quality of life and/or care of care home residents with dementia. The second is an observational approach, prominently dementia care mapping (DCM). The third source incorporates focus groups and interviews, some of which may include a questionnaire and/or rely on third party perspectives—primarily family carers (Nolan et al., 2003). Work that focuses specifically on the subjective experience of the person with dementia is a new fourth addition to the research portfolio (Clare et al., 2008). A brief overview of the first three sources of evidence will be offered before turning to reviewing work that is attempting to capture the resident's subjective experience in more detail.

Objective assessment of quality of life and care

Assessing quality of life among care home residents is a difficult task; it is a complex construct which is variously measured and evaluated. A number of scales do exist, several of which have been specifically developed for people with dementia such as the Quality of Life in Alzheimer's Disease scale (QoL-AD) (Logsdon et al., 1999; Hoe et al., 2005), the DEMQOL (Smith et al., 2005), and the dementia quality of life (DQoL) instrument (Brod et al., 1999). Although instruments vary considerably in nature and content, common domains include: physical functioning, cognitive abilities, ability to participate in meaningful activities, and mood.

A persistent challenge in evaluating quality of life is that there are often differences between the ratings of staff, carers, and residents. This appears to be a consequence of a difference in emphasis: a recent study found that residents' quality of life scores were most affected by the presence of depression and anxiety, whereas staff ratings were more associated with dependency and behaviour problems (Hoe et al., 2006). A full picture of quality of life may thus require a combination of measures, incorporating the observations of all three groups (Gaugler et al., 2004; Sloane et al., 2005).

Despite the difficulties associated with measurement, evidence to date suggests that quality of life in care homes is largely determined by the existence of mental health problems and subjective well-being (e.g. Smallbrugge et al., 2006). Systematic assessment of residents' needs, and consideration of whether or not they have been met, has been suggested as a means of improving quality of life. The Camberwell Assessment of Need for the Elderly (CANE: Orrell and Hancock, 2004) has been used towards this end.

When people are very dependent and live in a care home, quality of life becomes inextricably linked to quality of care (Brooker, 2008a). Good quality care depends on a range of macro-level factors, such as the financial stability of the provider, as well as micro-level factors such as staff's job satisfaction. Given the multifaceted nature of quality of care an approach that accommodates multiple methods is recommended, rather than relying on a single source of evidence (Innes and Kelly, 2007; Barnett, 2000). As will be discussed shortly, DCM has this capacity making it a popular instrument—if not strictly a 'measure'—for use in this field.

The use of research measures in assessing quality of life in people with dementia has been criticized for reflecting a traditional biomedical approach to understanding the condition (Warner et al., 2010). The limited capacity of most measures to accommodate the resident perspective is also an issue and one that needs to be addressed if they are to retain credibility (Szczepura and Clay, 2008). Further research in refining the development of instruments may be useful in providing greater consensus about what constitutes a reliable assessment of quality of life among residents with (often advanced) dementia. Also, which particular measures are most appropriate for specific settings and populations. After all, care home residents with dementia—much like any other group—are far from homogeneous. However good a single measure is, it is unlikely to be able to extend itself to accurately assessing quality of life in a range of different long-term care contexts and across all levels and types of dementia.

Observational methods

Structured observational methods developed specifically for evidencing quality in care settings have been around for many years. They provide an opportunity to include the perspective of the person with dementia by collecting data on their experiences in communal areas, how they spend their time, and how they are treated by staff and visitors.

The most widely used dementia-specific observational tool is DCM (University of Bradford, 2005). Kitwood, who developed the early prototype, described it as 'a serious attempt to take the standpoint of the person with dementia, using a combination of empathy and observational skill' (Kitwood, 1997: 4). DCM constitutes an observational approach where items recording residents' activity can be combined to calculate a dementia care index score (Brooker, 2007). It requires training to employ but even with a standardized training programme, the interrater reliability of practitioners using DCM in regular practice is not high; those who use DCM for research purposes can achieve good reliability (Sloane et al., 2005). That it is both an evaluative instrument and a vehicle for practice development places it in a unique position in terms of assessing quality of life among care home residents, including those with high levels of dependency (Brooker, 2005, 2008b).

A linked example of an observational tool is that developed for inspecting the standards of care in English care homes for people with dementia. The Short Observation Framework for Inspection (SOFI) draws heavily on DCM and involves structured observation of a sample of five residents in a communal area and over a lunch period, usually for a couple of hours (Commission for Social Care Inspection, 2008a).

This supplements interrogation of case records, staff interviews, and other aspects of inspection.

A 2007 CSCI inspection of care homes for people with dementia using SOFI found some excellent examples of one-to-one attention and care offered with warmth, understanding, and tolerance (CSCI, 2008b). However, it also identified widespread adoption of a functional impersonal approach to care. The report noted that quality of staff communication with residents—both verbal and non-verbal—had a significant impact on well-being. Positive communication that is warm and friendly results in the person with dementia feeling happy and relaxed. Conversely, negative or neutral communication—interactions that are impersonal and task focused—leaves residents feeling distressed, withdrawn, and at greater risk of developing challenging behaviour. Staff attitudes are also important. A recent study by Spector and Orrell (2006) found a correlation between 'increased hope in care staff' and improved resident quality of life. It is evident from CSCI inspections, and related research, that residents with dementia do not always receive person-centred care—care which is delivered in ways that promote independence and autonomy and which draw on the person's individual life course and experiences.

More recently, video and digital recordings have also been used in care settings. They can provide very fine-grained analysis enabling in-depth observation to occur (Cook, 2002; Murphy, 2007). Video evidence can be particularly valuable when working with people with very advanced dementia whose speech on first listening seems meaningless, but on repeated replay shows clear attempts at communication (e.g. Killick and Allan, 2006).

The extent to which selfhood or identity is preserved in people with dementia has been a key focus of observational studies (Hubbard et al., 2003; Mayhew et al., 2001). Research suggests that although the self is affected by dementia, manifestations of self-hood and identity persist even in late stages of the illness along with the capacity to develop positive therapeutic relationships (Edelman et al., 2005; Williams and Tappen, 1999). This is an issue the author returns to later.

Interviews and focus groups

Increasingly, accounts of living with dementia in a care home are gathered directly from interviews with residents themselves. This work challenges the widely held view that people with significant cognitive impairment are 'unsuitable' interviewees. A study by Mozley et al. (1999), for example, found that a large proportion of their sample with advanced dementia were able to answer questions about their quality of life. This, and related work, identified that increased engagement with the environment, better functional ability, and improved mood status are user-defined determinants of improved quality of life (Hoe et al., 2006). A study by Byrne-Davis et al. (2006), drawing on data from focus groups, found that people with moderate or severe dementia were able to talk about quality of life in meaningful ways. The key issues that participants emphasized were: social interaction, psychological well-being, religion/spirituality, independence, financial security, and health. As with video evidence, transcriptions of interview data can reveal emotional content and meaning that is missed during the interview. This approach dovetails with work on narrative and identity discussed below (Hyden and Orulv, 2009).

Both observational-based and interview-based research with care home residents identify recurrent issues of loss, communication difficulties, frustration, and sadness along with lack of meaningful occupation (Tester et al., 2004). Minimal levels of well-being are noted in many studies. Although these are particularly pronounced for people with the greatest dependency needs, it has been suggested that this may well be related to a third factor: the poorer quality of psychosocial care provided to this group (Brooker, 2008a). Interview-based research suggests that engagement levels tend to be higher among those residents whose relatives are encouraged to visit the care home often and with whom staff have ongoing communication (Hubbard et al., 2002).

In 2008, the Alzheimer's Society undertook a study of dementia care in care homes. Using a mixture of focus groups and questionnaires it gathered data from 4084 family carers, care home managers, and workers; residents were not directly included. The study found that people with dementia are not always afforded dignity and respect and that expectations of quality of life tend to be low (Alzheimer's Society, 2008). 'Dementia' had become a label which subsumes all other characteristics and needs and which renders other aspects of the person's identity and history redundant, or at least secondary (Warner et al., 2010). This tendency undermines the delivery of individual-ized care and encourages a regimented task-oriented approach. Lack of activity and stimulation were also highlighted with 54% of carers reporting that their relative was left in his or her room for hours with no attempt from staff to engage with them. These problems were particularly acute for people with more severe dementia. As the avail-ability of activities and opportunities for occupation is a major determinant of quality of life, this is a primary concern. Related work has identified the need to ensure resi-dents retain the right to make choices and are accorded some degree of autonomy over decisions that affect their daily life and well-being (Train et al., 2005).

The potential role of 'Talking Mats' to enhancing communication with people with advanced dementia, and thereby gaining additional insight into their experiences, is a noteworthy new development. The Talking Mat is a low-tech framework comprising a textured mat and visual symbols allowing residents with limited verbal skills to express their views. Although not a research or interview tool per se, early work sug-gests it can positively influence the quality of interaction between staff and residents and enhance staff's ability to communicate effectively (Macer and Murphy, 2009). It can also aid the involvement of residents in decisions about their life and care (Murphy et al., 2010).

Capturing the subjective experience of living with dementia

In the last few years, attempts to directly explore the subjective experiences of people with dementia in long-term care have been made. Two separate but linked interpretive methodological routes have been employed in this work: biographical methodology and phenomenology. Unlike most of the methods already reviewed, the key aim of these approaches is to explore the lived experiences of residents and see the world 'through their eyes' in an unscripted way. Although it has a link to improving care practice, its core focus is on extending understanding about the nature and dimensions of residents daily lives and how far their sense of self and identity is retained. It shares a number of dimensions of artistic interventions with residents, a point underscored in Chapter 4.

Biographical theories suggest that narrative, life history, and their expression through story telling are crucial in the development and preservation of self. Surr (2006) adopted an interpretive biographical approach to gathering data from a series of unstructured interviews with 34 care home residents in 2004–2005 (the sample was part of a larger dataset). This approach claims to provide insight into how individuals construct their lives; the aim is to gain an understanding of the person as an individual set within the context of their life and situation.

Surr's findings revealed that a number of key issues influenced residents' sense of self and well-being:

- *Relationships* with relatives, care home staff, and other residents (see Box 6.1 for two case vignettes),
- Having an *occupation or social role* within the home, for example one resident was encouraged to be involved in activities such as going shopping or to church where she felt useful and *was involved in a group activity*,
- Continuing to have a *family role* such as being a parent and taking pride in your children,
- Presenting oneself as *caring for others*, mainly relatives, and
- *Illness and being cared for by others.*

This study showed that participants—*regardless* of the severity of their dementia—were able to construct stories about their lives and selves (Sabat, 2001). As Surr states (2006): 'By recounting stories about their life, part and present . . . during the (unstructured) interviews, residents succeeded in presenting their self in a way that integrated

Box 6.1 Two Case Vignettes

Olga: Olga, who was of German origin, was ostracized by other residents because of her nationality. The social exclusion and stigmatization that resulted from this had a negative effect on Olga's sense of self, and in the 6 months she participated in the study, she never settled into the home. One staff member commented: 'She is very restless and won't sit still for long. She is very much a loner and this is because a lot of the other residents don't really like her' (p. 1725).

Ida: The care staff noticed that Ida began to display a new self when a male member of staff joined the team. One staff member commented, 'Ida has changed the way she acts . . . She flirts with him and does silly things she wouldn't normally do. She gets jealous if he talks to Lucy . . . Ida knows who he is and her face lights up when he enters the room' (p. 1725).

Source: Surr, C.A. (2006). Preservation of self in people with dementia living in residential care: a socio-biographical approach. *Social Science and Medicine, 62*, 1720–1730.

the whole of their life from the past to the present . . . demonstrating biographical continuity' (p. 1727). Overall, the study identified that relationships with family, other residents, and care home staff are significant in the preservation, or undermining, of selfhood. Although positive relationships were supportive of self, negative relationships served to undermine it. Ability to adopt desirable social roles, being 'allowed' to tell one's own story, and having it taken seriously by the listener, were all important elements of preservation of self.

Drawing on the same dataset, Clare et al. (2008) extended Surr's findings (2006). The research team adopted an interpretive phenomenological approach to (re)analyse interview data collected on 80 residents (Bowling, 2002). This explores individuals' lived experiences and how they make sense of their experiences by focusing on internal psychological meanings evident in their accounts; it is informed by descriptive and hermeneutic traditions. This tradition emphasizes the need to understand experiences from the perspective of the person being studied; it involves a set of procedures that include careful (re) listening to the participant's narratives, detailed coding of interview transcripts, and the emergence of 'codes' reflecting emerging themes (Bryman, 2004). The analytic process was supported by the use of a qualitative software programme.

Thematic analysis highlighted four interrelated experiences (see Box 6.2). Daily life was shaped by the losses resulting from dementia for most residents and distressing thoughts and feelings were common. The psychological impact of 'being in the home' was associated with a sense of uncertainty, lack of control, and limited self-determination. Fear of 'being along' and/or 'of being lost' were also dominant issues. Despite this, through their accounts, residents emerged as 'agents actively seeking to cope with their situation' (Clare et al., 2008: 718). Many found ways to contribute to daily life and focus on the positive aspects of being in a home, including having access to supportive and warm relationships. Such relationships appeared to be pivotal to

Box 6.2 Key Themes

Key themes that emerged from Clare et al.'s (2008) study were:

- *Nothing's right*—isolation, alienation, lack of choice, lack of control, fear, worthlessness
- *I'll manage*—making the best of things, valuing contacts and friendships, finding ways of continuing to be useful, being accepted as you are, having a friend in the home, having links with relatives/family, acknowledgement of getting older
- *I still am somebody*—part of coping, affirming one's sense of identity, managing well despite limitations
- *It drives me mad*—frustration and anger at the situation, confined, wanting more independence, boredom, lack of activity, annoying behaviour of other residents, uncertainty, fear, irritation.

Source: Clare, L., Rowlands, J., Bruce, E., et al. (2008). The experience of living with dementia in residential care: an interpretive phenomenological analysis. *The Gerontologist*, 48(6), 711–720.

maintaining a sense of well-being; their absence contributed to feelings of distress and alienation. This evidence dovetails with Surr's earlier analysis (2006).

Although participants displayed many constructive ways of coping, the effects of dementia-related changes, coupled with the context of institutional care, placed severe limitations on their expression of personal agency. Consequently, some residents experienced frustration, anger, and boredom, especially around minimal activity and daily occupation (Train et al., 2005). Lack of freedom and independence was experienced as 'restrictive' and communal living could give rise to considerable confusion. These two studies—and those adopting similar approaches—expose a rich seam of experiential evidence adding subjective depth to our understanding of 'care home life' and offering direction for investment in good practice with residents with dementia.

That this work also links to emerging research focused on narrative and identity in people with dementia is additionally interesting. Specifically, how people with advanced dementia use their remaining linguistic and cognitive abilities, together with non-verbal cues, as resources in communicating and negotiating identity in everyday narratives (Caddell and Clare, 2010; Hyden and Orulv, 2009). Despite the non-linear nature of much of the storytelling, early research suggests that 'fragments of autobiographical narrative' are evident and that this process is part of the user's identity work in the face of evolving disease (Hyden and Orulv, 2009: 212). That it can be supported by staff, for example they can provide 'scaffolding' in the form of dates or events, or begin a conversation that facilitates storytelling, is very important especially in the context of long-term care (Brown-Wilson et al., 2009). Further, that this approach has strong resonance with Kitwood's view that, 'attending carefully to what people with dementia say and do in the course of their ordinary life' is a notable strength (1997: 16).

Evidencing the perspectives of people with advanced dementia is a resource-rich activity. Ensuring that staff and residents are engaged with the research process takes considerable time and patience as does establishing a rapport with participants. The careful interpretation of what is being communicated is also demanding and requires attention to the individualized and nuanced nature of both verbal and non-verbal communication (CSCI, 2008). Immersion in the care home setting is often a prerequisite for appreciating the meaning of data; some knowledge of the residents' lives and situations is also an aid to effective analysis. If we are serious about addressing current deficits in care home provision, understanding the subjective experience of residents with dementia is a fundamental dimension of enhancing practice and improving both quality of life and quality of care.

Living with dementia in care home: assessing and understanding the experience

It is clear from the above review that current methodologies tend to focus on assessing residents' quality of life with a view to enhancing care practice, rather than focusing on the experience of living with dementia in a care home per se. Although there is little argument that quality of life intersects powerfully with quality of care, it is nevertheless a notable feature of this field of enquiry to date and one that characterizes much of the discourse.

There is a linked tension between the objective evaluation of quality of life and the broader conceptual issue of how quality of life is defined and understood by older people with moderate to severe dementia. This is reflected by the tendency for (most) quality of life measures to marginalize (or even exclude) the perspective of the person with dementia and instead rely on 'objective' indicators, for example level of challenging behaviours, or the proxy views of others. The role of observational methodologies—especially DCM—in taking account of the user experience has been considerable and more recent attempts to use interviews and focus groups indicate a conceptual shift towards greater, and more central, incorporation of the resident perspective. Work that attempts to explicitly gather evidence about residents' subjective experiences of living with dementia in a care home is the most recent addition to the evidence base. That these depend on experiential methodologies, that do not 'fit' easily alongside work that is underpinned by objective 'measures' or more traditional research methods (see Surr, 2006; Clare et al., 2008 above) is notable.

Discrepancies between the views of residents and carers about quality of life and/or how it is assessed by research instruments underscores the importance of taking account of the user view. For example, a recent study by Droes et al. (2006) with people with dementia and their carers identified a number of domains that were important to residents and not to carers. These included: financial situation, sense of aesthetics in the living environment, and being of use and/or having a purpose that gives life meaning. Additionally, residents identified a number of domains that were absent from the quality of life instruments used in the same study. These were: security, privacy, self-determination, and freedom (Droes et al., 2006). It is striking that the domains identified by residents tend not to be disease oriented (e.g. cognitive decline), but are broadly focused on social engagement, purposeful activity, self-determination, and well-being.

That assessment of quality of life is increasingly understood as being rooted in the subjective experience of the person with dementia is a pivotal conceptual shift (Warner et al., 2010). It is also now accepted that people with dementia—even those with advanced dementia—are able to communicate meaningfully about their life and experiences (Byrne-Davis et al., 2006). These twin trends not only lend weight to the argument that greater attention needs to be paid to incorporating residents' own perspectives but that it needs to be a core component of work exploring quality of life in care homes rather than an 'add on'.

Finding out what determines 'a good life' for older people in care homes is the focus of recent work by the National Development Team for Inclusion (2009) and Bowers et al. (2009). These studies echo existing work in noting that the voices of residents who need a lot of support tend to be marginal to discussion about quality of life and care. This not only means that their contributions are not taken account of but the fact that they are excluded (further) contributes to their loss of role, identity, and personhood; it also lowers self-esteem and confidence (Scourfield, 2007). Relying on others to 'speak for' the older person as a proxy also serves to disempower the older person and colludes with the belief that they are not reliable commentators on their own lives or experiences.

Drawing on fieldwork with residents with higher levels of dependency (some of whom had advanced dementia), the study identified six elements of, or 'keys' to, a good quality of life:

- Personal identity and self-esteem
- Meaningful relationships
- Home and personal surroundings
- Meaningful daily and community life
- Personalized care and support
- Personal control and autonomy (Bowers et al., 2009)

The dimensions of this model resonate with those in the 'Senses Framework' devised by Nolan et al. (2006). This framework was developed in work with care home residents with dementia and their paid and family carers and identifies six senses that underpin psychological well-being: a sense of security, continuity, belonging, purpose, achievement, and significance (Davies and Nolan, 2008).

Conclusion

People with dementia living in care home face enormous challenges (Fossey, 2008). In addition to their declining cognitive powers, residents have to cope with a new and often unpredictable environment. Additionally, frailty, communication difficulties, and dependency on others often mean that their needs are overlooked and their voices marginalized. Understanding more about the experience of living in a care home with dementia can make a critical contribution to improving both quality of life and quality of care (Clare et al., 2008). Research instruments, interviews, and observational methods have made a significant contribution to our appreciation of what is important to residents with dementia. More recent research that attempts directly to capture the lived experiences of residents is adding further to our understanding of 'what matters'. Specifically, residents tend to prioritize non-disease-related domains of quality of life such as social engagement, purposeful activity, self-determination, and well-being. These are at odds with those prioritized by carers and 'objective' measures which tend to privilege functional and cognitive deficits. Not only is it evident that residents are able to meaningfully describe their experiences and daily lives but they also appear to retain a sense of self, identity, and agency (Brooker, 2008a).

There is a distinctive need for work on assessing quality of life among residents with dementia that places their subjective experience at its core (Owen and NCHRDF, 2006). Excellence in dementia care begins with an understanding of what it is like to live with the illness throughout its trajectory (Phinney, 2008). As there is no doubt that residential care will continue to make a significant contribution to the care of people with advanced dementia in the future, increased emphasis on research that explores the dimensions of quality of life from the perspective of residents is a pivotal component of improving life quality and building effective care practice.

References

Alzheimer's Society (2008). *Home from Home*. London: Alzheimer's Society.

Barnett, E. (2000). *Including the Person with Dementia in Designing and Delivering Care: 'I Need to be Me!'* London: Jessica Kingsley Publishers.

Bowers, H., Clark, A., Crosby, G., et al. (2009). *Older People's Vision for Long Term Care*. York: Joseph Rowntree Foundation.

Bowling, A. (2002). *Research Methods in Health*. Bucks: Open University Press.

Brod, M., Stewart, A.L., Sands, L., & Watson, P. (1999). Conceptualisation and measurement of quality of life in dementia: the dementia quality of life instrument (DQoL). *The Gerontologist, 39*, 25–35.

Brooker, D. (2005). Dementia Care Mapping (DCM): a review of the literature. *The Gerontologist, 45*, 11–18.

Brooker, D. (2007). *Person-centred Dementia Care: Making Services Better*, University of Bradford. London: Jessica Kingsley Publishers.

Brooker, D. (2008a). Quality: the perspective of the person with dementia. In: M. Downs & B. Bowers (Eds.), *Excellence in Dementia Care: Research into Practice* (pp. 476–491). Bucks: Open University Press.

Brooker, D. (2008b). Person centred care, in mental health in care homes for older people. In: R. Jacoby, C. Oppenheimer, T. Dening, & A. Thomas (Eds.), *The Oxford Textbook of Old Age Psychiatry*. Oxford: Oxford University Press.

Brown-Wilson, C., Cook, G., et al. (2009). The use of narrative in developing relationships in care homes. In: K. Froggatt., S. Davies, & J. Meyer. *Understanding Care Homes: A Research and Development Perspective* (pp. 70–90). London: Jessica Kingsley Publishers.

Bryman, A. (2004). *Social Research Methods*. Oxford: Oxford University Press.

Byrne-Davis, L., Bennett, P., & Wilcock, G. (2006). How are quality of life ratings made? Towards a model of quality of life in people with dementia. *Quality of Life Research, 15*, 855–865.

Caddell, L.S. & Clare, L. (2010). The impact of dementia on self and identity: a systematic review. *Clinical Psychological Review, 30*, 113–126.

Clare, L., Rowlands, J., Bruce, E., et al, (2008). The experience of living with dementia in residential care: an interpretive phenomenological analysis. *The Gerontologist, 48*(6), 711–720.

Commission for Social Care Inspection (CSCI) (2008a). *See Me, Not Just My Dementia: Understanding People's Experience of Living in a Care Home*. London: CSCI.

Commission for Social Care Inspection (CSCI) (2008b). *The State of Social Care in England 2006–07*. London: CSCI.

Cook, A. (2002). Using video observation to include the experiences of people with dementia in research. In: H. Wilkinson (Ed.), *The Perspectives of People with Dementia: Research Methods and Motivations.* London: Jessica Kingsley Publishers.

Davies, S. & Nolan, M. (2008). Attending to relationships in dementia care. In: M. Downs & B. Bowers (Eds.), *Excellence in Dementia Care: Research into Practice* (pp. 438–454). Berkshire: Open University Press.

Dening, T. & Milne, A. (2009). Depression and mental health in care homes. Depression, suicide and self-harm in older adults. *Quality in Ageing, 10*(2), 40–46.

Department of Health (2008). *Living Well with Dementia: A National Dementia Strategy*. London: Department of Health.

Droes, R., Boelens-van der Knoop, E., Bos, J., et al. (2006). Quality of life in dementia in perspective. *Dementia, 5*(4), 533–558.

Edelman, P., Fulton, B.R., Kuhn, D., et al. (2005). A comparison of three methods of measuring dementia-specific quality of life: perspectives of residents, staff and observers. *The Gerontologist, 45,* 27–36.

Fossey, J. (2008). Care homes. In: M. Downs & B. Bowers (Eds.), *Excellence in Dementia Care: Research into Practice* (pp. 336–358). Berkshire: Open University Press.

Gaugler, J.E., Leach, C.R., & Anderson, K.A. (2004). Correlates of resident psychosocial status in long-term care. *International Journal of Geriatric Psychiatry, 19,* 773–780.

Hoe, J., Katona, C., Roch, B., et al. (2005). Use of the QOL-AD for measuring quality of life in people with severe dementia—the LASER-AD study. *Age and Ageing, 34,* 130–135.

Hoe, J., Hancock, G., Livingston, G., et al. (2006). Quality of life of people with dementia in residential care homes. *British Journal of Psychiatry, 188,* 460–464.

Hubbard, G., Cook, A., Tester, S., & Downs, M. (2002). Beyond words: older people with dementia using and interpreting nonverbal behaviour. *Journal of Ageing Studies, 16,* 155–167.

Hubbard, G., Tester, S., & Downs, M. (2003). Meaningful social interactions between older people in institutional care settings. *Ageing and Society, 23,* 99–114.

Hyden, L.-C. & Orulv, L. (2009). Narrative and identity in Alzheimer's disease: a case study. *Journal of Aging Studies, 23,* 205–214.

Innes, A. & Kelly, F. (2007). Evaluating long stay care settings: reflections on the process with particular reference to DCM. In: A. Innes & L. McCabe (Eds.), *Evaluation in Dementia Care.* London: Jessica Kingsley Publishers.

Killick, J. & Allan, K. (2006). The Good Sunset Project: making contact with those close to death. *Journal of Dementia Care, 14,* 22–24.

Kitwood, T. (1997). *Dementia Reconsidered: The Person Comes First.* Buckingham: Open University Press.

Logsdon, R.G., Gibbons, L.E., McCurry, S.M., et al. (1999). Quality of life in Alzheimer's disease: patient and caregiver reports. *Journal of Mental Health and Aging, 5,* 21–32.

Macer, J. & Murphy, J. (2009). *Training care home staff to use Talking Mats with people who have dementia.* York: Joseph Rowntree Foundation.

Mayhew, P.A., Action, G.J., Yuak, S., et al. (2001). Communication from individuals with advanced DAT: can it provide clues to their sense of self-awareness and well-being? *Geriatric Nursing, 22,* 106–110.

Milne, A. & Peet, J. (2008). *Challenges & Resolutions to Psycho-social Well-being for People in Receipt of a Diagnosis of Dementia: A Literature Review.* London: Mental Health Foundation and Alzheimer's Society.

Mozley, C., Huxley, P., Sutcliffe, C., et al. (1999). 'Not knowing where I am does not mean I don't know what I like': cognitive impairment and quality of life responses in elderly people. *International Journal of Geriatric Psychiatry, 14,* 776–783.

Murphy, C. (2007). User involvement in evaluations. In: A. Innes & L. McCabe (Eds.), *Evaluation in Dementia Care.* London: Jessica Kingsley Publishers.

Murphy, J., Oliver, T.M., & Cox, S. (2010). *Talking Mats Help Involve People with Dementia and their Carers in Decision-making.* York: Joseph Rowntree Foundation.

National Development Team for Inclusion (2009). *Finding Out what Determines 'A Good Life' for Older People in Care Homes.* York: Joseph Rowntree Foundation.

Nolan, M., Lundh, U., Grant, G., & Keady, J. (2003). *Partnerships in Family Care*. Berkshire: Open University Press.

Nolan, M., Brown, J., Davies, S., et al. (2006). *The Senses Framework: Improving Care for Older People through a Relationship Centred Approach*, Getting Research into Practice Series. Sheffield: University of Sheffield.

Orrell, M. & Hancock, G. (2004). *CANE: Camberwell Assessment of Need for the Elderly*. London: Gaskell.

Owen, T. & the National Care Home Research and Development Forum (2006). *My Home Life: Quality of Life in Care Homes*. London: Help the Aged.

Phinney, A. (2008). Toward understanding subjective experiences of dementia. In: M. Downs & B. Bowers (Eds.), *Excellence in Dementia Care: Research into Practice* (pp. 35–51). Berkshire: Open University Press.

Sabat, S. (2001). *The Experience of Alzheimer's Disease*. Oxford: Blackwell Publishing.

Scourfield, P. (2007). Helping older people in residential care remain full citizens. *British Journal of Social Work, 37*(7), 1135–1152.

Sloane, P.D., Zimmerman, S., Williams, C.S., et al. (2005). Evaluating the quality of life of long-term care residents with dementia. *The Gerontologist, 45*, 37–49.

Smallbrugge, M., Pot, A.M., Jongenelis, L., et al. (2006). The impact of depression and anxiety on well being, disability and use of health care services in nursing home patients. *International Journal of Geriatric Psychiatry, 21*, 325–332.

Smith, S.C., Lamping, D.L., Banerjee, S., et al. (2005). Measurement of health related quality of life for people with dementia: development of a new instrument (DEMQOL) and an evaluation of current methodology. *Health Technology Assessment, 9*(193), LIII–LIV.

Social Care Institute for Excellence (2009). *Personalisation Briefing: Implications for Residential Care Homes*. London: Social Care Institute for Excellence.

Spector, A. & Orrell, M. (2006). Quality of life in dementia: a comparison of the perceptions of people with dementia and care staff in residential homes. *Alzheimer's Disease and Associated Disorders, 20*(3), 160–165.

Surr, C.A. (2006). Preservation of self in people with dementia living in residential care: a socio-biographical approach. *Social Science and Medicine, 62*, 1720–1730.

Szczepura, A. & Clay, D. (2008). *Improving Care in Residential Care Homes: A Literature Review*. York: Joseph Rowntree Foundation.

Tester, S., Hubbard, G., Downs, M., MacDonald, C., & Murphy, J. (2004). Frailty and institutional care. In: A. Walker & C. Hagan Hennesey (Eds.), *Quality of Life in Old Age*. Bucks: Open University Press.

Train, G.H., Nurock, S.A., Mandela, M., et al. (2005). A qualitative study of the experiences of long-term care for residents with dementia, their relatives and staff. *Aging and Mental Health, 9*, 119–128.

University of Bradford (2005). *DCM 8: User's Manual*. Bradford: University of Bradford.

Warner, J., Milne, A., & Peet, J. (2010). *'My Name is not Dementia': Literature Review*. London: Alzheimer's Society.

Williams, C.L. & Tappen, R.M. (1999). Can we create a therapeutic relationship with nursing home residents in the later stages of Alzheimer's disease? *Journal of Psychosocial Nursing, 37*, 28–35.

Part 2

The outside view

Chapter 7

Regulation and quality

Rekha Elaswarapu

Abstract

Regulating care homes is a challenging task. In good part this is a consequence of the fragmented and diverse nature of the care home sector; homes differ considerably in terms of size, culture, funding patterns, and resident profiles. Although the UK's regulatory framework(s) have seen many changes in recent years, the fundamental principle of regulation remains the same: to ensure that people who use services are safe and receive high quality care in a personalized way that maintains their dignity and human rights. Given the complex nature of delivering effective care to older people with—often serious—mental health problems, the role of a robust regulatory framework in upholding standards and ensuring accountability is a key lever for quality improvement. This chapter reviews the role of regulation in supporting the delivery of quality care to older people with mental health conditions living in a care home and explores some of the challenges facing regulation now and in the future.

Introduction

Regulating the quality of care homes[1] is a challenging task. In good part this is because of the fragmented and diverse nature of the sector, the complexity of funding systems, and the variety of types and sizes of care homes. For smaller care homes meeting the requirements of the regulatory agency can place a substantial burden on their limited resources. By contrast, larger care homes may have their own internal assessment

---

[1] Throughout this chapter, 'care homes' refers to all types of care homes both residential and nursing homes. 'Residential homes' are homes registered to provide personal care only to residents. 'Nursing homes' are registered to offer nursing care to at least some residents. Part I, Section 3 of the Care Standards Act (2000) defines a care home as any home which provides accommodation together with nursing or personal care for any person who is or has been ill (including mental disorder), is disabled or infirm, or who has a past or present dependence on drugs or alcohol.

processes such as audits, and tend to be more prepared for the demands of regulation. There is an inherent tension among private providers between the need to adhere to regulations and the drive to make a profit.

Although regulation of the care home sector has witnessed significant change over the last decade, its fundamental aim remains the same: to ensure that service users are safe and receive care that meets defined standards of quality and maintains their dignity and human rights.

This chapter reviews the role of regulation in ensuring quality of care for older people with mental health problems living in a care home, how it has changed since the mid-1980s, and how it can improve quality.

Quality of mental healthcare in care homes

In recent years, a range of government policies have highlighted the importance of regulation in improving the quality of health and social care services. These include: the National Service Framework for Older People (Department of Health, 2001), Everybody's Business (Department of Health, 2005), High Quality Care for All (Department of Health, 2008a), No Secrets (Department of Health, 2000), Putting People First (Department of Health, 2007a), Our Health Our Care Our Say (Department of Health, 2006), and Transforming Adult Social Care Services (Department of Health, 2008b), and the NHS Constitution (Department of Health, 2010). Despite this policy emphasis, the quality of care, including mental health care, in care homes has routinely been identified as less than satisfactory (Tucker et al., 2007).

As mental health problems are a common feature of the care home population— over two-thirds of residents have dementia—ensuring good quality mental healthcare is a priority for those agencies tasked with regulation (Age Concern and the Mental Health Foundation, 2006).

Older people in care homes tend to have a range of comorbid conditions and complex needs. As at least two-thirds of care home residents have moderate to severe dementia and many have impaired communication skills, providing good quality care is a challenging task. Ensuring that this vulnerable—and often invisible—population receives high quality clinical and personal care, that their needs and preferences are fully taken care of, and that their dignity and privacy is promoted, is an overarching aim of regulation (Healthcare Commission, 2007). Two recent reports on dementia care have highlighted the important contribution played by strong leadership and a skilled workforce in delivering high quality care alongside inspection and regulation (All-Party Parliamentary Group on Dementia, 2009; National Audit Office, 2010).

Specific concerns have been identified around the provision of healthcare services and prescribing patterns. The provision of primary care and good quality specialist care to care home residents with dementia and/or depression can make a pivotal contribution to their health and well-being (Alzheimer's Society, 2007; Ames, 1990). There have long been concerns about uneven and fragmented primary care provision to the care home sector, an issue that has been highlighted by the Disability Rights Commission (2006) and Patterson (2008) and acknowledged by the General Medical

Council (2008) and the Department of Health (2007b). Similar concerns exist in relationship to specialist and community mental health services; their role in preventing some resident admissions to hospital has specifically been highlighted (Healthcare Commission, 2008).

Recent research into prescribing practices in care homes has also highlighted concerns about inappropriate use of antipsychotic drugs for residents with 'challenging behaviour'; these are primarily people with dementia (All-Party Parliamentary Group on Dementia, 2008; Barber et al., 2009; Department of Health, 2009a; Fahey et al., 2003; Joseph Rowntree Foundation, 2008). The Human Rights Act (HMSO, 1998) and the Mental Capacity Act (2005)—and in particular its section on Deprivation of Liberty Safeguards—has been instrumental in raising the need to ensure the protection of adults with mental illness who may lack capacity living in a care home. This includes decisions about treatment and medication (HMSO, 2005). Action on Elder Abuse, News, and Media (2010) has also reported many cases relating to potential abuse or very poor practice in relationship to the care of frail older people in care homes, including residents with dementia. This has contributed to the call for better systems of protection of care home residents.

In light of the complexities of the environment in which care homes operate, the role of robust regulatory processes in helping to ensure the welfare of the residents can be seen as a key lever for quality improvement.

What is regulation?

Regulation is often perceived as the panacea of poor practice and performance. This perception stems from lack of understanding of the regulatory function and its remit. Broadly defined, regulation is 'sustained and focused control exercised by a public agency over activities which are valued by a community' (Selznick, 1985). Although regulation can take a number of forms, the most common form in the health and social care sector is a policy requirement to meet a set of standards defined and devised by government.

A regulatory framework has the following key features:

- A *purpose* such as ensuring safety of service users, access to services particularly for those who are vulnerable due to illness or dependency, and/or value for public money by making service providers accountable. These aims may be in conflict with one another.

- The *regulatory* function is undertaken by *a regulatory body* with clearly defined powers laid down by the law as well as structures for accountability. This body is separate from service providers and their relationship is one of an independent assessor and provider.

- The *regulatory* body provides *clear and transparent processes* through which regulatory assessments are carried out; and finally.

- Clarity about the *organizations* that are required to be regulated.

Regulation is governed by a matrix of regulatory requirements. These are a mixture of mandatory policy guidance that is laid down by legislation, for example the National

Dementia Strategy (Department of Health, 2009b), and good practice materials, for example guidelines issued by the National Institute for Health and Clinical Excellence and Social Care Institute for Excellence (2006).

Although the regulatory function can be delivered in a number of ways, it tends to have a threefold purpose:

- *Improving performance* by ensuring a certain standard of quality of the services with a particular focus on poor performing organizations.
- *Inspecting services* with the aim of evaluating the welfare of service users and accountability of the providers.
- *Informing the public and stakeholders* on the performance of the regulated organizations by benchmarking them across the care sector and providing comparative information on performance to allow informed choices.

Regulatory bodies have enforcement powers to ensure the safety of users in a wide range of service settings including residents of a care home. This may take the form of initial registration and subsequent ongoing monitoring to seek assurance that the registered organizations are maintaining the required standard of care. The enforcement activity includes the possibility of de-registering a service or imposing certain conditions that the service has to meet in order to continue to practice, see the case studies (opposite) for an example.

Good regulation can play a crucial role in ensuring high quality health and social care services and can reduce the regulatory burden considerably by following the five principles of good regulation:

- Transparent
- Accountable
- Proportionate
- Consistent
- Targeted—only at situations or services where action is needed

The above functions are interrelated and should collectively lead to the ultimate goal of ensuring high quality service through the regulatory processes (Better Regulation Executive, 2009).

Regulatory framework for care homes: pre-1985 to present

The regulatory landscape for care homes has been subject to significant improvement over the last 20 years. Prior to 2002, the regulation was basically devolved to local health authorities and councils and was underpinned by locally defined standards. This resulted in considerable variability in the quality of services and how they were regulated. During this period, residential homes providing nursing as well as personal care were required to register with the health authority as 'nursing homes', whereas those providing only personal care had to be registered as a 'residential home' with the local authority. Although this dual registration allowed for better service provision due to individual in-depth focus on personal care and nursing care regulation, it also imposed a greater regulatory burden on registered homes (Joseph Rowntree

Enforcement

Case study 1: Care homes for older people: *ABC house*

The quality rating for this care home is: zero star—poor service.

This is a 30 bedded home for older people which includes people with dementia.

This is a report of an inspection to assess whether services are meeting the needs of people who use them. The legal basis for conducting inspections is the Care Standards Act (2000) and the relevant NMS for this establishment are those for *care homes for older people*.

Nutrition

Case notes for five people were tracked. We also spoke to the residents as well as observed the meal times.

What we found

There is no clear system of assessment of nutritional needs for the residents. Not all care plans identified the additional help that the frail residents needed with eating and drinking. During observation, it was noted that one resident who needed pureed food due to swallowing difficulties had been given un-pureed food. This could have been a potential safety issue. Staff were not seen to be providing assistance with food and drink for those whose care plan indicated this need. There was no adequate system of recording the food intake which did not demonstrate that the nutritional needs were being met. These issues have been identified in previous inspections.

In view of the ongoing failure to meet previous requirements to provide proper care and treatment to service users a Statutory Requirement Notice has been issued.

Statutory requirement notices

If a provider does not make improvements that we have asked them to make, we can send them a legal notice that describes:

- Which regulation is being broken

- What improvements they have to make

- How long they have to do it

- We will follow-up whether the improvements have been made. If they have not we will take further action, in line with the enforcement pathways.

Case study 2: Any town lodge

The quality rating for this care home is: zero star—poor service

This is a 10 bedded home for older people.

This is a report of an inspection to assess whether services are meeting the needs of people who use them. The legal basis for conducting inspections is the Care Standards Act (2000) and the relevant NMS for this establishment are those for *care homes for older people*.

What we found

Staff were not following the safeguarding protocols as they had not been trained on this aspect.

Condition

All staff to be trained on safeguarding protocol within 3 months from the date of registration.

Foundation, 1995). This subsequently led to the single registration process introduced under the Care Standards Act (2000).

A significant move towards having nationally driven standards and centrally directed regulation came about in 2002 (see Box 7.1). This shift is widely regarded as the foundation for the current regulatory framework. The advent of the National Care Standards Commission (NCSC), which was set up and given statutory status by the Care Standards Act of 2000, introduced a more streamlined structure to the regulation of care homes. However, NCSC was seen as rather resource intensive compared to its predecessors. The increased cost of regulation and the time sent on inspections were considered disproportionate and carried a potential risk of increase in registration fees for the service providers due to the raised administrative costs for the NCSC (Netten et al., 2004). NCSC was replaced by the Commission for Social Care Inspection (CSCI) in April 2004.

Box 7.1 The regulatory framework—post-2002

Regulatory framework

2003–2004
- National Care Standards Commission, an independent body with a range of enforcement powers to replace the existing local and health authority inspections
- Remit to register and inspect social care providers and commissioners of social care services

2004–2008
- Commission for Social Care Inspection became operational in April 2004. It was established with a remit to undertake announced and unannounced inspections of providers and commissioners of social care services
- Range of enforcement powers to take action about poor performance
- Periodic and thematic reviews on specific aspects of services

Key relevant legislation/policy
- Care Standards Act (2000)
- The National Care Standards Commission (Registration) Regulations (2001)
- Care Homes Regulation (2001)
- Care homes for older people: NMS* and the Care Homes Regulations— Care Home Regulations (2001) (as amended 18 February 2003)
- The National Care Standards Commission (Registration) (Amendment) Regulations (2003a)
- The National Care Standards Commission (Fees and Frequency of Inspections) Regulations (2003b)

- Health and Social Care (Community Health and Standards) Act (2003)
- Care homes for older people: NMS and the Care Homes Regulations— Care Home Regulations (2001) (as amended 18 February 2003)
- Care Standards Act (2000)
- Commission for Social Care Inspection (Fees and Frequency of Inspections) Regulations (2004)
- Commission for Social Care Inspection (Fees and Frequency of Inspections) Regulations (2007a,b)

Box 7.1 The regulatory framework—post-2002 (continued)

2009 to present

Care Quality Commission became operational in April 2009 with a remit to:

♦ Register, inspect, and regulate health and adult social care services;
♦ Protect the interests of people held under the Mental Health Act;
♦ Work with providers and commissioners of local services towards improving those services;
♦ Give individuals, families, and carers clear information about availability of care services and their quality;
♦ Take action where services are unacceptably poor; and
♦ Produce an annual national commentary on the state of health and social care services including the local commissioning arrangements.

♦ Health and Social Care Act (2008a,b)
♦ Health and Social Care Act (2008a,b) (Regulated Activities) regulations 2010
♦ NMS continue to apply until 1 October 2010 and then replaced by the new regulations on essential standards for quality and safety as prescribed by the Care Quality Commission (Registration) Regulations (2009a)

Source: Care Quality Commission (from various CQC sources).
*NMS: National Minimum Standards

Standards for quality and safety

The core aim of any form of regulation is to ensure that quality standards set for a care service are met by providers and commissioners. The Care Standards Act (2000)—and subsequent service specific regulations—laid the legislative foundation stones for regulating the care home sector. They also established minimum standards regarding the management of the care home, staff, premises, and general conduct of the agencies providing care home services. More specifically the roles include:

♦ Registration: what is required for a provider to be 'fit for purpose'
♦ Fees: how much it costs a provider to register with the regulator
♦ Basic requirements to run a service

The National Minimum Standards (NMS) (Care Standards Act, 2000), which came into force in 2002, (Department of Health 2003) were underpinned by the following basic principles of quality of care in a care home:

1 Focus on service users
2 Fitness for purpose
3 Comprehensiveness

4 Meeting assessed needs

5 Quality of services

6 Quality of workforce

They covered key aspects of user quality of life including:

1 Choice of home

2 Health and personal care

3 Daily life and social activities

4 Complaints and protection

5 Environment

6 Staffing

7 Management and administration

These standards were supported by guidance logs for inspectors and the service providers detailing CSCI's expectations of service providers with regards to compliance with each of the standards (Care Quality Commission, 2009b). The guidance also allowed service providers to self-evaluate their performance against the guidance. Although CSCI recognized that there are many ways care home providers can deliver 'good care' and 'good outcomes' for residents, they must all meet the minimum standards developed as a consequence of regulatory legislation. An example of how guidance can clarify what a specific NMS means is given in Box 7.2.

During the period of oversight of the CSCI (2004–2008), regulatory processes underwent substantial changes. These primarily related to a reduction in the number and frequency of inspections—which has been experienced by many care homes as

Box 7.2 Guidance relating to the NMS on meeting needs

Outcome
Service users and their representatives know that the home they enter will meet their needs.

All specialist services offered (e.g. services for people with dementia or other cognitive impairments, sensory impairment, physical disabilities, learning disabilities, intermediate or respite care) are demonstrably based on current good practice, and reflect relevant specialist and clinical guidance.

Guidance
Although some permanent residents may welcome short-stay residents as providing new company and variation to their lives, we have noted from feedback over time that many find frequent or high levels of turnover of short-stay residents to be unsettling, intrusive, and to encroach on their privacy. Providers considering offering intermediate or short-term care should bear this in mind and consult existing residents before offering it. Some homes which provide well-established short-term care do so by having a degree of separation of accommodation so that long-term residents are less affected.

Source: Care Quality Commission, Care Homes for Older People: Guidance Log (2009b).

rather 'top heavy'—and a shift to the development of proportionate and targeted inspections. These were based on annual risk assessments of how care homes were meeting the needs of residents. Also in 2007, a quality rating system was introduced which allowed inspections to be focused on those care homes where standards were not being met and quality was poor. Care Quality Commission will be using these ratings until October 2010 when the new regulations will become operational (Care Quality Commission, 2010a). In the period after October 2010, there will be a new set of ratings which will be in line with the new registration system introduced in October 2010. Detail on quality ratings is given in Box 7.3.

Box 7.3 The quality ratings system

In 2007, CSCI introduced a quality ratings system for each service. It was designed to give a more rounded assessment of the care services and include information on outcomes for service users rather than simply data on national minimum standards. Under the quality ratings system, services are classified as follows:

3 stars—excellent
2 stars—good
1 star—adequate
0 stars—poor

The rating of a service is based on the information received by the regulatory body from a number of sources, including:

- Feedback from interviews with staff and service users.
- Self-assessment information given to the regulator by the care service through annual quality assurance assessment (AQAA).
- The results of surveys filled in by people using the service, their relatives, and other professionals involved in their care.
- The findings of a key inspection, usually unannounced, which looks at every aspect of a service.
- Information held about the history of the service including NMS compliance.

Each type of adult social care service has its own set of national minimum standards, that the service is expected to meet. The scores awarded are:

1—Not meeting standard with major shortfalls
2—Not meeting standard with minor shortfalls
3—Meeting standard
4—Exceeding standard

All registered services had a baseline assessment and CSCI placed greater emphasis on incorporating views of service users in its judgements of the quality of care. Care homes with a 3 star rating had a full inspection at least once every 3 years to allow less intrusion from the regulators, whereas those with poor ratings were subject to full inspections more frequently. CSCI also carried out random inspections of a number of services each year, regardless of the quality rating of a service.

Source: Care Quality Commission, Quality Ratings for Care Services (2010a).

Besides the regular inspection process, the CSCI also undertook in-depth studies on specific topic areas such as dementia care (Commission for Social Care Inspection, 2008a). The development and use of observational tools such as SOFI (Short Observational Tool for Inspection) improved the inspection process as it enabled inspectors to collect evidence about the care of residents with dementia (Commission for Social Care Inspection, 2007a,b). Similarly, another initiative—Experts by Experience (Commission for Social Care Inspection, 2008b), whereby service users and/or their carers joined the inspection teams—significantly enhanced the richness of the evidence collected during inspections of care homes. These experts may visit care homes for older people and support the process by looking at what is happening in the care homes, see how everyone gets on together, and what the home feels like. They also talk to the residents to seek their feedback on their experience of living in the care home.

As from October 2010, the NMS and quality ratings were replaced by new regulations: the essential standards of quality and safety applicable to all health and social care organizations (Care Quality Commission, 2009c). There are 28 regulations altogether: 16 of these relate directly to standards on safety and quality and 12 relate to the routine management of a service. Some sample regulations and related outcomes are offered by way of an example in Box 7.4.

All care homes undertake regulated activities. All those providing nursing and/or personal care in a care home setting are required to register and provide evidence of compliance with registration requirements.

The Care Quality Commission is responsible for enacting the enforcement powers stipulated under the Care Standards Act (2000); it also has additional powers under the Health and Social Care Act (2008a,b). The differences between the two pieces of legislation are presented in Box 7.5.

Box 7.4 Regulation requirements relating to the essential standards of quality and safety

Regulation title	Summary of outcome	Requirement from the providers
Care and welfare of people who use services	People experience effective, safe, and appropriate care, treatment, and support that meet their needs and protect their rights	Assess the needs of people who use services Planning and delivering care, treatment, and support so that people are safe, their welfare is protected, and needs met Taking account of published research and guidance Make reasonable adjustments to reflect people's needs, values, and diversity Have arrangements for dealing with foreseeable emergencies

Box 7.4 Regulation requirements relating to the essential standards of quality and safety *(continued)*

Management of medicines	People who use services will have their medicines at the times they need them and in a safe way Where possible information about medicines being prescribed made available to them or others acting on their behalf	Handle medicines safely, securely, and appropriately Ensure that medicines are prescribed and given by people safely Follow published guidance about how to use medicines safely
Safeguarding people who use services from abuse	People are protected from abuse, or the risk of abuse, and their human rights are respected and upheld	Identify and prevent abuse from happening in a service by responding appropriately to a concern about possible or actual abuse Ensure staff have access to government policies and local guidance about safeguarding people Make sure the use of restraint is appropriate, proportionate, reasonable, and justifiable, and respects dignity and human rights Understand diversity beliefs and values that influence the identification, prevention, and response to the safeguarding concerns
Requirements relating to workers	People who use services are safe and their health and welfare needs are met by the staff who are fit, appropriately qualified, and are physically and mentally able to do their job	Have effective recruitment and selection procedures in place including carrying out relevant checks Ensure staff are registered with, and allowed to work by the relevant professional body/regulator

Source: Care Quality Commission, Essential Standards of Quality and Safety (2009c).

The new regulatory system promises greater emphasis on outcomes for service users. It intends to incorporate user and carer perspectives and experiences into all regulatory processes such as case tracking, use of observation tools (see SOFI mentioned earlier), and surveys asking residents their view of the care home in its inspections (Care Quality Commission, 2009d).

Box 7.5 Comparison of enforcement powers between the 'old' and 'new' regulatory regime

Power	Care Standards Act (2000)	Health and Social Care Act (2008a,b)
Issue a warning notice	✗	✓
Impose, vary, or remove conditions	✓	✓
Issue a penalty notice in lieu of prosecution	✗	✓
Suspend registration	✗	✓
Cancel registration	✓	✓
Prosecute for specified offences	✓	✓

Source: Care Quality Commission, Enforcement Policy (2009d).

Measuring what matters

One of the most effective outcomes for a regulator is the accurate assessment of 'what really matters' to service users in achieving high quality care. Although there have been a number of attempts to identify a set of indicators that reflect what is important to older people living in a care home, data on 'outcomes' tend to be limited and/or focused on a single home or group of homes (Owen and NCHRDF, 2006; Netten et al., 2010). Generalizing the findings of a single research project to the whole sector is challenging for reasons already discussed; genuinely incorporating the views of residents with dementia in evaluations of care home quality is especially difficult (see Chapter 6).

A salient feature of the new regulatory framework is the use of information to ensure proportionate and targeted inspections of services where inspection is required. This intelligence known as the 'quality and risk profiles'[2] based on specific indicators for each service provider will trigger an area of concern and a possible inspection which would be 'targeted' in a number of ways. For example, a full inspection of all aspects of care in a care home, or only a part inspection of the area of concern, such as medicines management for people with dementia. This approach reduces the regulatory burden on care homes and allows the inspection system to focus more effectively on those homes that are performing badly as and when this is identified. This is a change in inspection patterns. The approach used by CSCI included visiting care homes rated as excellent once every 3 years. Inspectors thus may have missed deterioration in performance between visits. Under the new system concerns raised in the quality and

[2] The Quality and Risk Profile (QRP) is a dynamic approach to combining a range of information from service users, together with information from regulatory activity, external bodies, and national datasets. The QRP indicates where there may be good performance or areas of concern based on the data items that it contains, it does not provide the judgement.

risk profiles can be addressed quickly rather than allowing bad practice to become embedded.

The impact of regulation on care home quality

> Now that regulators are asking about support for staff my manager will send me on training courses which is better for me to do my job'.
>
> A head cook in a care home for older people

Assessing the impact of regulation on improvement in service provision and/or better outcomes is complex as it is often difficult to prove direct causality between the two. Improvements in services or care practice may be a result of a combination of factors, regulation being one of them (Day et al., 1996). An increased competition and higher expectations among service users, and an increased need to ensure competence of the workforce, providers, and commissioners also play a role (Sparrow, 2000).

One of the ways the impact of a regulatory framework can be established is by examining to what extent has regulation succeeded in its primary functions. The three main functions of any regulatory framework are:

- To improve standards of safety and quality in care homes
- To inform the public about quality of services
- To improve outcomes for people who use services

Improving safety and quality

One of the ways improvement in quality and safety can be demonstrated is by looking at the compliance rates of service providers with the essential standards of quality and safety. An analysis of the performance of all care homes in England (see Box 7.6) for older people shows that there has been a substantial increase in compliance with key standards (including protection) since the introduction of the NMS in 2002 (Care Quality Commission, 2009e). However, the report also found that considerable improvement was still needed on standards relating to record keeping, service user plans, medication, and staff supervision. Additionally, a fifth of care homes for older people were found not to be meeting the standard on social activities—an important indicator of good quality care for older people with mental health problems.

Informing the public about quality of services

Regulation has a key role to play in facilitating informed decision-making for people using the services and their carers. A report commissioned by CSCI found a positive link between higher awareness about quality ratings for the care home and the choice of a home with a higher quality rating although this was not the sole deciding factor (Commission for Social Care Inspection, 2009).

One of the key commitments of the Care Quality Commission as the new regulatory body is to publish information widely thus helping people who use services, and their carers, to make informed decisions and effective choices.

Box 7.6 Improvement in percentage of care homes for older people meeting each standard since the introduction of NMS

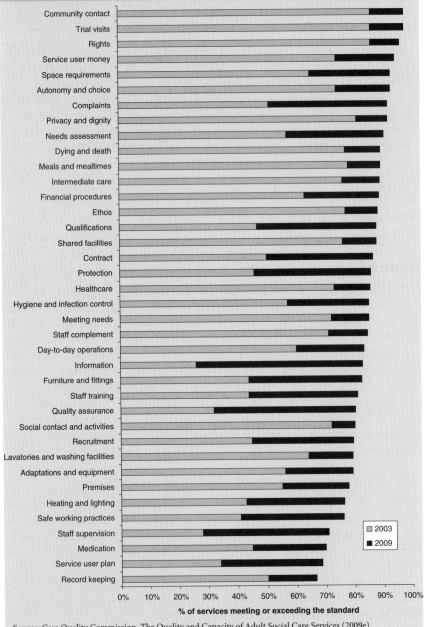

% of services meeting or exceeding the standard

Source: Care Quality Commission, The Quality and Capacity of Adult Social Care Services (2009e).

Improving outcomes for people who use services

This is the most challenging and difficult aspect of a regulatory process. Although regulation and inspection may have a positive impact on raising some standards in care homes, overall regulation is not a resource neutral process and can lead to negative impact for people using the service.

The costs of compliance fall disproportionately on smaller care homes and may, paradoxically, reduce user choice due to a reduction in the services provided (University of Portsmouth, 2005). Further, centrally driven regulatory processes have been criticized for being rigid and for curbing innovative developments that may improve care and quality of life for residents (Johnson et al., 1988). They may even contribute to a culture of care that encourages 'ritualistic compliance' with standards, especially when an inspection is due, at the expense of creative thinking, flexibility, and genuine bottom up improvements to care (Raleigh and Foot, 2010).

There are also ethical issues associated with the closure of a small care home due to poor performance. Although such an action may be entirely justified on safeguarding grounds, it also results in vulnerable residents being moved to a new environment. This causes considerable upheaval and distress to residents, especially those with dementia, and may well impact negatively on their well-being and quality of life (Owen and NCHRDF, 2006).

However, it is important to note that enforced closures of care homes are rare and only done in circumstances where there is no other alternative. In the majority of cases where standards are not met or there are concerns about care quality, the regulatory body works with the care home to improve the quality of care through action plans and signposting to good practice guidance and examples (Care Quality Commission, 2010b).

In contrast with the previous regulatory frameworks which focused on processes and systems, the new regulatory framework promises to be more outcomes-focused and its success in meeting this commitment will need to be evaluated in due course.

The future of regulation

We need to change the way we look at care and take a broader view. Where does social care stop and healthcare begin? It should all be seen as part of a continuum of care and support—and the overall quality should be viewed from the individual's perspective.

Carer of husband with dementia

The Health and Social Care Act (2008a,b) gave rise to a new regulatory system across the health and social care system, which, as noted above, will ensure greater focus on outcomes. Registration of all regulated activities is the cornerstone of the new regulation process; this is intended to ensure that all people using health and social care services in England can expect a certain standard of quality of care.

This new regulatory system faces a number of key challenges. Inspecting and regulating health and social care services under the one umbrella agency will be complex. There are significant differences between the health and social care sectors, services, personnel, systems, legal requirements, and user populations. The fact that health and social care services and agencies also vary in terms of size, structure, staff types and competencies, and funding arrangements is also an issue.

In addition, the downward trend in funding for public services coupled with a substantial growth in likely demand for care home places in the near future will put a substantial strain on resources. This will impact on the scope and scale of regulatory operations. In future, regulators will need to think 'smartly', including working in partnership with other regulatory and professional bodies and sharing information. The regulatory system needs to achieve two sets of balances simultaneously: that between needing to capture sufficient information about the quality of care provided by a home while reducing the demands of regulation on the homes themselves, and that between working with the care home sector to encourage gradual improvements in care quality while ensuring the protection of vulnerable residents from harm. There remains a need to evaluate what actually matters to care home residents especially those with dementia and improve the quality of data about social care provision. The upcoming survey of social care and the national minimum datasets for social care are a welcome contribution to achieving the latter goal (NHS Information Centre, 2010).

Conclusion

Regulation plays a crucial part in improving quality. The star ratings for adult social care in particular played a really important part in driving up standards in the care home sector. It also promotes self-evaluation mechanisms for the sector by providing guidance which in turn leads to improvement in adherence to the quality standards. The real improvements, however, are very much dependent on the relationship between a provider and the regulator. It has been noted that providers generally welcome the regulatory scrutiny where the intention is to work in partnership with a common goal of improvement in quality. In cases where regulation is seen as a stick there is a tendency towards tokenistic compliance. It is important for the regulator to identify and celebrate the good parts as well as tackle the not so good ones.

Regulation also has a key role in facilitating empowerment by involving people in regulatory processes and providing comparative information on performance across the sector for people who use services. Although both of these have been an integral aspect of regulation over the years, there is no evidence to prove that this has in fact led to the empowerment of service users. In addition, the quality of outcomes may be due to a combination of factors, regulation being one of them.

Regulation has been seen as a key lever for improvement and it has succeeded to some extent by shining a light on poor performance. However, the process itself is expensive and intensive. Although there are many challenges, there is also a growing support for the quality agenda aimed at facilitating quality in the care home sector.

Regulation has moved from being centred on systems and processes to outcomes for people in recent years. Regulatory process can be a proactive tool to help improve outcomes for people using the service by listening to what people want, helping to share good practice among providers, and moving the bar for quality and safety upwards as the sector develops. With the right information for better risk profiling and proportionate targeting, and improving the providers' confidence in self-assurance, the regulators can be seen as equal partners in the agenda to improve quality of care, including mental healthcare, for older people living in care homes.

References

Action on Elder Abuse, News, and Media (2010). Available at: http://www.elderabuse.org.uk (accessed 25 May 2010).

Age Concern and Mental Health Foundation (2006). *Promoting Mental Health and Well-Being in Later Life*. Available at: www.ageuk.org.uk (accessed 14 February 2011).

All-Party Parliamentary Group on Dementia (2008). *Always a Last Resort: Inquiry into the Prescription of Antipsychotic Drugs to People with Dementia Living in Care Homes*. London: Alzheimer's Society.

All-Party Parliamentary Group on Dementia (2009). *Prepared to Care: Challenging the Dementia Skills Gap*. Available at: http://www.alzheimers.org.uk (accessed 24 July 2010).

Alzheimer's Society (2007). *Home from Home: A Report Highlighting Opportunities for Improving Standards of Dementia in Care Homes*. London: Alzheimer's Society.

Ames, D. (1990). Depression among elderly residents of local authority residential homes, its nature and the efficacy of intervention. *British Journal of Psychiatry, 156*, 667–675.

Barber, N.D., Alldred, D.P., Raynor, D.K., et al. (2009). Care homes use of medicines study: prevalence, causes and potential harm of medication errors in care homes for older people. *Quality and Safety in Healthcare, 18*, 341–346.

Better Regulation Executive (2009). *Striking the Right Balance: BRE Annual Review 2009*. Available at: http://www.bis.gov.uk/assets/biscore/better-regulation/docs/10-578-striking-the-right-balance-bre-annual-review-2009.pdf (accessed 21 February 2011).

Care Standards Act (2000). (c.14). London: HMSO.

Care Homes Regulations (2001). SI 2001/3965. London: HMSO.

Care Quality Commission (Registration) Regulations (2009a). SI 2009/3112. London: HMSO.

Care Quality Commission (2009b). *Care Homes for Older People: Guidance Log*. Available at: http://www.cqc.org.uk/_db/_documents/20090105_Guidance_Log_Care_Homes_for_Older_People_v_001-09.doc (accessed 14 February 2011).

Care Quality Commission. (2009c). *Essential Standards of Quality and Safety*. London: Care Quality Commission.

Care Quality Commission (2009d). *Enforcement Policy*. London: Care Quality Commission.

Care Quality Commission (2009e). *The Quality and Capacity of Adult Social Care Services 2008/09*. London: Care Quality Commission.

Care Quality Commission (2010a). *Quality Ratings for Care Services*. Available at: http://webarchive.nationalarchives.gov.uk/20100611090857/http://www.cqc.org.uk/guidanceforprofessionals/adultsocialcare/inspection/ratingsandreports/qualityratingsforcareservices.cfm (accessed 21 February 2011).

Care Quality Commission (2010b). *Regulating for Better Care Edition 1*. Available at: http://www.cqc.org.uk/_db/_documents/20100224_Ambulance_Regulating_for_better_care__FINAL.pdf (accessed 24 May 2010).

Commission for Social Care Inspection (2004). *Fees and Frequency of Inspections: Regulations*. SI 2004/662. London: HMSO.

Commission for Social Care Inspection (2007a). *Fees and Frequency of Inspections: Regulations*. SI 2007/556. London: HMSO.

Commission for Social Care Inspection (2007b). *Guidance for Inspectors: Short Observational Framework for Inspection*. London: Commission for Social Care Inspection.

Commission for Social Care Inspection (2008a). *See Me Not Just Dementia—Understanding People's Experiences of Living in a Care Home*. London: Commission for Social Care Inspection.

Commission for Social Care Inspection (2008b). *Experts by Experience—How People who Use Services Help us Make Service Better*. London: Commission for Social Care Inspection.

Commission for Social Care Inspection (2009). *CSCI Quality Ratings Market Research Report*. London: Commission for Social Care Inspection.

Day, P., Klein, R., & Redmayne, S. (1996). *Regulating Residential Care for Elderly People: Social Care Research Findings Paper 78*. York: Joseph Rowntree Foundation.

Department of Health (2000). *No Secrets*. London: Department of Health.

Department of Health (2001). *National Service Framework for Older People*. London: Department of Health.

Department of Health (2003). *Care Homes for Older People: National Minimum Standards—Care Homes Regulations—As Amended 18 February 2003*. London: TSO.

Department of Health (2005). *Everybody's Business*. London: Department of Health.

Department of Health (2006). *Our Health Our Care Our Say*. London: Department of Health.

Department of Health (2007a). *Putting People First*. London: Department of Health.

Department of Health (2007b). *NHS-funded Nursing Care: Guide to Care Home Managers on GP Services for Residents*. Available at: http://webarchive.nationalarchives.gov.uk/+/www.dh.gov.uk/en/Healthcare/IntegratedCare/NHSfundednursingcare/DH_4000392.

Department of Health (2008a). *High Quality Care for All*. London: Department of Health.

Department of Health (2008b). *Transforming Adult Social Care Services*. London: Department of Health.

Department of Health (2009a). *The Use of Antipsychotic Medication for People with Dementia: Time for Action. A Report for the Minister of State for Care Services by Professor Sube Banerjee*. London: Department of Health.

Department of Health (2009b). *Living Well with Dementia—A National Dementia Strategy*. London: Department of Health.

Department of Health (2010). *The NHS Constitution for England*. Available at: http://www.dh.gov.uk/prod_consum_dh/groups/dh_digitalassets/@dh/@en/@ps/documents/digitalasset/dh_113645.pdf (accessed 24 May 2010).

Disability Rights Commission (2006). *Equal Treatment: Closing the Gap*. London: Disability Rights Commission.

Fahey, T., Montgomery, A., Barnes, J., & Protheroe, J. (2003). Quality of elderly residents in nursing homes and elderly people living at home—controlled observation study. *British Medical Journal*, *326*, 580.

General Medical Council (2008). *Conflicts of Interest*. Available at: http://www.gmc-uk.org/guidance/ethical_guidance/conflicts_of_interest.asp (accessed 24 July 2010).

Health and Social Care (Community Health and Standards) Act (2003). (c.43). London: HMSO.

Health and Social Care Act (2008a). (c.14). London: HMSO.

Health and Social Care Act (2008b) *(Regulated Activities) Regulations* 2010. SI 2010/781, London: HMSO.

Healthcare Commission (2007). *Caring for Dignity—A National Report into Dignity in Care for Older People in Hospital.* London: Healthcare Commission.

Healthcare Commission (2008). *Equality in Later Life—A National Study of Older People's Mental Health Services.* London: Healthcare Commission.

Human Rights Act (1998). (c.42). London: HMSO.

Johnson, N., Jenkinson, S., Kendall, I., Bradshaw, Y., & Blackmore, M. (1988). Regulating for quality in the voluntary sector. *Journal of Social Policy, 27*(3), 307–328.

Joseph Rowntree Foundation (1995). *Care Standards in the Residential Care Sector: Social Care Summary 6.* York: Joseph Rowntree Foundation.

Joseph Rowntree Foundation (2008). *Improving Care in Residential Care Homes.* Available at: http://www.jrf.org.uk (accessed 24 July 2010).

Mental Capacity Act (2005). (c.9). London: HMSO.

National Audit Office (2010). *Improving Dementia Services in England—An Interim Report.* London: TSO.

National Care Standards Commission (2001). *Registration Regulations.* SI 2001/3969. London: HMSO.

National Care Standards Commission (2003a). *Registration Amendment Regulations.* SI 2003/369. London: HMSO.

National Care Standards Commission (2003b). *Fees and Frequency of Inspections Regulations.* SI 2003/368. London: HMSO.

National Institute for Health and Clinical Excellence and Social Care Institute for Excellence (2006). *Dementia: Supporting People with Dementia and their Carers. Clinical Practice Guidelines.* London: NICE.

Netten, A., Williams, J., Dennett, J., Wiseman, J., & Fenyo, A. (2004). *Social Care Regulation: Resource Use. Final Report.* Discussion Paper 2042/4, PSSRU. Canterbury: University of Kent.

Netten, A., Beadle-Brown, J., Trukeschitz, B., et al. (2010). *Measuring the Outcomes of Care Homes: Final Report.* Discussion Paper 2696/2, PSSRU. Canterbury: University of Kent.

NHS Information Centre (2010). *Putting People First User Experience Survey.* Available at: http://www.ic.nhs.uk/services/social-care/news-and-events/putting-people-first-user-experience-survey (accessed 24 July 2010).

Owen, T. & the National Care Home Research and Development Forum (NCHRDF) (Eds.) (2006). *My Home Life: Quality of Life in Care Homes.* London: Help the Aged.

Patterson, M. (2008). *Can we Afford the Doctor? GP Retainers and Care Homes.* London: English Community Care Association.

Raleigh, V.S. & Foot, C. (2010). *Getting the Measure of Quality—Opportunities and Challenges.* London: The Kings Fund.

Selznick, P. (1985). Focusing organisational research on regulation. In: R. Noll (Ed.), *Regulatory Policy and Social Sciences* (pp. 363–368) . Berkley: University of California Press.

Sparrow, M. (2000). *The Regulatory Craft: Controlling Risks, Solving Problems and Managing Compliance* (p. 288). Washington, D.C.: The Brookings Institution.

Tucker, S., Baldwin, R., Hughes, J., et al. (2007). Old age mental health services in England: implementing the National Service Framework for older people. *International Journal of Geriatric Psychiatry, 22*(3), 211–217.

University of Portsmouth (2005). *Regulation of Adult Social Care (RASC) Research Project.* Report on Phase 1 Finding: Executive Summary. Portsmouth: University of Portsmouth.

Chapter 8

Funding: paying for residential care for older people

Theresia Bäumker and Ann Netten

Abstract

This chapter reviews funding for residential and nursing home care for older people in the United Kingdom. Future demand for long-term care, and commensurate expenditure, are projected to rise substantially in the next decades with the significant growth in the number of very old people. The financing of long-term care has, and continues to be, an issue of considerable debate. One of the core issues relates to achieving an appropriate and equitable balance between public and private responsibility for funding. The authors first consider local authority funding and the nature of the eligibility criteria which targets this support, before discussing the National Health Service (NHS) as a relatively small but growing source of funding. The chapter then discusses private funding of care home places, such as spending down of assets including selling of homes, and concludes by offering a brief overview of the future of long-term care funding.

Introduction

The cost of caring for individuals in care homes is substantial and rising. This is due to the intensive nature of the support required for residents with multiple and complex health problems and to the growth in the number of elderly residents with this level of need. As at April 2009, total demand for care home places for older people (and younger adults with physical disabilities) was estimated to be 472,600. This is an increase of 1.3% over the previous year's figure. Prior to that, demand had been in decline for 12 successive years (Laing and Buisson, 2009a). The estimated value of the care home sector is just over £13 billion, of which private (for-profit) care homes account for £9.4 billion and not-for-profit homes a further £1.9 billion. In comparison, spending on community-based care services was estimated to be £7.52 billion in 2007/2008 (Laing and Buisson, 2009b). The public sector funds the majority of long-term care for older people.

Eligibility for public support

There are national regulations for the receipt and funding of care home places. Currently, each local authority sets eligibility criteria for services, based on national guidelines. New, revised national guidance *Prioritising Need in the Context of Putting People First* (Department of Health, 2010a) was introduced in February 2010 to replace the existing *Fair Access to Care Services* guidance (Department of Health, 2003) introduced in 2003. This incorporates the new approaches developed as part of the government's personalization agenda and has been applicable since April 2010. Once an individual has been assessed as eligible for care in a care home, local authorities will determine the user charges depending on the user's financial means. The exception is in circumstances where the accommodation is provided as part of the after-care package of services under Section 117 of the Mental Health Act 1983 (Age Concern, 2010). The means test takes account of the person's income and assets. Local authorities must adhere to statutory guidance in the government document *Charging for Residential Accommodation Guide* (CRAG) (Department of Health, 2010b), which is written in support of *The National Assistance (Assessment of Resources) Regulations 1992 (SI 1992/2977)*. CRAG is updated each April.

For the financial year 2010/2011, individuals with capital exceeding £23,250 (or with a weekly income greater than the sum of the care home fees and a Personal Expenses Allowance of £22.30) receive no public financial support (Department of Health, 2010c). Individuals with capital no greater than £23,250 are able to receive financial support for their care by the appropriate local authority, but must fully contribute their weekly assessed income except for a Personal Expenses Allowance and any Pension Savings Disregard (similar to Pension Savings Credit received when living in one's own home). No account is taken of capital or savings below £14,250. Capital between £14,250 and £23,250 will be assessed to show an assumed or 'tariff' income of £1 per week for every £250, which the individual must pay from their capital. Capital can be in a variety of forms including savings, investments, and property. With respect to income, local authority calculations will assume that income available from social security benefits such as the State Pension, Pension Credit, etc. is being claimed. For individuals receiving financial support for their care, Attendance Allowance and the care component of Disability Living Allowance entitlement will usually stop 4 weeks after placement. The income and assets of spouses, children, and other relatives are not taken into account, though spouses may be asked to make a contribution (Comas-Herrera et al., 2004).

In April 2009, 52% of independent sector care home residents were estimated as having their fees fully, or partly, paid by local authorities. Central government funds allocated to local authorities are thus very important to the care home sector, particularly in less affluent areas where the local authority funding share is higher. The Treasury has recognized that paying for the support needs of older people is a major challenge faced by society, but the government, and the 2009 Green Paper, did not give any indication as to its intention for the size of the social care (including care homes) funding envelope. The 2009 budget revised downwards the government's forecast for annual real increases in total government spending on public services and benefits from 2010/2011, from 1.1% (as forecast in the pre-budget report 2008) to

0.7% (Laing and Buisson, 2009b). Social care funding remains non-ring fenced within local authority spending, and its future prospects are unclear. The negative effects of very tightly constrained local authority budgets might be somewhat moderated by the continued small decrease in local authority placements, which could create headroom for fees to at least keep pace with inflation (Laing and Buisson, 2009b). This will put further pressure on occupancy, but in recent years the gap has been filled by rising demand from self-funders and demand from the NHS (see later in chapter).

In July 2009, the government's Green Paper, *Shaping the Future of Care Together* (HM Government, 2009), was published. It returned to the question of the appropriate and sustainable balance between public and private funding of long-term care, which the government's response to the 1999 Royal Commission had failed to resolve. A key recommendation of the Royal Commission on Long Term Care (1999) was that the nursing and personal care components of care home fees should be met by the state—without a means test—and financed out of general taxation. The Scottish Executive decided that both nursing care and personal care would be publicly funded, for both institutional-based care and community-based care (Community Care and Health (Scotland) Act, 2002). In part, the rationale for this was to ensure that personal care was provided free to individuals with all types of chronic health conditions, not just some. The National Assembly for Wales and the Northern Ireland Assembly decided to publically fund only nursing costs, as in England.

Although the recommendation to publically fund all personal care was not accepted in England, from October 2001 'free nursing care' has meant that the nursing component of care home costs is met by the state. The NHS is a growing source of funding for care homes (Laing and Buisson, 2009b). Its share increased from 10% of nursing care residents in 2007 to 16% in 2009, although this represents only 7% of all care home residents (as no one in receipt of personal care only is NHS funded). From October 2001 to October 2007, residents receiving nursing care provided through care homes were assessed and funded on the basis of three bands: high, medium, and low. In March 2010, the Department of Health announced that the single rate for NHS-funded nursing care contribution for the financial year 2010/2011 is £108.70 per week in England. Those on the low or medium band prior to October 2007 will have been moved onto this flat rate payment. This payment for the care provided by a registered nurse is paid directly to the care home, and is deducted from the local authority contribution to fees. It does not reduce the resident's assessed financial contribution or any third party contribution to the costs of personal care (Counsel and Care, 2010). Those residents on the higher band (now £149.60 per week) will remain on this until reviewed, where depending on the outcome, they may either: (i) receive the flat rate if their needs have reduced, (ii) remain in the higher band if their needs fall between the two levels, (iii) have funding removed if they are no longer in a care home that provides nursing care, or (iv) receive NHS continuing healthcare if their needs have increased.

NHS continuing healthcare

NHS continuing healthcare is care wholly funded by the NHS, that is, non-means tested assistance with costs for the care home resident. It is applicable where the resident's needs are regarded as 'a primary health need'. This is a controversial issue and previous legal judgements and reports by the Parliamentary and Health Service Ombudsman have highlighted areas where eligibility criteria for this funding were too narrowly defined (Age Concern, 2010). It is against this backdrop that the *National Framework for NHS Continuing Healthcare and NHS-funded Nursing Care* was introduced in October 2007 and revised in July 2009 (Department of Health, 2009a). Department of Health statistics confirm a rapid rise in the number of people in England receiving NHS-funded continuing healthcare. Across the United Kingdom, as a whole the number of NHS fully funded care home residents is estimated at 26,000 in 2009, with the prospect of more being added (Laing and Buisson, 2009b). Potential drivers of growth are the new national eligibility criteria, and increased NHS outsourcing of continuing care to the independent sector as the NHS's own in-house provision of long stay hospital beds for elderly and mentally ill people continues its long-term decline.

Currently, the strict eligibility criteria still mean that overall few people qualify, and even those who do are reassessed regularly. Moreover, it seems that the availability of free care at the point of delivery still depends not on individual need, but on where individuals live, despite Ombudsman intervention establishing national guidance for primary care trusts (PCTs). This process raised the question of how many residents may have been wrongly denied fully funded NHS care and in 2003 the Ombudsman recommended that the NHS carry out retrospective reviews of continuing care funding decisions. According to the Department's figures, in 20% of the 12,000 cases reviewed, full or partial restitution was awarded at an estimated cost of £180 million. Losses to the individuals previously denied NHS continuing care funding included the sale of their homes. The Department of Health subsequently issued a letter to ensure 'that the correct process is being used to differentiate between people who receive fully funded NHS continuing care and the high band of NHS-funded nursing care' (Department of Health, 2005). The individuals most likely to be unfairly treated seem to be those with high level care needs that have been deemed not to meet the test of 'primary health need'.

Self-funding

Older people may arrange and pay privately for their own residential care without involving either the local authority or the NHS. In April 2009, about 40%—or an estimated 155,000 of older and physically disabled residents—of independent sector care homes were self-funded, receiving no state funding other than their universal social security entitlements (Laing and Buisson, 2009b). A larger proportion of the older population are falling into the self-funding category due to the increase in home ownership, which usually disqualifies people from local authority support. It may also be due to more rigorous investigation of situations where individuals have disposed of assets in order to qualify for public support. If the local authority finds evidence of deliberate, or intentional, 'deprivation of capital' such as the transfer of property, the individual will be treated as having 'notional capital' to the value of the capital disposed of (Department of Health, 2010b). If the sum of notional capital and actual capital exceeds the upper capital limit of £23,250, the local authority may assess the individual as responsible for the full costs of the care under Section 22 of the National Assistance Act 1948.

Growth of home ownership means that, as at 2008, almost 75% of retired households in England owned their own home (CLG Table 803, 2008). Given that only 40% of care home residents are currently self-funding (as noted above), it is likely that a substantial number have divested themselves of assets by the time they enter a care home (Laing and Buisson, 2009a). Homeowners can release funding tied up in their property either by downsizing to a smaller house, or freeing up capital while continuing to live in their home through commercial equity release schemes. It is notable that the recent sharp decline in house prices has dampened the market for these schemes (King's Fund, 2009). If bought early, equity release is unlikely to be used to fund community-based packages of care, or to leave resources available to pay care home fees. It is notable that the Wanless Social Care Review (Wanless et al., 2006) demonstrated that the income and wealth of those over 60 correlates inversely with dependency. In other words, those most in need of care and support tend to have fewer private resources; they are less likely to be homeowners or have occupational pensions.

Capital from property sales is the most important source of private funding for nursing and residential care. However, selling one's home to fund care home fees is a major commitment, and it has been the focus of much public and policy concern over the past 20 years. This concern has fuelled, in part, the introduction of a number of initiatives aimed at increasing the flexibility and/or reversibility of care home admission (Netten et al., 2005). Capital assets tied up in people's homes are disregarded for the first 12 months of admission; this includes self-funders who have been permanently in a care home for more than 12 weeks and whose savings run down to less than £23,250 (Department of Health, 2009b). Also, long-term loans known as 'deferred payment agreements' were introduced in October 2001, under section 55 of the Health and Social Care Act 2001. These allow councils to offer residents who cannot, or do not, want to sell their own homes the opportunity to defer payment of care costs to a later date, and have a charge levied by the council on their property value (Department of Health, 2000, 2001). Local authorities have discretion about whether to offer deferred payments, but the Local Authority Circular LAC(DH)(2009)3 (Department of Health, 2009b) states that it is unlawful for councils to operate a blanket policy to refuse applications on the grounds of, for example, insufficient council funds. They are required to consider each application on its own merits. With the credit crunch and weak housing market, many older people in need of care are unable to sell their homes to release funds to pay for care home fees (Passingham, 2009). In turning to the local authority for financial support, some individuals have found none. Instead of offering them the option of a deferred payment against their property, some local authorities with restricted budgets have encouraged individuals to build up a private debt with their care home provider.

Spending down of assets

There is widespread resentment among older people and their relatives that they should be required to spend down their 'hard earned' assets to the capital limit to meet expensive care home costs. With care home fees averaging £479 per week and nursing home fees at £669 per week, the sums needed to cover costs can deplete a lifetime's savings in a very short period of time. A study by the Personal Social Services Research Unit (PSSRU) in 2002 (Netten et al., 2002) examined the length of time for which self-funders would be able to fund the shortfall between their income and care home fees from their assets, before these were reduced to £16,000 (the capital limit at that time). Sixty-four per cent of residents were estimated to have sufficient assets to fund the shortfall for more than 5 years, while 10% would spend down their assets to the capital limit after only 1 year. For residents with average levels of income, the rate of reduction in the level of their assets was estimated to be substantial. In 1999, the government rejected the Royal Commission's recommendation to increase the upper capital limit to £60,000, because of the impact on public expenditure. However, the government did commit to reviewing the limits every year to keep them broadly in line with inflation. Care homes supported the modest increases, because a higher capital disregard would have meant an increase in the proportion of public funded residents paying the lower local authority determined fees (as discussed below).

Research has shown that self-funded residents tend to be charged more than publicly funded residents (Laing, 1998; Netten et al., 1998, 2001; CSCI, 2008). Local authorities have considerable market power to negotiate care home fees in their area as they are often the major purchaser of places. As one of their main goals is cost containment they exert relatively constant downwards pressure on fees and on the sector. The average uplift in baseline fee rates set by the UK local authorities was 2.6% in 2009/2010; this is just above the 2–2.5% that Laing and Buisson (2009b) estimate is needed to keep pace with care homes cost inflation. Since staff payroll is the main cost item, care home fee inflation should ideally track above wage inflation. One of the main mechanisms which care homes utilize to respond to cost pressure and the downwards pressure on margins exerted by local authority purchasers is to charge higher fees to self-funders. Fees of self-funders are typically £50–£100 higher than the fees paid by a local authority for a similar service (Laing and Buisson, 2009b). Laing and Buisson (2009b) predict that the polarization of public and private fees will continue to be a feature of the care home market in the future, with the caveat that some slowdown in private pay fee inflation may be experienced due to the economic downturn, a weak housing market and pressure on disposable income.

Effectively, self-funders are subsidizing publicly funded residents and are not in a position to negotiate fees downwards, nor do they receive support in doing so. There is a tendency for local authorities to focus their tightly constrained budgets on individuals who have passed the means test, and leave self-funders to 'fend for themselves'. For example, a 2002 survey of self-funders found that although the local authority had assessed half of the residents as in need of care home placement, in only 9% of cases had they negotiated fees on their behalf (Netten et al., 2002). Additionally, few self-funders are offered the opportunity to discuss their care options with social services (CSCI, 2008) or given advice about financial arrangements (Wright, 1998, 2003; Netten et al., 2002). In the long run, this neglect may have significant cost consequences. As discussed, self-funders tend to pay higher fees, not only because they cannot negotiate fees downwards, but because they often choose 'nicer' homes where fees tend to be higher. It is likely that self-funders will increase as a proportion of the total number of care home residents in the future. The economic downturn is not expected to signifi-cantly affect the volume of self-funded demand for a needs-driven service. Once this group has spent down their assets, they will then transfer to the, now much larger, group of residents funded by local authorities with a corresponding increase in costs.

There is often an assumption that one of the main reasons for high care home costs is the substantial profits being made by private providers. It is interesting to note how-ever, that the policy intention underpinning the drive to increase the use of independ-ent sector homes introduced in the 1980s was precisely the opposite. In fact, in the late 80s and early 90s, local authority managed homes were considerably more expensive than those in the independent sector, and the policy objective was to deploy market forces to increase efficiency and deliver value for money to both the state and the self-funder (Department of Health and Department of Social Security, 1989; Darton and Muncer, 2005).

The role of housing

One of the most difficult issues in debates around long-term care funding concerns the fact that many older people are obliged to sell their homes to pay fees. There is a widely expressed sense of indignation about taking the value of a house into account when assessing a resident's ability to pay. The right to leave property as an inheritance to the next generation is viewed by many as fundamental to a home owning democ-racy. The rules regarding the means testing of housing assets tend to strongly influence eligibility. If the value of the house was not included in the means test, research sug-gests that about 95,000 of the UK care home residents (24% of the total) would become eligible for public funding (PSSRU, 2006). It is interesting to note that if the value of the older person's house was taken into account in financial assessments of community-based care, around 175,000 domiciliary care users (12% of the total) would lose public funding (Hancock et al., 2007).

Although many older people are anxious about losing their home, their home is protected all the time that it is lived in by a close relative. Local authorities also have discretionary powers to exclude the value of homes from calculations if it continues to be the residence of a 'former carer or other type of person', or to offer deferred pay-ment agreements (as discussed above). However, individuals are often not informed of this discretion; also some local authorities choose not to use these powers. This results in considerable local variation in the number of users who are obliged to pay for care home fees and is at odds with the welfare principles of equity and universality. Robust estimates of how many homes are sold annually to fund care are not available. In part, this is a consequence of information not being collected centrally, for example the number of older people deferring care home payments. An estimate frequently quoted by politicians and the media—possibly derived from work on housing equity and inheritance—is that 40,000 homes a year are sold to fund care home fees (Hamnett, 1995, 1997). In the government's response to the Health Committee Report on Continuing Care in July 2005, the 12-week disregard of property from the means test for residential care was said to benefit around 30,000 people a year (HM Government, 2005).

Since 2004, the government has stimulated growth of the 'extra care housing' market through the Department of Health's Extra Care Housing Initiative Fund. Although there is no universal definition of extra care housing, Laing and Buisson (2009b) suggest that it is characterized by the fact that it is primarily for older people; the accommodation is largely self-contained; care can be delivered flexibly, usually by a team of staff based on the premises; support staff are available on the premises 24 hours a day; domestic care, communal facilities, and related services are available; meals are usually available and charged for when taken; it aims to enable self-care and independent living; and it offers security of tenure. Extra care housing has been viewed as a possible alternative to care home provision, and is a model which enables people to safeguard their capital by purchasing or part-purchasing their accommodation. However, the volume of extra care housing is limited and there seems to be no current plans to extend the Department of Health's Fund beyond 2010. During the 2010 General Election campaign, neither Labour nor the Conservatives had specific policies on extra care housing.

The Green Paper *Shaping the Future of Care Together* (HM Government, 2009) proposed—as is the case in extra care housing—to separate out the cost of accommodation from the cost of care and support in residential care or nursing home provision. However, the purpose in this was to apply the options for long-term care funding reform only to the costs of people's care, rather than to ensure that individuals were able to preserve their capital as with extra care housing. In fact, Hirsch (2009) suggests that by separating out accommodation costs from the support packages that would be provided to people requiring residential or nursing home provision, the Green Paper proposals seems further to disengage housing from care issues. This emphasis is at odds with the goal of linking housing with health and care as set out in the housing for an ageing society strategy, *Lifetime Homes, Lifetime Neighbourhoods* (Department for Communities and Local Government, 2008; Counsel and Care, 2010).

The future of social care funding

The degree to which the costs of care are borne by individuals as private citizens or by the state will depend on the nature of government policy both now and in the future. The current system for funding adult social care has been criticized as unfair, complex, and financially unstable. The need for reform was recognized as early as 1998, when the government established the Royal Commission on Long Term Care, whose recommendation for free personal care it did not accept (Royal Commission on Long Term Care, 1999). In 2009, the government set out options for consultation in the Green Paper, *Shaping the Future of Care Together* (HM Government, 2009). Other proposals were published in the White Paper *Building the National Care Service* (Department of Health, 2010d) in March 2010, just weeks before the general election.

The White Paper sets out an ambitious plan for reform towards a National Care Service, including minimum national standards and entitlements; it aims to directly address issues of inequity and the so-called 'postcode lottery' (Department of Health, 2010d). It intends that local authorities will no longer set their own eligibility and charging criteria and that individuals will receive care and support based on their individual level of need, rather than their postcode. It also proposes a cap on the costs of residential care from 2014 onwards, at an initial cost to the state of £800 million, so that service users' homes and savings are protected from care charges after a period of 2 years (paid through freezing inheritance tax thresholds, increasing the statutory retirement age of 65, and by greater efficiencies in the care system). It estimates that this will affect around 55,000–60,000 individuals. However, the White Paper lacks detail on funding, and the long timescale for implementation means changes in the system are unlikely to be in place before 2016. The 2010 change in government has heralded more uncertainty and further delays, as reviews of the previous administration's policy decisions are inevitable. The key question is whether the White Paper proposals will survive. Although the Conservatives have pledged to 'reform social care', their manifesto contrasts sharply with developing a National Care Service. They reject compulsory payment in favour of a voluntary one-off insurance premium of around £8000, which would protect people's homes from being sold to meet the costs of residential care. The Liberal Democrats, criticizing the voluntary insurance scheme as unworkable, had previously shown a preference for a partnership model—where the state and the individual both contribute to the costs of long-term care—but in their manifesto the party retreated from outlining any details, promising instead to 'immediately' establish an independent commission to develop future proposals for long-term care (King's Fund, 2010). Now that the country has a hung parliament with power shared between Conservatives and Liberal Democrats, the direction of policy on long-term care is likely to be a combination of these two proposals.

Conclusion

Future funding for long-term care will almost certainly continue to be a composite of contributions from the local authority, the NHS, and the individual and their family. However, the balance of 'who pays for what' and in 'what proportion' will most likely shift towards the individual to a greater degree than hitherto as a consequence of public funding cuts. To date, increases in public funding have not kept pace with rising demand for care services, a picture unlikely to change in the short or medium term. Demographic changes, notably an ageing population and an increase in the number of people with chronic ill health and/or disability, will continue to exert pressure on the whole care sector particularly long-term care. Privately funded demand for residential care is projected to track demographic change and it is unlikely that the inequities that characterize care home funding at the present time will be resolved in the near future. Recently, the government (HM Government, 2008) recognized that 'people find the current means testing system unfair' (p. 26) and that 'the system of social care (appears to) penalize those who save for their old age' (p. 14). Although this acknowledgement of public concern is an important policy marker, addressing the major issues of social care underfunding, the rising costs of supporting highly dependent individuals in care homes, and meeting increased demand for long-term care, is a significant and complex challenge. The role that funding plays in decision-making will be pivotal and the need to address it with robust evidence, a commitment to equity, and a view to the long-term cannot be overstated.

References

Age Concern (2010). *Paying for Permanent Residential Care: Factsheet 10*. London: Age Concern.

CLG Table 803 (2008). *Household Characteristics: Economic Status of Household Reference Person, by Tenure*. Available at: www.communities.gov.uk/housing/housingresearch/housingstatistics/housingstatisticsby/householdcharacteristics/livetables (accessed 10 May 2010).

Comas-Herrera, A., Wittenberg, R., & Pickard, L. (2004). Long-term care for older people in the United Kingdom: structure and challenges. In: M. Knapp, D. Challis, J. Fernandez, & A. Netten (Eds.), *Long-Term Care: Matching Resources and Needs* (pp. 17–30). Aldershot: Ashgate Publishing Ltd.

Commission for Social Care Inspection (CSCI) (2008). *The State of Social Care in England 2006–2007*. Newcastle Upon Tyne: Commission for Social Care Inspection.

Community Care and Health (Scotland) Act (2002). *Community Care and Health (Scotland) Act 2002* (2002 asp 5). Edinburgh: HMSO.

Counsel and Care (2010). *Care Home Fees: Paying them in England*. London: Counsel and Care.

Darton, R. & Muncer, A. (2005). Alternative housing and care arrangements: the evidence. In: B. Roe & R. Beech (Eds.), *Intermediate and Continuing Care: Policy and Practice* (pp. 183–203). Oxford: Blackwell Publishing.

Department for Communities and Local Government (2008). *Lifetime Homes, Lifetime Neighbourhoods. A National Strategy for Housing in an Ageing Society*. London: Department for Communities and Local Government.

Department of Health (2000). *The NHS Plan: A Plan for Investment, A Plan for Reform*. Cm 4818-I. London: HMSO.

Department of Health (2001). *Charges for Residential Accommodation—CRAG Amendment No. 15. LAC (2001) 25*. London: Department of Health.

Department of Health (2003). *Fair Access to Care Services: Guidance on Eligibility Criteria for Adult Social Care*. London: Department of Health.

Department of Health (2005). *Ensuring that all Recipients of High Band NHS-funding Nursing Care have been Correctly Considered against Eligibility Criteria for Fully Funded NHS Continuing Care: 28 November*. London: Department of Health. Available at: http://www.dh.gov.uk/en/Publicationsandstatistics/Lettersandcirculars/Dearcolleagueletters/DH_4125309 (accessed 4 June 2010).

Department of Health (2009a). *The National Framework for NHS Continuing Healthcare and NHS-funded Nursing Care (revised)*. London: Department of Health.

Department of Health (2009b). *Charges for Residential Accommodation—CRAG Amendment No. 28. LAC (DH) (2009) 3*. London: Department of Health.

Department of Health (2010a). *Prioritising Need in the Context of Putting People First: A Whole System Approach to Eligibility for Social Care—Guidance on Eligibility Criteria for Adult Social Care, England 2010*. London: Department of Health.

Department of Health (2010b). *Charging for Residential Accommodation Guide (CRAG): March 2010*. London: Department of Health.

Department of Health (2010c). *Charges for Residential Accommodation—CRAG Amendment No. 29. LAC (DH) (2010) 2*. London: Department of Health.

Department of Health (2010d). *Building the National Care Service*. Cm 7854. London: HMSO.

Department of Health and Department of Social Security (1989). *Caring for People: Community Care in the Next Decade and Beyond*. Cm 849. London: HMSO.

Hamnett, C. (1995). Housing equity release and inheritance. In: I. Allen & E. Perkins (Eds.), *The Future of Family Care for Older People* (pp. 163–180). London: HMSO.

Hamnett, C. (1997). Housing wealth, inheritance and residential care in Britain. *Housing Finance, 34*, 35–38.

Hancock, R., Wittenberg, R., Pickard, L., et al. (2007). *Paying for Long-Term Care for Older People in the UK: Modelling the Costs and Distributional Effects of a Range of Options*. PSSRU Discussion Paper No. 2336. Canterbury: Personal Social Services Unit, University of Kent.

Hirsch, D. (2009). *The Green Paper and Care Funding: On the Brink of a Sustainable Settlement?* York: Joseph Rowntree Foundation.

HM Government (2005). *Response to Health Select Committee Report on Continuing Care*. Cm 6650. (Presented to Parliament by the Secretary of State for Health). London: HMSO.

HM Government (2008). *The Case for Change: Why England Needs a New Care and Support System*. London: Department of Health.

HM Government (2009). *Shaping the Future of Care Together*. Cm 7673. London: HMSO.

King's Fund (2009). *Funding Adult Social Care in England: Briefing*. London: King's Fund.

King's Fund (2010). *Social Care: What has been Achieved?* London: King's Fund.

Laing, W. (1998). *A Fair Price for Care? Disparities Between Market Rates for Nursing/Residential Care and What State Funding Agencies will Pay*. York: York Publishing Services Ltd.

Laing & Buisson (2009a). *Care of Elderly People UK Market Survey 2009*. London: Laing & Buisson.

Laing & Buisson (2009b). *Laing's Healthcare Market Review 2009–2010*. London: Laing & Buisson.

Netten, A., Bebbington, A., Darton, R., Forder, J., & Miles, K. (1998). *1996 Survey of Care Homes for Elderly People. Final Report*. PSSRU Discussion Paper No. 1423/2. Canterbury: Personal Social Services Research Unit, University of Kent.

Netten, A., Bebbington, A., Darton, R., & Forder, J. (2001). *Care Homes for Older People: Volume 1. Facilities, Residents and Costs*. Canterbury: Personal Social Services Research Unit, University of Kent.

Netten, A., Darton, R., & Curtis, L. (2002). *Self-funded Admissions to Care Homes. A Report of Research Carried Out by the Personal Social Services Research Unit, University of Kent on Behalf of the Department of Work and Pensions*. Department of Work and Pensions Research Report No. 159. Leeds: Corporate Document Services.

Netten, A., Darton, R., & Williams, J. (2005). Care homes and continuing care. In: B. Roe & R. Beech (Eds.), *Intermediate and Continuing Care: Policy and Practice* (pp. 204–221). Oxford: Blackwell Publishing.

Passingham, A. (2009). *Finding and Financing Care in Hard Times: The Top Issues Reported to Counsel and Care's Advice Service in 2008*. London: Counsel and Care.

Personal Social Services Research Unit (PSSRU) (2006). *Paying for Long-Term Care for Older People in the UK: Modelling the Costs and Distributional Effects of Range of Options*. Research Summary. Canterbury: Personal Social Services Unit, University of Kent.

Royal Commission on Long Term Care (1999). *With Respect to Old Age: Long Term Care—Rights and Responsibilities. A Report by the Royal Commission on Long Term Care (Chairman: Professor Sir Stewart Sutherland)*. Cm 4192-I. London: HMSO.

Wanless, D., Forder, J., Fernàndez, J., et al. (2006). *The Wanless Social Care Review: Securing Good Care for Older People—Taking a Long-term View.* London: King's Fund.

Wright, F. (1998). *Continuing to Care: The Effect on Spouses and Children of an Older Person's Admission to a Care Home.* York: York Publishing Services Ltd.

Wright, F. (2003). Discrimination against self-funding residents in long-term residential care in England. *Ageing and Society, 25*(5), 603–624.

Chapter 9

Legal aspects

Amanda Keeling

Abstract

The main legal aspect surrounding the issue of mental health in care homes is the change in the law around mental capacity. Prior to the Mental Capacity Act (MCA) 2005, the law governing how we make decisions regarding the care, welfare, and finances of those who lack the capacity to make them themselves was relatively vague, reliant on a few cases which were slowly developing principles. The advent of the MCA 2005, which came into force in 2007, and the supplementary legislation of the recent Deprivation of Liberty Safeguards (DoLS), have dramatically changed the landscape for how we deal with individuals in our care, who cannot make decisions for themselves. This chapter aims to outline this legislation, and the impact it has on those caring for adults who lack capacity.

Introduction

Historically, the law around mental health referred only to those who were detained in institutions under the Mental Health Act (MHA). However, those who have mental disorders are not always in such hospitals, but also in care homes, where the MHA does not apply. However, there are clear mental health issues to be dealt with in care homes. These issues normally revolve around the fact that, due to their mental condition, the residents often lack capacity to make various decisions, from managing their finances to deciding what they want to wear that day, and a decision must be made on their behalf by their carer.

Up until recently, the law in this area was defined solely by the courts and their judgements. Although principles had begun to develop throughout that case law, there were inconsistencies, and it was felt that a clear, statutory footing for mental capacity law was required. The first steps in this area were taken by the Law Commission in its 1995 report on mental capacity.[1] Further consultation on the issues resulted in

---

[1] Report No. 231 (28 February 1995).

the Mental Capacity Act 2005, which takes the principles developed in the case law, particularly in medical and other welfare cases, and puts them in a statutory framework to provide guidance for those involved in the lives and decision-making of those who lack mental capacity in some areas of life.

In addition to the MCA itself, there now is supplementary legislation in the Deprivation of Liberty Safeguards. The DoLS legislation has designed a procedure, albeit a rather complex one, which allows for a deprivation of liberty, where it is necessary for the care and treatment of the individual to be authorized, monitored, and reviewed, and which can be appealed to the Court of Protection.

There is, therefore, a good deal of 'law' governing how we must treat those with mental health or capacity issues in care homes, which is designed to help guide those caring for these individuals to make good decisions regarding their welfare and financial decision-making. Yet the issue of how to help people who are having difficulty making decisions for themselves is something many carers find challenging. The national charity Counsel and Care, which works with older people and their families and carers to provide advice and information, has noted a marked increase in the calls they receive from concerned families and carers as to the support, of lack thereof, available to their older relatives or friends who are starting to find it difficult to manage their finances or are struggling to make decisions about their care and support by themselves.

The aim of this chapter is to outline the mental capacity legislation, how it works, and how it can be implemented. There is no denying that this area of law is complicated, and we must preface this chapter with a caution that such a short space is nowhere nearly enough to cover the topic in detail. Indeed, with regards to the DoLS specifically, it must be emphasized that it may sometimes be necessary to take legal advice as to whether or not individuals in a home's care are being deprived of their liberty and how best to proceed. However, we hope to provide an overview which will clarify matters somewhat, and provide a signpost for further information on the subject.

The Mental Capacity Act 2005

The MCA 2005 was a huge step forward for the law, and therefore practice, relating to how we care for people who lacked mental capacity to make various decisions. The MCA put down in statute many principles of decision-making which had previously been developed through a variety of different case law, and which had not always been clear or consistent. It also made clear that these principles could, and must, be used not only by the courts, but also day to day by those caring for people without capacity. Finally, and perhaps most importantly, it brought together in one piece of legislation powers to make decisions with regards to finance and welfare, and gave that power to those involved in the day-to-day lives of adults who lacked capacity, where previously such a power belonged only to the court. The scope of the MCA is thus wide ranging, touching on almost every aspect of the day-to-day life of someone who lacks capacity, making it an immensely important piece of legislation for all those involved in their care.

The theory at the heart of the MCA is respect for individual autonomy; people who are able to make decisions for themselves, who are deemed to have capacity, should be allowed to do so. This is underlined throughout the general principles in Section 1 of the Act, which require that a person be presumed to have capacity until it is proven otherwise, that all steps must be taken to try and enable the person to have capacity to make the decision themselves and that an unwise decision should not be considered to be one made without capacity.[2] This deference to an individual's autonomy is reflected in other areas all through the legislation, not least in the concept of 'best interests'. Best interests builds in a respect for the individual, requiring that we take account of the individual's past and present wishes and feelings, religious or other beliefs, and how the individual themselves would have made the decision, had they had the capacity to do so. Autonomy is also seen in the creation of the 'lasting power of attorney' (LPA) and 'advance directives'. The former allows a person to determine how they wish to be treated or cared for, or how they want their finances to be dealt with, and to give the power for making these decisions to another individual when they no longer have the capacity to do so themselves. The latter, often incorrectly called 'living wills', when created properly enable individuals to make advance decisions regarding medical treatment—including over matters which an LPA cannot bestow, such as refusing life-sustaining treatment.

The aim of the MCA is not to be paternalistic, but to recognize individuals' limitations, enable them to make the decision themselves and, where they cannot, to provide a framework which enables us to make the decision for them in a way which is best for them in as objective a fashion as possible, and to still include them in the process to the greatest extent possible.

The following sections will look at the key aspects of the MCA, in particular at how capacity must be assessed, what is meant by 'best interests', and other surrogate decision-making mechanisms, such as lasting power of attorney and court-appointed deputies.

Capacity

The MCA forms a two-step test for determining whether an individual has capacity to make a decision. Firstly, the individual must be shown to have a disturbance or impairment of their mental functioning, and secondly, that this causes them to be unable to make a decision. The MCA does not provide a definitive 'answer'; at some point, a value judgement must be made, but it certainly provides a firm framework within which to make those judgements.

An impairment or disturbance of the mind is a wide phrase, which covers some mental disorders such as dementia and intellectual disabilities, but also those who are concussed or suffering the symptoms of alcohol or drug abuse.[3] Without such an impairment or disturbance, an individual cannot be shown to lack capacity.

---

[2] Section 1 of the Mental Capacity Act 2005.
[3] See Mental Capacity Act 2005 Code of Practice (London: TSO), p. 44.

Once it is established that the individual has a disturbance or impairment of mind, it must be shown that they are also unable to make a decision. According to the test set out by the MCA, an individual is unable to make the decision if his/she is unable to:

(a) understand the information relevant to the decision,

(b) retain that information,

(c) use or weigh that information as part of the process of making the decision, or

(d) communicate his or her decision (whether by talking, using sign language, or any other means).[4]

However, in determining whether or not an individual is able to make a decision, the presentation of the information and method of communication is highly important. It is vital to consider the fact that an individual may be able to make a decision if the information is presented in a different manner, and other methods of communication are considered. Things such as easy-read formats and memory aids to assist in helping retention of information, and other forms of communication are all extremely useful in increasing an individual's capacity for decision-making.

It is important to note that an assessment for capacity is not general, but time and issue specific to the relevant decision, for example 'Where do I want to live?' and 'Can I take that decision myself?' at this point in time. That an individual lacks capacity to make a specific decision does not mean he/she lacks capacity to make all decisions, and capacity should be assessed each time. This is something which must borne in mind by those making decisions about a person's capacity; there has been criticism from enquirers to Counsel and Care about the content of the 'capacity assessment' in relation to the questions asked during the assessment, which seem to bear little relation to the specific issue at hand (i.e. where a person wants to live).

Best interests

The MCA demands that when making decisions for people who lack mental capacity, we must do so in their 'best interests'. It is a concept which is not simple to grasp and, as with determining capacity, there certainly isn't a straightforward answer as to what is in someone's best interests. The idea of 'best interests' decision-making is to balance the individual's opinions and views with those of their carers, family, or health or social care professionals involved in their care or welfare where it relates to the decision which has to be made, and come to an objective decision as to the course of action.

The concept was formally established in the case of *Re F(Mental Patient: Sterilisation)*,[5] which stated that medical treatment (in the instant case, sterilization of a young woman with intellectual disabilities) could be given when the patient was unable to consent where it could be shown that such treatment was in the patient's 'best interests'. In *Re F*, it was determined that what was in the patient's best interests was determined by the common law doctrine of necessity, in this case the medical necessity of the

---

[4] Section 2(1) Mental Capacity Act 2005.

[5] [1990] 2 AC 1.

operation placed against the psychological harm it was felt would result from her lack of understanding of both the biological processes of pregnancy and childbirth, and her inability to look after a child. Such treatment would not be considered negligent provided it complied with the *Bolam* test for negligence.[6]

This early invocation of the concept founded on medical necessity, and what medical practitioners felt was required in the 'best interests' of the person's health and medical welfare changed over the following 15 years to the point at which the MCA was passed into law. The concept of best interests was used to permit caesarean sections,[7] blood transfusions,[8] other cases of sterilization,[9] and tissue donation,[10] but by the early 2000, the scope of 'best interests' was widened, to apply to non-medical cases, such as parental contact[11] and place of residence of individuals with intellectual disabilities.[12]

What the MCA has attempted to do is to take the principles which have been developed in the case law and set them down in statute. This is done in Section 4 of the Act, but it must be emphasized that this section does not provide a definition of 'best interests'. Section 4 provides a list of factors which must be considered by the decision maker when they are deciding the best course of action. The decision cannot be based purely on the individual's appearance or age, or on their behaviour. Account must be taken of past, and present, wishes and feelings, beliefs and values, and anything else the individual would have taken into account. The decision maker must consult those named by the individual, those caring for him or her, and officially appointed LPAs or deputies.

The difficulty is that, while providing what Lewison J has described as a 'structured decision-making process',[13] the MCA still requires value judgements to be made; essentially, there is no straightforward answer, even after legislation. It should be noted, however, that the Court of Protection has a best interests jurisdiction in relation to disputes that cannot be resolved, for example disputes over residency between family and social services, and can make these decisions.

One particular issue which presents a great problem in determining best interests is how much weight should be given to the individual's current wishes and feelings. This is something which callers to Counsel and Care have brought up frequently as a concern, many of whom worry about their relatives or friends being able to receive appropriate care, in a setting of their choice, and are often worried about situations where the wishes and wants of the older person seem to be disregarded in favour of the

---

[6] The *Bolam* test stipulates that such treatment, even if harmful, is not the result of negligent action provided that the individual has acted '*in accordance with a practice accepted as proper by a responsible body of medical men skilled in that particular art*'.

[7] *Re MB* [1997] 2 FLR 426.

[8] *Re T* [1993] Fam 95.

[9] *Re S* [2000] 2 FLR 389 and *Re A* [2000] 1 FLR 549.

[10] *Re Y* [1997] Fam 110.

[11] *Re G* [2004] EWHC 2222 (Fam).

[12] *Re S* [2003] EWHC 1909 (Fam).

[13] *Re P* [2009] EWHC 163 (Ch).

opinions of professionals (or sometimes other family members), once the older person has been assessed as having lost mental capacity for all decision-making.

The MCA requires in Section 4 that when considering what is in someone's best interests, the person's past and present wishes and feelings must be taken into account, along with their beliefs and values and any other factors the individual would have considered if they were making the decision themselves. There are several things to be said here; first, what an individual's wishes and feelings may be in the present will often conflict with past opinions and where they do not, may still seem unwise or harmful. Second, it must always be remembered that, while wishes, feelings, beliefs and values, and other factors must be considered, they do not have to be determinative.

It is worth discussing some of the case law, as this issue has been dealt with in some detail by the courts. The facts of these cases vary, from a woman's sexual contact with a man who would seem to be violent,[14] to contact with an abusive father,[15] and to bestowal of a lifetime's fortune on a seemingly undeserving and untrustworthy individual.[16]

In *M, ITW v Z*,[17] Munby J noted that the individual's wishes and feelings will always be a significant factor, but that the weight attached will vary with each case and the facts thereof. In addition, he notes that there is no hierarchy of the factors in s.4(2), and therefore while significant weight will be given to the individual's present wishes and feelings, equally they must be borne out by all relevant circumstances. These include, he lists (a) the level of incapacity, (b) the strength and consistency of the views, (c) the impact on the individual should his or her wishes be ignored, (d) the extent of rationality or irrationality of the views and possible implementation of this, and (e) whether these desires can be accommodated within the overall realm of 'best interests'.

This issue has been reconsidered very recently, in a matter that has immediate relevance to care homes. *Dorset County Council v EH*[18] concerned the removal of an elderly woman with dementia to a care home against her wishes. The court concluded that EH did not and was not able to understand the seriousness of her illness and the subsequent risks she faced living alone. On this basis, her objection to moving into a care home could not be given considerable weight.

What must ultimately be remembered in this process is that, while the decisions being made are about a real person with real feelings and wishes, a best interests decision is not a 'substituted judgement' test.[19] That is, we are not trying to make the decision *as they would have*, had they had the capacity. A best interests decision is a balancing act, with their wishes, and how they would have made the decision as factors to be considered, but equally must in the end be a decision which results from an

---

[14] *Local Authority X v MM (by her litigation friend, the Official solicitor), KM* [2007] EWHC 2003 (Fam).
[15] *Re G* [2004] EWHC 2222 (Fam).
[16] *Re M, ITW v Z, M and others* [2009] EWHC 2525 (Fam).
[17] Ibid.
[18] [2009] EWHC 784 (Fam).
[19] *Re P* [2009] EWHC 163 (Ch) para. 37.

objective consideration of all factors. However, it is a value judgement, and will never be simple. The MCA serves to provide clear principles to guide the decision maker, but it is not a definition or an answer book.

Lasting power of attorney, court-appointed deputies, and advance directives

There are some decisions concerning individuals who lack capacity to make decisions for themselves, which must be made by a specific person. This is either because the individual, prior to losing capacity, bestowed on a a specific person the power to make the decisions on his or her behalf, or because the Court of Protection has made an order bestowing the power to make such a decision on a specific person subsequent to his or her application to the court for such a power.

The first type of situation is the bestowing of a LPA. That the individual is to be granted this power must be recorded on specific forms, which must then be registered with the Office of the Public Guardian. There are two different types of LPA, one for financial affairs and a second for welfare (care, medical procedures, etc.).[20] Prior to the LPA, the previous framework of enduring power of attorney (EPA) covered property and financial affairs only; the LPA framework allows for individuals to make specific decisions about how they want their welfare to be determined once they lack capacity, as well as how their estate be managed.

Where there is a need for ongoing decisions to be made, but there is no LPA or EPA giving anyone such a power, the Court of Protection may appoint a 'deputy' with the appropriate power. This is a position which can be applied for, or the court may make the decision to appoint a deputy during other proceedings.[21]

Both deputy and attorney must always act in the individual's best interests[22] and only within the parameters given to them by either the LPA or the Court of Protection. The most important restriction on both an attorney and a deputy is that they are not permitted to refuse or cease life-sustaining treatment; this is something which must be directly applied for at the Court of Protection.[23]

The only way an individual can refuse life-saving treatment is to record that wish in an 'advance directive'. These are often incorrectly called 'living wills'. This is incorrect, because they are not, unlike a will, unlimited in scope, but refer only to a very specific circumstances regarding medical treatment. An advance directive can refuse the administration, or continuation of specific treatment, including life-sustaining treatment.[24] This previously was a power only the courts could employ, and has been particularly controversial. However, it is important to emphasize that an advance directive cannot command specific treatment (particularly euthanasia). It can only

[20] Mental Capacity Act 2005, s. 9(1).

[21] Mental Capacity Act 2005, s. 16.

[22] Mental Capacity Act 2005, s. 9(4)(a).

[23] Mental Capacity Act 2005, s. 11(8). Section 11 also outlines other restrictions on the donee of a LPA, which primarily concern the conditions under which a donee may authorize an act intended to restrain the individual.

[24] Mental Capacity Act 2005, s. 24(1).

require that a specific treatment does not begin, or that an existing treatment must cease at a particular point. Advance decisions do not have to be written down, except in cases which concern life-sustaining treatment, when it must be written and signed by both the individual and a witness in each other's presence.

The Deprivation of Liberty Safeguards (DoLS)

The DoLS take the form of schedules A1 and 1A of the MCA 2005, and establish a framework by which care homes and hospitals may apply for authorization to deprive individuals, who lack capacity to make decisions over their care or treatment, of their liberty.

The safeguards are a direct response to a judgement by the European Court of Human Rights (ECtHR) in *H.L. v United Kingdom*, in which the court was highly critical of the way in which adults who lacked capacity to decide over their treatment or care were being deprived of their liberty. The ECtHR criticized both the lack of procedure by which individuals were deprived of their liberty and the inadequate appeal mechanisms which existed to contest that deprivation. The DoLS create a detailed procedure which aims to allow for deprivation of liberty in an individual's best interests in a non-arbitrary fashion.

Potentially, the DoLS legislation could have a huge impact on how care homes must manage the care of individuals with mental capacity issues. What constitutes a deprivation of liberty is not completely clear (see section 'Making the application'), but what is obvious is that the DoLS may well cover a significant proportion of care home residents. To keep the care and treatment of residents within the law, it is vitally important that care homes are aware of how the legislation operates and will impact on them, and that they may require legal advice in some individual cases. There are concerns from callers to Counsel and Care that the process of seeking to move an individual to a care home begins before the case is examined in detail and consideration is given to whether there is a 'less restrictive option' available. In some cases reported to Counsel and Care, the mental capacity of the older persons has not been formally assessed before the process of trying to move them to the care home begins. Although the emphasis with DoLS is that it should only be used where there is no other option, it seems to some enquirers to Counsel and Care that the opposite is happening, whereby the option of possibly employing DoLS is seen as a way of 'persuading someone that it would be best to move to a care home'.

Making the application

If the care home or hospital where an individual is resident, or is due to be resident (termed in the legislation as a managing authority), feel that it is necessary to deprive an individual of his or her liberty, they must apply to the relevant supervisory body for a standard authorization. If the person is to be cared for in a care home, the supervisory body will be the local authority where the individual is normally resident; if it is a hospital, the hospital must apply to the primary care trust. The request for standard authorization must be completed on 'Form 4', outlining the purpose and reasons for the deprivation.

In cases where the managing authority believes the need to deprive liberty is a matter of urgency, it is possible for the managing authority to issue an urgent authorization (on Form 1 of the DoLS official forms). This must be immediately submitted to the supervisory body, along with a request for standard authorization on Form 4.

Qualifying requirements and assessments

In order for a request to be granted, six qualifying requirements must be met. When an application for standard authorization is received by a supervisory body, it will commission assessments to determine whether the qualifying requirements are met. For this, there is a timescale of 21 calendar days for a standard authorization application and 7 calendar days for those standard requests received in conjunction with a notification of an urgent authorization.

The six requirements are:

1 *Age*: the individual must be shown to be over 18.
2 *Mental capacity*: it must be shown that the individual lacks the mental capacity to make the relevant decision with regards to treatment or care.
3 *Mental health*: it must be shown that the individual is suffering from a mental health disorder under the criteria outlined in the MHA 1983 (as amended by the MHA 2007).
4 *No refusals*: it must be shown that there is no valid advance directive refusing the treatment, or an EPA/LPA with the power to refuse such care or treatment.
5 *Eligibility*: the individual must not be subject to orders under the MHA 1983, nor *should* they be subject to detention under those provisions.
6 *Best interests*: it must be shown that (a) the proposed authorization amounts to a deprivation of liberty and (b) this deprivation would be in the individual's best interest.

After the assessments

Once all the assessments are complete, if all six requirements are met, the supervisory body will review all the documentation, and determine whether or not to authorize the deprivation of liberty. They will also decide on any conditions which will apply if the deprivation is authorized, (for example requiring that the individual be accompanied out three times a week), and appoint an official representative, which may be either a family member, close friend, or a paid professional.

From this point, the managing authority is under an obligation to monitor the individual for any changes to the qualifying requirements, and if such a change is noticed, to request a review of the authorization by the supervisory body. This point is particularly relevant for care homes, as they must continue to make sure that the qualifying requirements are met, particularly whether the person continues to lack capacity to make the relevant decision. Managing authorities must also be aware that the person themselves, or their representative, may also request review if they feel that any of the qualifying requirements are no longer met, including whether or not the deprivation continues to be in the individual's best interests. In addition, they also have leave of appeal against decisions to the Court of Protection.

What is a deprivation of liberty?

The DoLS legislation does not have a statutory definition of 'deprivation of liberty'. This is because, according to the minister then responsible for the legislation, the government wished to remain true to the case law of the ECtHR, which has frequently resisted attempts to define deprivation to a specific set of circumstances. This means that determining the existence of a deprivation of liberty is very much a legal question of balancing previous case law and keeping up to date with new case law.

The ECtHR has consistently held that deprivation of liberty should be considered in the 'classic' sense of physical liberty,[25] though it must be emphasized that this is more than just freedom of movement.[26] The initial approach of determining the existence of a deprivation is to look at the 'concrete situation' of the case at hand,[27] taking into account a range of criteria, including type, duration, effects, and manner of implementation of the measure in question.[28] However, it was emphasized in *Guzzardi v Italy* that, while these factors are important to take into account, the difference between a restriction and a deprivation of liberty is not one of nature or substance, but of degree or intensity of the action.[29] Thus, no particular activity is, of itself, automatically a deprivation of liberty, but rather it is the intensity with which the action is performed that can lift it above restriction to become deprivation. It is this fact which has meant that there is no 'deprivation of liberty' definition, but rather the 'degree and intensity' of the action must be assessed on a case-by-case basis.

A good example of the degree and intensity principle is the case of *Ashingdane v United Kingdom*.[30] The case concerned an inmate at Broadmoor Hospital whose request for transfer to a more open mental health institution had been rejected due to the stance of nurses at that hospital against those patients who were detained as a result of criminal activity. At the ECtHR, he argued that he was being deprived of his liberty by being forced to remain at Broadmoor, but the court found that the restrictions at the open institution were not of less enough a degree and intensity to fall below the threshold of deprivation. Therefore, there was no legitimate reason for him to move institutions, as he would still remain deprived of his liberty in either place.

What tipped the balance in *H.L. v United Kingdom*, the case which led to the DoLS reforms, was the 'complete and effective control' which was exercised over HL's care and movement. In this case, the court determined that the 'concrete situation' was that he was '*under continuous supervision and control and was not free to leave*', and that

---

[25] *Engel and others v The Netherlands Application no. 5100/71; 5101/71; 5102/71; 5354/72; 5370/72),* 8 June 1976.

[26] This is made clear in Engel at paragraph 58, emphasizing that there is an Optional Protocol to the Convention (Protocol No. 4) which deals with freedom of movement specifically.

[27] Ibid.

[28] *Guzzardi v Italy (Application no. 7367/76),* 6 November 1980, para 92.

[29] Ibid., para 93.

[30] *Ashingdane v United Kingdom* (Application no. 8225/78), 28 May 1985.

the intensity of this control was such that it amounted to a deprivation of liberty. It is this aspect of being control over someone's life which obviously has most application when considering deprivation of liberty in the context of a care home. Residents are dependent on their carers for many aspects of day-to-day life, and therefore the power to prevent an individual from doing something he/she wants to do is often in the hands of the carer. Care homes must, therefore, be very careful to assess how much control they are exercising over an individual's life; who they can see and when, what they can do and when, where they can go and when.

Interface with the Mental Health Act 1983

One particular challenge for those involved in making applications for DoLS is whether to use DoLS or the provisions for detention under the MHA 1983. The interface between the MHA and DoLS revolves around an individual's eligibility for deprivation of liberty under DoLS. An individual will be ineligible for deprivation of liberty under DoLS, if he/she is currently subject to any provisions under the MHA (detention under Sections 2 or 3 and leave therefrom, community treatment orders and guardianship) or should be subject to such provisions. The former part is easy to check, the latter part presents more of a problem.

Generally, in a care home, the MHA is not an option, and therefore cannot be used. However, in homes where it can be used, there is a careful decision to make. The test for determining which regime should be used has two stages.

First, it must be shown that the individual falls within the scope of the MHA. This means that he/she meets the criteria for detention set out in Sections 2 and 3 of the MHA. It is important to note that where the individual does fall within the scope of the MHA, the decision maker does not have a 'choice' between DoLS and the MHA. If the second part of the test is met, the MHA must be used.

The second part requires that (a) for the individual to be ineligible for DoLS, the 'relevant instrument' (i.e. the standard authorization) authorizes the individual to be a mental health patient and (b) that the individual objects to being a mental health patient.[31] If the standard authorization applied for would authorize the individual to be a mental health patient, and the individual is objecting to being a mental health patient, then the MHA must be used. If an individual is not a mental health patient, or is not objecting, then the deprivation of liberty can be authorized under DoLS.

The test for establishing whether or not the individual is a mental health patient is a 'but for' test; 'but for' the treatment the individual was receiving for any physical ailment, would he/she need to be deprived of the liberty? For example, an individual with dementia being treated for pneumonia is being treated for the physical illness, not the dementia. The individual needs to be deprived of their liberty because he/she does not understand the necessity for the medical treatment of the physical illness, not in order to treat dementia.

As has been emphasized, the situation in most care homes is simply a case of ensuring that individuals are not already subject to any MHA orders. Importantly, the fact

---

[31] Paragraph 5, Schedule 1A, Mental Health Act 2007.

that they might be objecting to the care or treatment is also not necessarily a barrier to an authorization under DoLS. There have been concerns expressed by callers to Counsel and Care that the use of DoLS is prevailing, as a deprivation under DoLS does not entitle individuals to free aftercare under Section 117 of the MHA, as they would have if they had been detained under Sections 2 or 3 of the MHA. If this is the case, it is not so much an issue of the interface between DoLS and the MHA as poor practice within services, and needs close examination.

Conclusions

The legal landscape affecting those who care for adults who lack capacity has changed significantly over the last 10 years, with the MCA 2005 representing the culmination of almost a decade of attempts at legislative consultation and reform. With the addition of the DoLS, there is now comprehensive legislation governing the actions of care homes, and careful consideration must be given to these provisions when making decisions regarding the care and treatment of adults who are not able to make those decisions for themselves. Although the legislation employs some difficult concepts, it has established a clear framework which can be negotiated with training and, in difficult cases, good legal guidance, and most importantly will allow for good decisions to be made on the behalf of those who are not able to do so for themselves.

Acknowledgements

The author would like to thank Counsel and Care and their Advice Team for their valuable comments, suggestions, and contributions to this chapter.

Further reading

Bartlett, P. (2008). *Blackstone's Guide to the Mental Capacity Act 2005*, 2nd Edition. Oxford: Oxford University Press.

Donnelly, M. (2009). Best interests, patient participation and the Mental Capacity Act. *Medical Law Review*, *17*(1), 1–29.

Dunn, M.C., Clare, I.C.H., Holland, A.J., & Gunn, M.J. (2007). Constructing and reconstructing 'best interests': an interpretative examination of substitute decision-making under the Mental Capacity Act 2005. *Journal of Social Welfare & Family Law*, *29*(2), 117–133.

Dunn, M.C., Clare, I.C.H., & Holland, A.J. (2008). Substitute decision-making for adults with intellectual disabilities living in residential care: learning through experience. *Health Care Analysis*, *16*, 52–64.

Fennell, P. (2007). *Mental Health: The New Law*. Bristol: Jordans.

Hope, T., Slowther, A., & Eccles, J. (2009). Best interests, dementia, and the Medical Capacity Act 2005. *Journal of Medical Ethics*, *35*, 733–738.

The Mental Capacity Act 2005 Code of Practice (2005). London: TSO.

Social Care Institute for Excellence's Mental Capacity Act Resources. Available at: http://www.scie.org.uk/publications/mca/index.asp. (accessed 01 March 2011)

Chapter 10

Abuse in care homes for older people: the case for safeguards

Hilary Brown

Abstract

Abusive or neglectful practice of older people can develop insidiously. Most caregivers do not choose to harm others; they intend to do good work but find themselves in situations they are unable to manage. Most abuse results from poor practice within a care home rather than from the deeds of one 'bad' individual. Its causes are thus issues such as lack of training and/or leadership, acceptance of embedded poor practice, and lack of appreciation of staff rather than individual pathology. Preventing and responding to abuse require clear standards so that abusive practice can be readily identified and responded to. This chapter advocates that any suspected abuse should be reported to the Safeguarding system and investigated to uphold high standards. The emphasis must be on preventing abuse by improving standards of practice. This requires honest dialogue between managers and care staff about the difficult challenges that can arise in working with older people with complex needs, especially dementia. It is inevitably stressful but with good leadership and training it can be a motivating and positive experience. Safeguarding should be seen as an integral part of good care, not an optional extra or an unnecessary imposition.

Safeguarding and personalization

This chapter explores what is meant by the terms 'abuse' and 'safeguarding' and what we understand about the causes of harm in care homes for older people and the means of preventing it. The origins of safeguarding come from concerns about the abuse of vulnerable older people, including care home residents, culminating in the publication of *No Secrets* in 2000 (Department of Health, 2000). *No Secrets* forms the basis of the current Safeguarding[1] arrangements for vulnerable adults. Further legal protection is provided by the *Mental Capacity Act 2005*, which contains safeguards against deprivation of liberty, either in care homes or hospitals. Although additional powers have been proposed by recent reviews of *No Secrets* (Department of Health, 2008a) and adult social care legislation, these have not been implemented as yet (Law Commission, 2008).

Recent policy emphasizes choice and personalization—for example self-directed support and personal budgets—alongside early intervention and more flexible use of resources (Department of Health, 2007, 2008b). The ideological aspiration is to move away from 'batch' care and institutionalized provision, to extend community-based living for older and disabled people and their family carers, but it is important to acknowledge that they are underpinned by an economic imperative.

On the face of it, it may appear that arguments for independence and choice are at the opposite end of the spectrum from safeguarding, but this is not so. The key argument in this chapter is that safeguarding complements the facilitation of personal independence and choice for vulnerable people by ensuring that they are protected from harm. 'Choice' is not an *alternative* to safeguarding or protection but rather they are complementary and necessary elements of both policy and practice.

Safety without overprotection: a balanced approach to risk

Several serious case reviews[2] have focused on individuals who refused care services when they were at risk of abuse or when their mental health problems made it difficult for them to engage with paid carers or professionals (Keywood, 2010). These reviews have recommended that practitioners look beyond the 'rejection of help' to whether the person has communication difficulties, has mental incapacity, and/or understands the consequences of refusing services for their health and well-being. Workers in mental health outreach teams are familiar with these dilemmas and about the importance of clear principles for assessing when intervention is in the person's best interests. This helps us to view Safeguarding as a way of *assuring* not *overriding* the right of people who use care services to protection alongside liberty and agency.

The word 'risk' may be used in contradictory ways in these discussions. Some people argue that risk is an essential ingredient of a valued lifestyle, while others become anxious about the possibility of catastrophic outcomes or liability. We all accept risk as an essential part of daily life in a free society: if not, we would never leave home, play sport, or take a chance on friendship or love. We also take precautions by locking our front doors, avoiding rough areas late at night, purchasing insurance, and not opening our doors to strangers. Some people thrive on excitement and spontaneity, while others prefer routine and order, tending to avoid too much change or challenge.

---

[1] Safeguarding with a capital S is used to refer to the formal system for protecting vulnerable adults.

[2] Serious care reviews for adults are not enshrined in law as they are for children but are seen as good practice in relation to vulnerable adults, for example, Association of Directors of Adult Social Services (2005).

Caution is often a feature of the lives of older people who draw in their horizons as their ability to cope with change lessens. In some cases, such as frontal lobe dementia, people may become more inclined to take risks or behave positively recklessly!

So while 'protection' may seem restrictive or unnecessary, a person's ability to keep control over the degree of risk they allow into their lives is often central to maintaining their chosen lifestyle. Protecting our property, feeling safe in our relationships, managing our personal space and bodily functions are aspects of our adult lives that we take for granted; when our abilities in these areas falter it feels like a significant loss. This may be a particularly acute loss when an older person moves into residential care because this marks a transition from managing independently to becoming dependent on others.

Nevertheless, although we *all* attend to risk in our lives, a focus on safeguarding vulnerable people is often perceived as overprotective. The evidence of rising allegations of abuse suggests that this is not the case (Cambridge et al., 2006; Kalaga and Kingston, 2007). Instead, in reality, older people are often put in situations that carry *more* risk than others would find tolerable, at times when they are *less* able to apply the kind of caution that other citizens would exercise. For example, older people receiving a domiciliary care service may be very frail but their homes are regularly open to people they may not know. They rely on the goodwill and professional and honest conduct of those people and the agencies that employ them. A cruel worker, who abuses their trust, takes their property or carries out care tasks in an insensitive or neglectful way will have a profound impact on their sense of well-being and personal safety. Many people would not allow a stranger to enter their homes, particularly to perform intimate tasks such as bathing. Attending to protection, over and above what seems ordinary, is therefore justified in these, and similar, circumstances. Most people do not ask their friends to submit to a Criminal Records Bureau check or fill in 'risk assessment forms', but there again most people do not live in accommodation that has no locks on the doors, nor do they have to rely on unfamiliar people to help them intimately in their bathrooms or bedroom as is the case in a care home. See Case Study 10.1 for an example of a relatively common situation of risk that an older person living in the community (or a care home) may face.

Case study 10.1

Mrs Bolton lives in her own home near an estate with a high number of young people using drugs and out of work: her grandson visits regularly but he often takes money from her purse and can become threatening if she tries to reason with him. She tends to downplay the impact of these outbursts but is visibly upset by them. Domiciliary care staff who visit Mrs Bolton daily have difficulty coming to a decision about whether she would be better off if her grandson stopped coming, or if this is a risk worth taking so that she can continue to see him as she is very fond of him. In this case, there is a clear choice to be made between risk and a valued relationship. But usually people do not find themselves at risk as a result of such an explicit dilemma. They are more likely to find themselves gradually exposed to indifferent care, or withdrawing as a result of anxiety or confusion, or not coping because those involved are not noticing gradual changes and making timely adjustments.

So the aim of safeguarding is not to curtail vulnerable people from living interesting or full lives, it is to achieve a level of safety that would be considered *normal* for other citizens. Keeping a vulnerable person safe may involve *heightened* alertness and *more* rigorous planning or management of risk. The outcome should look ordinary but the inputs may need to be more concentrated and focused than would be required for someone less vulnerable. For example, the Office of the Public Guardian acts to protect the financial affairs of older people who lack capacity through a framework of supervision, involving either a power of attorney or an appointed deputy (Office of the Public Guardian, 2008). This allows someone close and trusted, or someone professional and experienced, to monitor the person's assets and to spend money in ordinary ways on his or her behalf. The extra scrutiny is not designed to interfere unnecessarily but to ensure assets are appropriately and safely used.

Safeguarding does not set out to be restrictive but to create an environment in which vulnerable people can be helped to live as ordinary a life as possible while having their care provided safely and sensitively. Sometimes there is a difficult balance to strike (see Case Study 10.2). A typical 'risk' scenario in a care home includes an older person being:

- left sitting in wet incontinence pads until he or she gets pressure sores because no one has attended to his or her needs,
- deliberately ignored as a response to challenging behaviour or aggression,
- given the wrong medication because a staff member was too busy or was not concentrating,
- unable to prevent a stranger from taking the engagement ring that reminded him or her of a much loved and missed partner, and/or
- in debt because his or her savings have been mismanaged or diverted by others.

Vulnerability to abuse

The term 'vulnerable adult' refers to someone who '*is or may be in need of community care services by reason of mental or other disability, age or illness* **and** '*who is, or may be unable to, take care of himself or herself, or unable to protect himself or herself against significant harm or exploitation*'.

Case study 10.2

Mrs Smith is incontinent and suffers from frequent urinary infections. Amy, an inexperienced care assistant, is convinced that she wets herself to annoy or detain her at the end of a shift. She has received no induction or supervision. When Mrs Smith wet herself shortly after Amy had changed the sheets she lashed out at her and threatened her saying she was 'an evil old witch'. Good continence care would have avoided this situation and appropriate training and supervision could have put Amy straight before she allowed her frustrations to spill over into abusive conduct. Mrs Smith cannot get away from Amy and she may also not be able to report her cruelty to the manager of the service. Her dependency makes her especially vulnerable to abusive or neglectful practices.

This two part definition means that the safeguarding process is managed in different ways depending on the ability of the person to take action on his or her own behalf. Many people receiving community care services can manage their own safety and use mainstream services to protect themselves, especially if they are given advice or sign-posting to sources of help. Mrs Bolton, for example (see Case Study 10.1), was encouraged to discuss her grandson's behaviour with the local community support officer and the police advised of the options available to her. She was then left to decide if she preferred putting up with her grandson taking money from her purse and continuing to see him or not seeing him at all. The community support officer came in the afternoon when Mrs Bolton was most alert; she sat with her for an hour, and worked hard to put her at her ease. The officer had attended training on abuse of vulnerable adults so she understood the issues and could provide an appropriate level of support and advice. Mainstream services such as the police need to be mindful of the needs of older people, and be willing to support them to make a complaint, access specialist services, or even prosecute an abuser.

Individuals with dementia in a care home may not be able to make their own decisions in circumstances of risk, abuse, or exploitation; nor can they act to remove themselves from harm or request that abusive or difficult people be taken out of their lives. They need public agencies to act decisively on their behalf; this responsibility is reflected in the guidance *No Secrets* (Department of Health, 2000).

Understanding a wide range of abuses

No Secrets (Department of Health, 2000) was a response to over a decade of campaigning and research that had revealed the nature and extent of abuse against older people, particularly physical and financial abuse by their families and neglect in institutional care (Brown and Seden, 2003). *No Secrets* defines abuse as single acts rather than as embedded in ongoing relationships or care contexts. It classifies abuse as being physical, sexual, psychological or financial, or as neglect, and it acknowledges that abuse could happen in the person's own home, in a care home, or in public places. Although it has been a helpful policy in raising awareness about different types of abuse, its perspective that abusive incidents are disconnected acts has contributed to *patterns* of abuse being missed and to the complex dynamics that give rise to abuse and/or neglect being unacknowledged. It reflects, to a large extent, the nature of the evidence base about abuse at that time but it also set the tone for future research and monitoring exercises (Brown and Stein, 1998).

More recent research suggests that there are clear patterns of abuse within particular relationships and in certain contexts (Brown and Seden, 2003). For example, abuse of an older person by a co-resident relative, particularly a spouse, shares many of the risk characteristics of domestic violence; characteristics that are amplified by age and frailty (Beach et al., 2005). In community settings, a perpetrator may move in on a vulnerable person, using their space, taking their food and refusing to leave. Another pattern is of predatory abusers who target and groom visibly vulnerable people, usually in relation to financial or sexual abuse.

Thus, describing instances of abuse as disembodied 'acts', without regard to their context, tends to obscure patterns of abuse and context-specific risks. This is also true of abuse occurring in long-term care settings, sometimes referred to as 'institutional abuse'. A recent analysis of safeguarding alerts to a local authority in southern England showed that half of these concerned incidents occurred in residential care (or supported living) (Mansell et al., 2009). Analysis further suggests that abuse in care homes tends to be multifaceted and is often a function of a number of interrelated factors: resources, knowledge, work-related stresses, and features of a particular staff team (Cambridge et al., 2006).

Abuse in care homes

Evidence about institutional abuse of older people suggests—as might be expected—that the commonest perpetrators of abuse are those care home staff routinely involved in their day-to-day care (Kalaga and Kingston, 2007; National Center of Elder Abuse, 2005). Staff in care homes are often overworked and highly stressed; many are dissatisfied with their work and feel 'put upon' by the home, residents, and a society that does not value their work or efforts. Furthermore, their work is ill-paid and they often have scant employment protection, benefits, or status (Poinasamy and Fooks, 2009). Some individual staff members may simply be temperamentally unsuited to working with older people; they may lack patience, empathy, interest, or restraint for reasons of their own. For example, if someone has experienced violence in his or her own life it can be difficult for him or her to empathize with vulnerable others. Such individuals may be prone to lash out verbally or physically when overwhelmed or tired. Occasionally, individuals are so damaged that they carry inside them a *compulsion* to hurt others and in rare instances they may actively seek opportunities to control or harm vulnerable people (Bentovim and Williams, 1998). There are now various screening mechanisms to prevent such unsuitable individuals from working in the care sector. These include professional regulation and accreditation, Criminal Records Bureau checks, and seeking references from previous employers, but also removing someone from the register if he or she commits abuse, or entering the name onto a legally regulated register such as that operated by the Independent Safeguarding Authority. Using these safeguards properly are key elements of good recruitment.

However, abuse and neglect are more often a consequence of a care home 'regime and culture' (National Center of Elder Abuse, 2005: 14) rather than a 'bad' or inadequate individual. Treating residents as a homogeneous 'batch' rather than as individual people and being obliged to prioritize functional care tasks over social interaction are noted risk factors. In part, these mechanisms operate to distance the staff from the people they care for: to defend them against the pain and anxiety of dealing with very frail, often demented people (Menzies-Lyth, 1959). For young, poorly supported care staff—often young women looking after old women—they come face to face with their future selves and they do not like what they see. Unless there is strong leadership, a supervision system, and training in place to counter the fear and disgust that hands-on care for older people with dependency needs can engender, such feelings can turn into anger, blame, and resentment. These, in turn, can encourage an approach to care that condones, or at least ignores, abuse, violence, neglect, and the routine humiliation of residents (Smith and Brown, 1992).

Sometimes it appears as if the regime itself is oppressive and impersonal or negligent and hazardous. Incidents may occur that hardly seem anyone's 'fault' but are then repeated. For example, a resident chokes but nothing is done to assess the swallowing or how to feed that resident more safely; someone slips from a hoist but the injuries are explained away and no training is provided to ensure it does not happen again. An incident may initially arise as a result of ignorance only to turn into several similar incidents that demonstrate more conscious negligence. This need to balance support for an inadequate service, with enforcement against a deliberately uncaring one, tests the resolve of Safeguarding workers when investigating a failing care home. For example, in one service, several older people had carpet burns on their heels where they had been dragged into a chair or bed rather than lifted properly. This may have been accidental when it first happened but, after this harmful practice was identified, the care home was asked to ensure staff received training on lifting and handling. When this was not implemented a year later, and the poor practice still continued, the injuries to residents could be seen as part of a wider problem and as deliberately harmful and neglectful.

In some ways, abuse can be thought about as a virus. Much like a virus, abusive practice can seep gradually and invisibly into the culture of a care home, and 'infect' the values of staff, allowing standards of care to deteriorate. Staff may forget that the person they are changing or dressing is a human being, they may stop referring to them by name, or looking at them respectfully; they may leave the toilet door open instead of closing it, or make jokes about appearance or behaviour. These poor practices may start out as lapses but where such issues are not challenged or changed, they simply become the cultural norm. 'Culture' in this context (National Center of Elder Abuse, 2005: 14) means both the informal relationships and atmosphere in a home and its formal policies, guidelines, and ways of organizing care. This includes how individual staff are assigned to work with individual residents, how they divide their time between care priorities, and how they address service users. While staff may use jokey or sarcastic banter to help them cope with their stressful roles, it can undermine the dignity and essential humanity of each resident, particularly if they have dementia. It can contribute to the development of uncaring practice which can, in time, slide into abuse and neglect.

Occasionally, a new member of staff will challenge what they see, only to be told 'this is the way we do things around here, they don't mind'. Once standards have slipped below a certain level there is no anchor to counter the acceptance or deepening of poor practice. Staff are tempted to cut corners, turn a blind eye to cruelties such as rough handling when carrying out personal care tasks, accept open criticism of older people who wet the bed or have other accidents, or help themselves to residents' belongings. Staff receive a message from the service that these things are unimportant and learn to ignore the policies that should protect residents. Formal guidance has limited power in a working environment of this kind.

The policies and procedures governing daily practice in a home are of course important but, if there is a huge gap between the goal of idealized care and the actual reality, staff tend to 'turn off' and resort to their own ways of doing things even if these are ill-informed, insensitive, or outside the bounds of professional practice (Wardaugh and

Wilding, 1993). Morale may also be low, as staff may feel that policies simply exist to protect managers and to please inspection agencies, rather than to help them do a difficult job well. This can be compounded by a lack of acknowledgement from colleagues and management about the challenges of care home work. Formal guidance can also be overly complicated.

In summary, vulnerability to abuse is a product of a number of intersecting factors, primarily the complexity and multiplicity of need among residents/patients, their marginal or low social status, *and* the care context. Key problems that deepen vulnerability are poor physical health, communication problems, and difficulties in performing activities of daily living; the combination of issues that tend to accompany advanced dementia pose particular challenges. Negative attitudes towards older people and the low value attributed to caring for them, inside and outside care home settings, contribute to a denigration of their experiences and the experiences of care home staff. A recent inquiry into poor practice and abuse in a hospital ward for older people identified nine contributory factors (Commission for Health Improvement, 2003). These were mostly environmental and cultural rather than individual, challenging the 'scapegoat' approach to early abuse inquiries. This analysis has been used as a reference point in later inquiries and underpins care home and hospital regulation (see Box 10.1).

Preventing abuse

Dealing with abuse starts with prevention. Once abuse has been identified reporting concerns promptly is a first step, followed by assessing the problem thoroughly and identifying specific improvements that can be implemented to reduce the risk of it being repeated in future. No care home can be immune against an individual member of staff who sets out to be abusive, but all homes are responsible for abuse that arises out of poor management, leadership, values, or practices.

Box 10.1 Factors that contributed to abuse on Rowan Ward

- ◆ Poor environment
- ◆ Low levels of staffing
- ◆ High use of bank staff
- ◆ Little staff development
- ◆ Poor supervision
- ◆ Lack of knowledge about how to report incidents
- ◆ Closed and inward looking culture
- ◆ Weak management at ward and board level
- ◆ Geographical isolation (Commission for Health Improvement, 2003)

Prevention is often regarded as having three levels:

- *Primary prevention* reduces the likelihood of abuse from happening in the first place, for example good staff training, support, and supervision; clarity about how to manage care tasks and challenging behaviours; careful recruitment and sensible policies.

- *Secondary prevention* refers to willingness to acknowledge difficulties and report them promptly, so that formal processes of investigation and review can be instituted. This is the equivalent to early diagnosis and prompt intervention in dealing with an illness. However, in a bad service, this does not readily occur and poor practice can persist over many years until it is regarded as the norm (Kalaga and Kingston, 2007: 23).

- *Tertiary prevention* is about minimizing the damage to those affected, for example giving them time and space to get angry and/or offering counselling to aid recovery. The aim should be to help the abused person(s) get back their sense of self and build trust. It includes acknowledging the extent and nature of the abuse or neglect difficulties, not denying it. This might involve saying to someone, '*I know you suffered in this way and we will take this into account when we allocate staff to you in future and arrange your care in this placement . . .*' Reparation should also be concerned with restoring a service to stability and safe practice.

Given what has been said about the origins of abuse, prevention must operate at several different organizational levels. It is also important that it happens at different stages: our aim should be to prevent abuse from happening at all (primary prevention), but if poor practice slips through the net we need to detect it quickly (secondary prevention) and help the vulnerable adult(s) affected recover and get back to a situation of safety (tertiary prevention) by embedding lessons and improvements back into practice. Service failures *can* and should be used to improve care standards.

In preventing abuse, above all, staff need information because although a few people seem instinctively to know what to do, caring is not 'natural' or 'easy' or just a matter of using common sense. Mental health problems, especially dementia, are often complicated and idiosyncratic, so individual care staff may struggle to appreciate how a service user's behaviour is affected by his or her illness. Without accurate information, staff can be drawn into feeling angry and retaliatory. In their work, they are being asked **not to** act normally in the face of challenging behaviour, incontinence, aggression, irrationality, changing moods, and inconsistent attitudes. In ordinary life, these things provoke a response that has to be suspended; and if staff do not have information and training they cannot suspend their 'normal reactions' and abuse may follow. Staff need a range of supports, including regular, face-to-face supervision; team meetings; shadowing experienced staff; teaching from senior colleagues; professional advice; and written information. More formal training, such as dementia care mapping (see Chapter 21), can be valuable in attending to the particular needs of certain residents. As well as this, care in the home needs to be underpinned by careful regular assessment and properly delivered care plans.

Certain problems are especially challenging. Aggressive behaviour requires careful and sensitive handling, which requires a clear understanding about its function for the person. For example, residents with dementia may feel overwhelmed and may shout or lash out as a way of asking staff to leave them alone, but this is often labelled as 'seeking attention'. This can set off a chain of actions, including depriving them of attention to 'teach them a lesson' which then exacerbates the problem. It may also lead to punitive responses that are cruel and unnecessary. So, unless they understand the causes and nature of challenging behaviour, staff tend to fall back on simplistic 'common sense' notions borrowed from ordinary life. As noted above, these may lead to poor practice or abuse.

Another important issue in preventing abuse is the management of personal care, especially incontinence. This topic is often neglected by written guidance but nonetheless can occupy a lot of staff time. It is sometimes as though two worlds co-exist in a care home (Lee-Treweek, 1994): a sanitized 'front of house' world where everything is clean and ordered, and formal ways of operating rule the day, and a 'back-stage' world where all the real work is done behind closed doors by staff of lowly status, unacknowledged, and unrewarded. Bringing these worlds together is the role of team leaders and care home managers. Otherwise, a major part of the home's activities may lie outside any formal supervision or scrutiny and yet it is here that abuse tends to flourish (Cambridge and Carnaby, 2000).

Addressing these issues at the level of the service is not an alternative to tackling individuals about unacceptable practice but is an essential backdrop to doing so. In a good service, a cruel individual will be identified and dealt with quickly. Good workers will not be afraid to ask about areas of care that they find difficult or perplexing and seek advice or help. But in a service where practice varies and falls below an acceptable standard, the whole staff team becomes implicated in poor practice: staff are more likely to 'let things go' without challenging them, until acting unprofessionally or 'doing the bare minimum' becomes the norm. Attending to good practice in these difficult areas of care is an essential part of prevention. Good practice makes a clear commitment to treating residents as human beings whose dignity will be respected and their rights upheld. This may be done through training, guidance, and supervision but should also be modelled through good leadership and teaching by example.

Taking action against abuse

If abuse is suspected or reported, the first responsibility lies with the care home to decide how serious the situation or incident is. This can be illustrated by a case study described in Case Study 10.3.

This situation illustrates the power imbalance between her and the care worker. Elsie's inability to protect herself from harm and her dependency on the care staff for survival makes her acutely vulnerable to abuse. It is no wonder that she decides to downplay her abusive experiences. These facts would need to be taken into account in any investigation and decision-making, if Elsie did pursue an allegation of abuse. Although any consideration of Elsie's future care should prioritize what she herself wants, considerations of what is in her 'best interests' also need to be taken into account. A responsible provider cannot leave it to a vulnerable person who has been victimized

Case study 10.3

An older woman resident, Elsie, finds a particular care worker Ruth, rough and rude. Ruth gets more abrupt and short tempered towards the end of her shift and on several occasions she has threatened Elsie. She assumes that Elsie is being deliberately obstructive when actually she cannot control her body movements or aid the worker when she is being dressed. Once Ruth even hit Elsie because it took so long to get her changed and Ruth was in a hurry. Ruth wanted to leave on time to meet her boyfriend and there was no one else around for her to hand over to. Elsie recognizes that some of Ruth's behaviour is due to overwork and stress because there are never enough staff on duty at any one time, but she is frightened and wants to say something about her fears before Ruth does anything worse.

However, reporting Ruth to the manager would be fraught with difficulties. Elsie has several conflicting questions in her mind:

◆ Would it make things better or worse?

◆ Could Ruth be fired?

◆ Maybe it isn't really her fault and I am just being a nuisance?

◆ Might Ruth be angry and even rougher in future?

◆ Might Ruth develop a grudge and take things from my room in future or get her family to come round and break things as she once threatened?

◆ What if no one believes me or I can't make myself properly understood? Might they just think I am making things up or being difficult?

As I have nowhere else to go, I need to carefully weigh up whether complaining is a good idea or not.

to decide what course of action to take in the wake of abuse by a member of staff or as a result of neglectful practice. Moreover, if other vulnerable people are at risk from the same person, the home has to act on behalf of them all and not just Elsie. The analysis of why this happened, and the planning of corrective action has to be handled by those with a formal Safeguarding mandate. A systematic approach to considering how abuse has arisen can also be useful (Box 10.2). Another way of locating the cause of abuse is shown in Figure 10.1, which indicates the relationship between perpetrators, their intentions, and the types of action that may be required.

In summary, therefore, staff should be encouraged to report any concerns even if uncorroborated; any hint of abuse in a care home should be taken seriously, and agencies that have a formal Safeguarding role must regularly monitor the quality of care provided in all care homes. It is to the roles and responsibilities of these agencies that we now turn.

Formal safeguarding

Safeguarding arrangements vary across England, Wales, and Scotland, but all jurisdictions require concerns about abuse of a vulnerable adult to be reported to (adult) social services so that an investigation and resolution process can be initiated. The Safeguarding system has both an infrastructure, usually with a Safeguarding Adults Board to bring key agencies and individuals together strategically, and a 'practice arm'

Box 10.2 Questions to ask when diagnosing where abuse has come from

- Did this lapse in our policies occur only in relation to this resident?
- Was poor care delivered only by this one member of staff?
- Was this lapse in our usual standards of care only happening on one manager or shift leader's watch?
- Was there a line and did this staff member knowingly cross it?
- Was there a muddle, and did this person find the best way through it?
- Do we have policies or guidelines that are relevant to this situation?
- Are our policies and guidelines care inadequate in relation to this resident?
- Are our policies and guidelines adequate in relation to all residents and to all the primary areas of care?
- Do we know what standards we are working to but the resources are not sufficient to deliver to this standard consistently?
- Are we being asked to do contradictory things by our commissioners and regulators?

that deals with individual cases. The functions of a Safeguarding Board include audit and training, anticipating and planning for risk consequent on service changes, and monitoring concerns about failing services. It also monitors how individual cases are handled and deals with any problems in the system, for example blocks to communication between and within agencies.

Individual cases are managed through formal meetings that allow information to be shared across agencies and decisions to be taken. Concerns may be reported to social

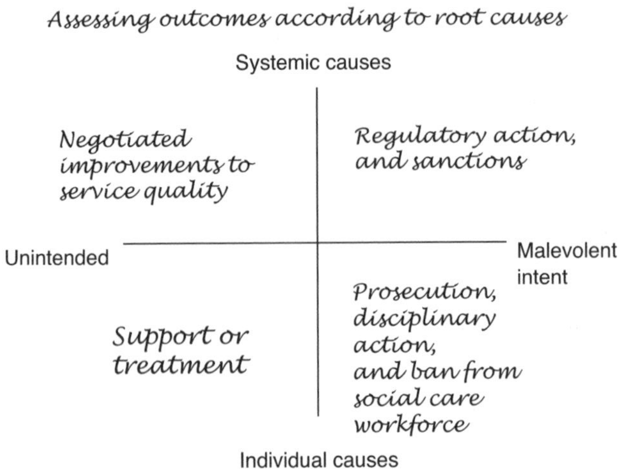

Assessing outcomes according to root causes

Systemic causes

Negotiated improvements to service quality | *Regulatory action, and sanctions*

Unintended — | — Malevolent intent

Support or treatment | *Prosecution, disciplinary action, and ban from social care workforce*

Individual causes

Fig. 10.1 Locating the cause of the abuse.

services via any agency. Initial referrals (alerts) are processed via a sequence of decision-making meetings (strategy or planning meetings, followed by a case conference). The first meeting, sometimes referred to as a planning meeting, strategy meeting, or professionals' meeting, initiates the investigation. In some ways this resembles a police investigation with interviews, witness statements, and reviews of documents or computer records. The investigation then proceeds using the mechanisms of care planning or regulation. A concern about poor practice may lead to a request for a care planning review to be conducted by adult social services and/or for the Care Quality Commission to undertake an unannounced inspection of a care service and/or for the local authority commissioners to meet with the service provider about contract compliance.

The aim of these inquiries is to establish a clear picture of the facts, but if there is insufficient evidence those responsible have to form a view about the likelihood and seriousness of the original allegation before it can be set aside. Cambridge et al. (2006: 61) reported that in one area of southern England about 40% of cases (alerts) reported to social services were confirmed, 40% had insufficient evidence to be pursued, and 20% were considered unfounded. Of course, as is often the case with child abuse and domestic violence, forensic evidence is rarely available. It is also appropriate that a high threshold of proof is required as a person's livelihood and reputation may be at stake when allegations are made. Nonetheless, the professionals involved must gather enough information to reach some conclusions about what happened, and create a protection plan to ensure the future safety of a vulnerable adult. The plan may focus on the vulnerable person, in which case it will be drawn up as an individual protection plan, and/or it might focus on the perpetrator of the abuse, in which case it will be handled through a disciplinary hearing or capability procedure or through the criminal justice system. Or it might examine what went wrong at the service level, for example in the care home, in which case it will be formulated as a service improvement plan.

As an example, social workers in a hospital team were concerned about a particular care home—Fairview Court[3]—because several residents had been admitted with severe pressure sores. One nurse complained that an employee of the care home was verbally abusive to her when she rang for some information about one patient. When the person investigating the concerns went to the home staff members were evasive about who had spoken on the phone. This apparent collusion raised the investigator's level of concern as it suggested a culture in which staff 'stuck together' and resisted any challenge to their practice. Meanwhile, the health professionals were clear that pressure sores were occurring unnecessarily. It was decided to review all Fairview Court residents on a three monthly basis and to record and report all pressure sores once they reached a specified level of seriousness. The home manager was asked to implement a series of changes and the local district nurse specialist offered to provide two training sessions, mandatory for all staff around the avoidance of bed sores. Thus, although the original allegation was not proved, underlying concerns were addressed, a higher level of scrutiny was established and improvements in resident care were monitored over a year, to ensure that a more professional culture was developing.

---

[3] Not a real place name.

Several long-standing night care workers left shortly after this intervention, and new employees were offered induction training by the home manager and the nurse specialist with a view to establishing high standards of care from the outset.

In some abuse cases concerns are not fully resolved but may nevertheless result in learning for the home that is useful. For example, post discharge a relative complained to the management of his mother's (ex) care home that when she was there she had been subjected to racial harassment. As the incident(s) occurred in the past the investigation could neither prove nor disprove the allegations. It did however leave staff unhappy at the unresolved implication that they were racist. A review was held including several debriefing meetings to discuss issues of cultural competency and to hear from staff from ethnic minorities about their experience of working in the service and of handling racism on a day-to-day basis from relatives as well as occasionally from colleagues. These debriefings acted as an intermediate response to the unresolved situation and helped to embed a culture of awareness about racism and what to do to address it.

In very serious cases, or where interagency working has failed, the local authority may undertake a *serious case review*, a formal investigation of how the case was handled, what actions were recommended, and how these were implemented. The purpose of the serious case review is to revisit an investigation that may have been unsatisfactory or where there is family or public disquiet about the outcome of the case. For example, following a case where a resident accidentally choked to death, the serious case review led to 'improvement plans' being drawn up across all the agencies concerned (Association of Directors of Adult Social Services, 2005; Brown, 2009; Manthorpe and Martineau, 2009). At the very top end of the scale of inquiry is the public inquiry. A prominent example is that into the death of David (Rocky) Bennett (Norfolk, Suffolk, and Cambridgeshire Strategic Health Authority, 2003) during an episode of control and restraint. This inquiry led to national recommendations about the use of physical restraint and triggered a major programme of work in the National Health Service (NHS) about racism in mental health services.

As discussed above, abuse is a multidimensional issue; different patterns of abuse each require a different set of responses and engagement with different professional networks and regulatory frameworks. The Safeguarding response also varies, to some degree, according to the nature and severity of the abuse involved. Its main aims are to understand the individual case but also to learn from the incident for the benefit of other vulnerable people in the future and to disseminate that learning. Table 10.1 shows how the outcomes can be conceptualized according to the perspectives of those involved.

An independent safeguarding system

The main reasons for having an external and formal Safeguarding system is to ensure that diagnosis of where the problem lies is thorough (in the NHS, inquiries use an approach called 'root cause analysis'); it is also an acknowledgement that analysis is often a complex time-consuming process requiring input from many generic and specialist agencies. For example, social services commissioners may review the

Table 10.1 Outcomes at different levels

For the victim	Immediate safety
	Long-term protection
	Redress
	Support for recovery
For the perpetrator	Criminal justice system
	Employment law/disciplinary
	Barring from workforce
	Other enforcement, for example injunction
	Extra help or enhanced care package if family member
	Extra help, training, or supervision if staff person
For the service	Improved practice
	Increased funding
	Increased professional advice and consultation
	Scrutiny or regulatory action
	Regulatory enforcement
	Closure
For the commissioning network	Changes to contract
	Change of funding
	Re-provision
	Change to interagency support
For national policy or legislative agenda	Serious case review, SUI, or public inquiry
	Acknowledgement of gaps in powers or duties

Source: Adapted from Brown, H. (2009). The process and function of serious case review. *Journal of Adult Protection, 11*, 38–50. Printed here with permission from Piers Professional.

specifications, contract, and pricing of a service at the same time as the police prosecute individual offenders or an agency that has breached health and safety legislation.

Another important consideration is that, without independent external review, it can be difficult to establish lines of responsibility and where failures may occur in investigating an allegation of abuse lie. For example, an individual constable may not have followed up a complaint with a view to investigating the theft of an older person's jewellery from a residential home. But this might have been an express instruction from his superior officer who, in turn, may be neglecting her responsibilities to attend the Safeguarding Adults Board on behalf of the police service.

Another example relates to the manager of a care home where there are inadequate staffing levels. The manager requests additional staff from head office but is given no further resources, indeed staff are removed and sent to another service managed by the same organization. Who is then responsible for ensuring that adequate care is provided to residents? If abuse occurs during that day's shift, is it the chief executive of the organization who should be held to account, the manager of the care home, or an overstretched staff member working an extra shift who failed to attend to a resident in need? There is a risk in these circumstances that senior staff avoid being held to account for abuses caused by lack of resources and front-line care staff are 'scapegoated' instead. Serious case reviews (see Brown, 2009) often uncover situations in which the least powerful individuals, such as agency workers or low paid care staff, have been held responsible for abuses inside very powerful and profitable organizations who have failed to resource the service adequately and have put profits before meeting the needs of residents. Locating responsibility for abuse at the feet of the least powerful members of the staff team is not only failing to analyse the causes of abuse adequately, but also reduces what is often a complex situation to the actions of a single individual. Even if this individual is, in part responsible, removing them and replacing them with a new person fails to coherently address the systemic causes of abuse leaving vulnerable residents at (more or less) the same level of risk as they were in before the abusive incident.

Conclusion

This chapter has explored how abusive or neglectful practice can develop—often unnoticed and unchallenged—inside care home settings. It can happen insidiously with acceptable standards of good practice gradually slipping from view. Most caregivers, whether paid or unpaid, do not choose to harm those they are looking after; they set out to do a good job but find themselves in situations beyond their limits or in which they feel pressured to react rather than responding thoughtfully and with care. This risk is deepened in situations where a care home's culture colludes with poor practice, does not offer training or leadership to staff, and expects staff to work in challenging situations without acknowledging how difficult their job is or appreciating their efforts. Preventing and responding to abuse requires clarity about what good practice is so that when abuses occur they can be identified, challenged, and addressed. Care home managers need a systemic understanding of how abusive practices may have developed or been allowed to continue. Reporting any abuse through the Safeguarding system is a third strand. This demonstrates a willingness to put things right and the chance to explore the root causes of the problem. Do the causes lie in the care home regime, in routine care practices, and/or is a rogue member of staff to blame? How far are inadequate resources responsible? Are there lessons about how residents are admitted to the home or the way staff are recruited and inducted? As this chapter shows, there is usually a complex interaction between these factors. Getting the 'diagnosis' wrong means that vulnerable people remain in high risk situations and individual staff members are erroneously held responsible for whole system deficits without lessons being learned.

However robust a Safeguarding system is, it is reactive; emphasis must be on preventing abuse by improving standards of practice. This requires honest dialogue between managers and care staff about the difficulties they experience and a realistic acknowledgement of the inevitable challenges of working with people with complex needs, especially dementia. Good leadership and robust training can contribute much to developing a positive care home culture and to helping staff find their work rewarding. Rather than an optional extra or unnecessary imposition, safeguarding needs to be viewed as an integral part of any care home's commitment to providing good care and reducing the risks of abuse or neglect to vulnerable older people.

References

Association of Directors of Adult Social Services (2005). *Safeguarding Adults: A National Framework of Standards for Good Practice and Outcomes in Adult Protection Work.* London: Association of Directors of Adult Social Services.

Beach, S., Schultz, R., Williamson, G., Miller, L., Weiner, M., & Lance, C. (2005). Risk factors for potentially harmful informal caregiver behavior. *Journal of the American Geriatric Society, 53*, 255–261.

Bentovim, A. & Williams, B. (1998). Children and adolescents: victims who become perpetrators. *Advances in Psychiatric Treatment, 4*, 101–107.

Brown, H. & Stein, J. (1998). Implementing adult protection policies in Kent and East Sussex. *Journal of Social Policy, 27*(3), 371–396.

Brown, H, (2009). The process and function of serious case review. *Journal of Adult Protection, 11*, 38–50.

Brown, H. & Seden, J. (2003). *Managing to protect.* In: J. Seden & J. Reynolds (Eds.), *Managing Care in Practice.* (pp. 219–248). Milton Keynes: Routledge and the Open University.

Cambridge, P. & Carnaby, S. (2000). *Making it Personal: Providing Intimate and Personal Care for People with Learning Disabilities.* Brighton: Pavilion Publishing.

Cambridge, P., Beadle-Brown, J., Milne, A., Mansell, J., & Whelton, B. (2006). *Exploring the Incidence, Risk factors, Nature and Monitoring of Adult Protection Alerts.* Canterbury: Tizard Centre, University of Kent.

Commission for Health Improvement (2003). *Investigation into Matters Arising from Care on Rowan Ward, Manchester Mental Health and Social Care Trust.* London: Stationery Office.

Department of Health (2000). *No Secrets: Guidance on Developing and Implementing Multi-agency Policies and Procedures to Protect Vulnerable Adults from Abuse.* London: HMSO.

Department of Health (2007). *Putting People First: A Shared Vision and Commitment to the Transformation of Adult Social Care.* Ministerial Concordat issued 10 December 2007.

Department of Health (2008a). *Transforming Social Care.* Local Authority Circular 9337. Available at: http://www.dh.gov.uk/en/Publicationsandstatistics/Lettersandcirculars/LocalAuthorityCirculars/DH_081934 (accessed 15 February 2011)

Department of Health (2008b). *Safeguarding Adults: A Consultation on the Review of the 'No Secrets' Guidance.* London: Department of Health.

Law Commission (2008). *Adult Social Care: Scoping Report.* London: Law Commission.

Lee-Treweek, G. (1994). Bedroom abuse: the hidden work in a nursing home. *Generations Review, 4*, 2–4.

Kalaga, H. & Kingston, P. (2007). *A Review of Literature on Effective Interventions that Prevent and Respond to Harm Against Adults.* Edinburgh: Scottish Government Social Research.

Keywood, K. (2010). Vulnerable adults, mental capacity and social care refusal. *Medical Law Review, 18*(1), 103–110.

Mansell, J., Beadle-Brown, J., Cambridge, P., Milne, A., & Whelton, B. (2009). Adult protection: incidence of referrals, nature and risk factors in English local authorities, *Journal of Social work, 9*(1), 23–38.

Manthorpe, J. & Martineau, S. (2009). *Serious Case Reviews in Adult Safeguarding*. London: King's College Social Care Workforce Research Unit.

Menzies-Lyth, I. (1959). The functions of social systems as a defence against anxiety: a report on a study of the nursing service of a general hospital. *Human Relations 13*, 95–121; reprinted in *Containing Anxiety in Institutions: Selected Essays, Vol. 1*. Free Association Books, 1988, pp. 43–88.

National Center of Elder Abuse (2005). *Nursing Home Abuse: Risk Prevention Profile and Checklist*. Washington, DC: National Center of Elder Abuse.

Office of the Public Guardian (2008). *Office of the Public Guardian and Local Authorities: A protocol for working together to safeguard vulnerable adults*. London: Office of the Public Guardian.

Poinasamy, K. & Fooks, L. (2009). Who Cares? *How Best to Protect UK Care Workers Employed through Agencies and Gangmasters from Exploitation*. Oxford: Oxfam.

Smith, H. & Brown, H. (1992). Inside out: a psychodynamic approach to normalisation. In: H. Brown & H. Smith (Eds.), *Normalisation: A Reader for the Nineties* (pp. 84–99). London: Tavistock/Routledge.

Wardaugh, J. & Wilding, P. (1993). Towards an explanation of the corruption of care. *Critical Social Policy, 37*, 4–31.

Chapter 11

Long-term care: an international perspective

Ricardo Rodrigues and Frédérique Hoffmann

Abstract

This chapter presents a comparative overview of the heterogeneous picture of institutional care across Europe. As the concept of 'ageing in place' has become central to care policies in Europe, only a minority of older people reside in care homes. Residents are increasingly older, not only due to population ageing, but also because the development of community-based care has delayed the need for admission. Residents are further characterized not only by the prevalence of dementia, but also by the over-representation of women as they are at higher risk of institutionalization for socio-economic reasons. A number of recent policy developments impact on care home developments in Europe. These include the introduction of market-based mechanisms to enhance choice and efficiency of care services; the drive to improve quality of care in care homes; and the blurring of the boundary between institutional care and 'alternatives' such as housing with care provided in the community.

Introduction

Long-term care for dependent older people finds itself at the centre of a process of welfare change across Europe and North America. For some countries, this means taking the first step towards setting up long-term care as a set of separate social programmes, even going as far as recognizing it as a new social risk or a 'fifth pillar' of their social protection systems. For others, the modernization process means introducing profound reforms to the way long-term care has been organized and paid for, for example, opening the provision of care to private sector providers and introducing market-like arrangements. Yet for some countries in Europe, long-term care still remains relatively undifferentiated from general social assistance and is treated as a core dimension of public welfare provision.

Set against this background of change, this chapter seeks to provide an overview of facts, figures, and policy trends in long-term care, focusing mainly on Europe. By way of providing context, the chapter begins by outlining the balance of care between institutional-based and community-based services before profiling the characteristics and health profiles of care home populations. It concludes with an overview of some of the key issues that dominate the current debate about the nature, organization, and funding of long-term care in Europe.

Providing an overview of long-term care is a complex task; this is due to the diversity of models and range of settings, the differences between welfare and insurance systems, the history of provider patterns, eligibility thresholds for admission to a care home, and cultural traditions. This diversity is compounded by policy changes that have blurred the distinctions between institutional care and community-based care, for example housing with extra care. A primary challenge in comparing trends and profiles relates to differences between how states define long-term care or institutional care as well as how and what they collect in terms of data. As it is beyond the remit of this chapter to conduct secondary analysis of primary data, the authors have been obliged to rely on what is currently collected and collated by (mainly) government departments in each country and also regional reports such as those produced by the European Union (EU). It is additionally noteworthy that as it is a relatively young subject (Marin et al., 2009), systems for collecting, analysing, and publishing data on long-term care are still in development, even in countries with more sophisticated long-term care systems.

In the context of this chapter, long-term care refers to care that is provided to frail or dependent older people who reside permanently in institutional settings (Organisation for Economic Cooperation and Development (OECD), 2005). It includes nursing homes where professional nursing care is provided; residential/retirement/older people's homes where help with Instrumental Activities of Daily Living (IADL) is provided; and facilities that combine help with IADL with a greater degree of independence and a home-like environment, that is, supported housing, housing with extra care, and/or assisted living. Although the majority of older people living in long-term care are very frail and dependent, in some countries people may be admitted for 'social reasons' such as isolation, living in extreme poverty. In Portugal for example, which only recently implemented a network of long-term care services, around one in four users cited 'isolation' or 'family conflicts' as the main reason for being admitted to a care home (Nogueira, 2009: 23).

The authors begin by reviewing the balance of care between care homes and community-based care before moving onto profiling the primary characteristics of users of long-term care, with a particular focus on age, gender, and functional limitations. They conclude by offering an overview of some of the key issues that dominate the current debate around long-term care in the developed world. These include: the introduction or enhancement of user choice mechanisms and improvements in the quality of care, especially for people with dementia.

Care at home versus care homes

The policy discourse regarding long-term care is predicated on the assumption that dependent older people wish to remain in their own homes for as long as possible.

A recent Eurobarometer survey (2007) suggests that there is widespread support for encouraging 'ageing in place' across most EU Member States (OECD, 2005). This model relies heavily on the availability and willingness of family carers to provide informal (or unpaid) care and although some countries, for example the United Kingdom, offer limited welfare benefits to family carers of working age, this in no way compensates for lost earnings. The recent introduction of personal budgets (and/or self-directed support) or cash-for-care benefits in a number of European countries such as the United Kingdom, the Netherlands, the Czech Republic, Austria, and Germany,[1] is an additional driver to facilitating the development of community-based services to help older people remain at home for longer (OECD, 2005; Ungerson and Yeandle, 2007). The positive emphasis on ageing in place is also influenced by a negative image of institutional care. Although cases of abuse and neglect have occasionally hit the headlines, examples of poor quality care are relatively commonplace; these have contributed to the poor public image of institutional care and to the almost universal view that care at home is better than care in a care home (Leichsenring, 2004). In reality however, how much has the 'balance of care' changed in the past decade across Europe?

The figures presented in Table 11.1 reflect the proportion of the population aged 65 years and older (i.e. the older population) that received care at home versus in institutional settings between the mid 1990s and 2004/2007 (Huber et al., 2009).

As can be seen, for most countries, the proportion of older people in institutional care today is approximately the same as it was in the mid-1990s. It remains confined to a minority of the older population; the unweighted average across the EU countries in Table 11.1 suggests that it applies to only about 3.3%. It is noteworthy that the proportion has remained almost the same despite the total number of older people in the European population increasing substantially as has the number of those admitted to a care home in absolute terms. For example, an additional 16,000 older people in Austria and 182,000 in Germany were admitted during the last decade. In fact, as identified by the OECD (2005), age-specific rates of nursing home admission may actually be decreasing once the effect of population ageing is taken into account.

Nevertheless, within this overarching trend, there are significant differences between individual countries. Sweden, Norway, Ireland, England, Denmark, and Iceland have witnessed a reduction in the absolute number of people living in care homes, albeit starting from relatively high figures in the mid-1990s. These countries represent those where community-based care policies and an emphasis on independence were most vigorously pursued. In Denmark for example, the building of new care homes was actually outlawed (Leichsenring, 2004). In the United Kingdom and Sweden, reducing the number of care home users was part of a shift towards targeting intensive care services on the relatively small number of elderly people with severe and/or intensive care needs. This trend was accompanied, in the case of the United Kingdom at least, by a reduction in the number of private providers in the care home market, driven by a combination of rising labour costs and a reduction in publically funded long-term

---

[1] In Austria and Germany, beneficiaries of 'the long-term care allowances' can use the benefits to pay for formal (services) as well as informal carers to help older people remain at home.

Table 11.1 Comparison of the 'balance of care': mid-1990s vs. most recent date, by country

Country	Mid-1990s		Year	Most recent date	
	Home care (%)	Institutions (%)		Home care (%)	Institutions (%)
Austria*	13.2	2.8	2006	14.4	3.3
Czech Republic[†]	8.0	3.4	2006	7.2	3.5
Denmark	20.0	4.1	2007	25.1	4.8
Estonia	1.5	1.2	2005	1.0	1.6
Finland	15.6	5.1	2005	16.6	5.5
France*	2.5	2.4	2007	4.9	3.1
Germany	7.3	3.3	2006	6.7	3.8
Hungary*,[†]	2.0	1.8	2005	1.9	2.2
Iceland	19.2	11.6	2005	21.1	9.3
Ireland	5.6	4.4	2004	6.5	3.6
Italy	1.8	2.2	2004	2.8	2.0
Latvia[†]	0.3	1.4	2007	1.9	1.5
Lithuania	0.8	0.7	2007	0.6	0.8
Luxembourg			2006	5.9	4.3
Israel	14.0	4.5	2004	16.9	4.6
The Netherlands			2006	21.1	6.5
Russian Federation[†,‡]		0.6	2001	3.9	0.7
Norway	18.2	5.7	2007	19.3	5.3
Poland*		0.5	2006	0.0	0.7
Portugal[†]			2007	3.9	3.4
Slovak Republic*,[†]		1.9	2005	2.3	1.7
Slovenia[†]	8.5	4.0	2007	9.0	4.0
Spain[†]	1.1	2.8	2006	4.2	4.1
Sweden	12.0	8.4	2007	9.7	6.0
Switzerland			2006	12.4	6.6
United Kingdom (England)	14.2	3.9	2006	12.6	3.5
Ukraine[†,‡]		3.1	2000	1.7	1.5

*The age threshold is the 60 years and older.
[†]May include those younger than 65 (Hungary only for institutional care).
[‡]The age threshold is the 55 years and older.
Source: Adapted from Huber et al. (2009). Facts and Figures on Long-term Care-Europe and North America.
  Vienna: European Centre for Social Welfare Policy and Research, p.72.

care fees (Netten et al., 2005). A blurring of the boundaries between what constitutes a 'care home' and what is termed 'assisted living', 'supported housing', or 'housing with extra care' complicates the picture further as these facilities are included in the definition of institutional care in some countries and not others despite the resident profile often being similar (Huber et al., 2009).

In Southern European countries on the other hand, the increase in the number of users of institutional care reflects the low overall availability of community care services, and a policy context in which 'policy makers strive, first of all, for a quantitative increase' (Leichsenring, 2004: 42). With the introduction of its long-term care social insurance system, Germany also saw an increase in the number of users of institutional care. This arose partially as a supply-side response to the introduction of a demand-driven system (i.e. entitlement to benefits follows the needs assessment regardless of income). The amount older people were entitled to receive to pay for institutional care was much higher than payments for community-based care, particularly for those assessed as being in the 'lower levels of need' category (Rothgang and Igl, 2007).

Finally, in several Eastern European countries institutional care remains an important part of care services for older people. This is partly due to the transition away from the 'Semashko model', which placed an emphasis on inpatient and specialist healthcare at the expense of health promotion, disease prevention, and primary care (Zoidze et al., 2007). Hospitals were key providers of 'social care' for the elderly during Soviet times. Since the early 1990s many have been 'converted' into nursing homes, although such institutions often remain underfunded and ill-equipped with poorly trained staff. At the same time, many of the financial and social supports which the elderly were entitled to (subsidies for food, housing, and transportation) have been eliminated or reduced in size and scope, or have deteriorated in quality. To some degree, this had the effect of reinforcing dependency on institutional care (Tobis, 2000). Moreover, scarcity of funding has meant that the development of home care services has been slow in some countries.

Care home residents' profile

The data displayed in Table 11.2 support the proposition that welfare policies have sought to support older people with dependency needs in their own homes, and target institutional care on the very elderly, dependent, and/or frail. Although overall, care home residents are likely to be aged over 80 years, this is less prominently the case in those countries that have only recently developed long-term care systems, such as Spain and countries in Eastern Europe. The profile of care home residents is not only younger in these countries but they also tend to be less dependent; as noted above, triggers for admission may sometimes be 'social'. These are also the countries where community-based services, especially home care, are less available, for example in Hungary or Poland.

Countries for which it is possible to construct a time-series continuum confirm that the care home population itself is ageing; in other words, ever-older cohorts of elderly people are admitted to long-term care (see Table 11.3). This suggests that community-based care services are allowing a greater number of frail older people to remain in

Table 11.2 Age distribution of care home residents by country

Country	Year	Users aged 65–79 in percentage of that same age group	Users aged 80 and older in percentage of that same age group	Users aged 80 and older in percentage of total old-age users
Denmark	2007	1.6	13.5	76.1
Estonia	2005	1.0	4.2	50.4
Finland*	2006	1.3	10.7	88.2
France†	2004	1.1	5.7	77.0
Germany	2006	1.2	12.2	74.8
Hungary	2005	1.6	6.4	41.8
Iceland	2006	3.2	26.1	74.3
Ireland	2006	1.6	11.5	69.5
Italy*	2004	0.5	3.7	85.6
Lithuania	2007	0.4	2.1	53.2
Luxembourg	2006	1.3	14.3	76.0
Israel	1999	1.6	15.0	72.0
The Netherlands	2006	2.1	19.8	76.3
Norway	2007	1.8	14.1	81.7
Poland*	2006	0.4	1.2	58.1
Slovenia	2007	1.3	12.1	63.8
Spain‡	2006	1.7	12.2	68.0
Sweden	2005	1.9	16.7	81.7
Switzerland	2005	1.8	18.8	79.9
United Kingdom (England)*	2006	0.6	4.2	87.7

*Age groups are 65–74 and 75 and older.
†Age groups are 60–74 and 75 and older.
‡Age groups are 65–80 and 81 and older.
Source: Adapted from Huber et al. (2009). Facts and Figures on Long-term Care-Europe and North America. Vienna: European Centre for Social Welfare Policy and Research, p.95.

their own homes for a longer period. Moreover, initiatives such as aids and adaptations, for example adapted showers and purpose-built accessible housing, are having a direct impact on the need for care home admission (OECD, 2005). For example, in the Netherlands approximately one-third of those aged over 55 years live in 'stairless' accommodation (Van Campen, 2008: 55). This trend can also be seen as supporting existing evidence about the compression of morbidity in later life, that is, many older people enjoy relatively good health until they are aged 75 years or older and then develop a range of conditions over a relatively short period of time. These combined factors contribute to delaying or even preventing institutionalization of many older people, a remarkable achievement in the context of an ageing population.

Table 11.3 Age profile of long-term care residents by country (percentages of the total number of residents)

Country	Year				
Ireland		1997	2000	2005	2007
<65		5.1	5.4	5.6	7.8
65–74		14.7	14.3	13	12
75–84		42.5	42.4	39.7	36.4
85+		37.7	38.0	41.5	43.9
The Netherlands*	1985	1990	1995	2000	2005
<65	0.9	0.5	0.4	0.2	0.5
65–74	10.2	7.4	6.5	5.5	5.9
75–84	48.8	44.3	39.9	36.5	36.5
85+	40.1	47.7	53.2	57.8	57.1
Sweden			1998	2004	2007
65–74			9.2	8.3	8.3
75–79			14.3	12.2	11.4
80–84			23.5	23.8	22.1
85+			53.0	55.7	58.1
Iceland		1993	1995	2000	2005	2006
<65		4.4	3.8	2.3	2.3	2.3
65–74		12.6	11.2	11.6	12.7	9.1
75–84		38.6	39.3	42.3	38.2	37.4
85+		44.3	45.7	43.7	46.8	51.3

*Only nursing homes are included.
Source: Department of Health and Children, Annual Survey of Long-stay Units; Statistics Canada, Residential Care Facilities Survey; Statistics Iceland; National Board of Health and Welfare (Sweden); CBS StatLine.

In terms of gender, women form the majority of residents. This is partly explained by the fact that they tend to live longer than men and in some countries, including Poland, Lithuania, Estonia, and the Slovak Republic, the proportion of older women in care homes is a direct reflection of the demographic profile of that country. In other countries, particularly in Western Europe, the proportion is greater than would be expected (see the odds ratio[2] in Table 11.4). This is likely to be a reflection, not of

[2] The odds ratio provides a measure of one event (institutionalization) taking place in one group (women) versus another group (men). Values of the odds ratio significantly below 1.0 mean that women are disproportionately represented in the profile of institutional care populations compared with their prevalence in the older population. Values of the odds ratio equal to 1 reflect a gender distribution of care home users that mirrors that of the older population.

Table 11.4 Gender distribution of long-term care residents by country

Country	Year	Percentage of older women	Odds ratio*
Estonia	2005	68.7	0.92
Finland	2006	74.8	0.49
France	2003	77.0	0.40
Germany	2006	79.7	0.35
Hungary	2005	68.6	0.72
Iceland	2006	64.2	0.65
Ireland	2006	68.5	0.57
Italy	2004	76.5	0.43
Israel	1999	72.0	0.51
Lithuania	2007	70.0	0.82
Luxembourg	2006	78.9	0.37
The Netherlands	2006	75.4	0.42
Poland	2006	60.6	1.00
Slovak Republic	2005	67.7	0.80
Slovenia	2007	77.4	0.45
Spain	2006	69.6	0.58
Sweden	2007	70.4	0.53
Switzerland	2005	75.4	0.44

*Values of the odds ratio significantly below 1 mean that women are disproportionately represented in the profile of institutional care population compared with their prevalence in the older population. Values of the odds ratio equal to 1.0 reflect a gender distribution of care home users that mirrors that of the older population.
Source: Adapted from Huber et al. (2009). Facts and Figures on Long-term Care-Europe and North America. Vienna: European Centre for Social Welfare Policy and Research, p.92.

dependency or health status per se, but of socio-economic situation. For example, a growing number of older women live alone, especially in the oldest old age groups, placing them at enhanced risk of care home admission. The most common living arrangement for older men is the couple-only household. This means that older men tend to have wives who provide care when they become ill, protecting them from being admitted to residential care. This is not the case for their female widowed counterparts (Huber et al., 2009: 91). Additionally, older women tend to have fewer financial resources to draw on to facilitate alternative choices to care home admission, for example private housing with care (Marin and Zolyomi, 2010).

In terms of other characteristics of care home users, evidence suggests that dementia is an overarching trigger for admission across Europe (Alzheimer Europe, 2006). As is known, the prevalence of dementia is strongly correlated to the age profile of a population. Therefore, those countries with a relatively large number of very old people have a higher incidence of dementia and a greater number of care home admissions of people with the condition. It is axiomatic that the proportion of people in care homes with dementia is high. It ranges from 70% to 80% in Sweden (SALAR, 2009), through 62% in the United Kingdom (Matthews and Dening, 2002), to around 42% in Finland (THL, 2009). Data on dementia prevalence in Eastern European countries are very limited.

The prevalence of dementia among care home residents is influencing the nature of long-term care in a number of Western European countries. The Netherlands and Sweden for example, have established a number of small institutional units for people with dementia. These are considered best suited to deliver higher quality specialist care and emphasize the need to offer supervision to residents alongside managing instrumental activities of daily living (IADL) (Boer, 2006). There have also been a number of initiatives that encourage people with dementia to remain for a longer period in the community. For example, recent reforms in the German long-term care insurance system entitle those diagnosed with dementia to receive payments to purchase community-based services with the aim of delaying, or even preventing, care home admission (BMG, 2009).

The changing picture of long-term care

Given the heterogeneous nature of populations across Europe and the different economies and cultures it can hardly be surprising that the profiles of care home populations differ significantly as do the priorities of each welfare state. In Western Europe key foci include the enhancement of choice and quality and the development of specialist care for people with long-term conditions (most notably dementia). In Eastern European contexts where public care for older people is relatively underdeveloped, governments are more concerned with establishing an infrastructure of care services for frail older people, including care home provision (Glendinning, 2009). Nevertheless, there are a number of overarching policy developments that can be distilled which are likely to shape the future profile and nature of long-term care across Europe.

Maintaining dependent and frail older people at home for longer periods—where the majority would rather be—is one such policy. This has required investment in domiciliary and other community-based care services and has, in many Western countries at least, been very effective at reducing the number of older people who would otherwise need admission to a care home. One of the consequences of this policy drive is that the population who do live in a care home, particularly those who require public funding, are very frail indeed; many have dementia and most have multiple and complex needs.

Another facet of recent policy development has been the blurring of boundaries between institutional care and care provided in the community, often through housing-related initiatives such as housing with extra care. These are popular 'alternatives' to a care homes for most elderly people as they tend to be able to offer choice, independence, and privacy. Although there have been much recent investment in these models of care in many European countries, this is now slowing down as a result of the recession. The fact that it is not a cheap alternative is also relevant.

A push to improve the quality of care offered in care homes and enhance the status of care home residents has been a prominent focus of recent care-related policy. In addition to establishing 'care standards' around issues such as levels of cleanliness, medicines safety, and access for residents' relatives, environmental improvements such as all residents having their own bedrooms have become increasingly common. In Sweden and Norway for example, this is now the rule rather than the exception (Marin et al., 2009). Even where a single room cannot be guaranteed, it has been articulated in policy statements or 'care charters' such as the German Charter of Rights for People in Need of Long-term Care and Assistance (DZA, 2005: Article 3). It is now widely recognized that the quality of care offered in a home profoundly impacts on the residents' quality of life and well-being and that this is linked not only to the issues we have identified but also to staff training and retention, the quality of managerial leadership in the home, and the provision of relationship-centred care where quality of life for residents, relatives, and staff is valued (Nolan et al., 2008).

The development of quasi-markets in welfare provision is relatively well established in Western Europe. The argument that the market can deliver increased efficiency, value for money, and choice is a prominent aspect of market-related rhetoric. Although specific arrangements vary between states, the opening up of the 'care home market' to independent providers is a common feature of most European countries. This is the case even when, historically, care homes have been publically funded and provided, for example in Sweden. Other ways in which the market has been introduced into welfare regimes includes the separation of the roles of provider (supplier)—which is open to the market—and commissioner (purchaser) which is the role retained by public authorities. The shift towards increased user choice and empowerment has recently taken a step further. Mechanisms that allow users to become direct purchasers of their own services—via a range of schemes including vouchers, cash benefits, and/or personal budgets—are now becoming established in a number of countries, including the United Kingdom, the Netherlands, and the Czech Republic.

Introduction of the market into the care home sector in the 1990s has strongly influenced the balance of 'who provides' care with an increasing proportion of the overall being provided by private or for-profit homes in many countries (Glendinning, 2009: 11) (see Table 11.5). Differences between countries can be explained, to a considerable degree, by the extent of public provision that was established before the quasi-market was introduced. In some countries, such as Spain, private providers make up the majority as there are a very limited number of care homes provided by public agencies. Other countries, such as Austria and Germany, have a more diverse range of providers as a consequence of having a well-established pool of care homes run by large not-for-profit organizations. In Sweden, the care home sector has historically been dominated by public providers. In order to foster greater diversity, in particular private development, separation of the 'assessment' and 'purchaser' functions within municipal departments was introduced. Competitive tendering for the contracting of services, such as the provision of care homes in a given area or for a specific group of users, was also established. This process has been criticized for replacing one monopoly (public) for another (public or private), as the provider that is selected through the tendering process is the sole provider of services in a given area.

Table 11.5 Distribution of providers of long-term care by country

Country	Year	Public	Private	
			Non-profit	For-profit
Austria	2007	55%	24%	21%
Belgium	2006	33%	33%	35%
Czech Republic	2007	91%	9%	
Finland	2007	90%	10%	
France	2007	54%	28%	17%
Germany	2006	7%	55%	38%
Iceland*	2006	74%	20%	7%
Lithuania*	2007	62%	38%	
Spain	2005	24%	76%	
Sweden	2008	85%	15%	
Switzerland*	2006	32%	68%	
United Kingdom†	2001	16%	54%	19%

*Number of institutions.
†Figures refer to England and do not add up to 100% as 'dual registered' places are not included.
Source: Statistisches Bundesamt; Leichsenring, K. (2009a); Leichsenring, K. (2009b). Ministry of Labour and Social Affairs (Czech Republic); IMSERSO; DRESS, enquête auprès des établissements d'ébergement pour personnes âgées; INAMI-RIZIV; National Board of Health and Welfare (Sweden), THL (Finland); Department of Health (UK); Huber et al. (2008). Statistics Iceland; Statistics Lithuania; Bundesamt für Statistik (Switzerland).

The establishment of quasi-markets in care has also resulted in an increase in the regulatory mechanisms used to monitor the purchasing systems deployed to buy care home services and the efficiency and quality of care home provision itself (Huber et al., 2008). This has called for public authorities to develop new competencies in tendering, purchasing, and cost accounting, for example in Sweden. The introduction of market-based mechanisms also prompted new kinds of relationships to develop between regulators and providers. In Germany, up until the introduction of market mechanisms, not-for-profit providers had a close-knit relationship with local authorities, based on trust and a common setting of objectives. This was replaced by the establishment of a purchaser/provider split, one based on ensuring that the care home provided both quality and value for money for the local authority (Leichsenring, 2009a). The market also encouraged providers to seek independent evidence of the quality of their services, for example via certification processes (Nies et al., 2010).

Although an increase in private provision is widespread, Sweden and England have witnessed a particularly notable concentration of care home provision in the private sector. This raises the question of whether the market has worked as a mechanism to increase diversity and offer greater choice of care home to older users. Moreover, the evaluation of the competitive tendering process in Sweden by the National Board of Health and Welfare revealed only negligible differences in price and quality between private and public providers (Trydegård, 2004). In light of growing budgetary pressures, cost minimization rather than quality has become the main driver of competition in many cases (Huber et al., 2008); commissioners have used their monopoly power to lower prices, thus pressuring providers to cut costs at the expense of quality (Kendall et al., 2003; Nies et al., 2010).

User choice, market competition, and a greater emphasis on regulation have contributed to an increased level of transparency about the nature and quality of care home provision. In the Netherlands for example, care homes have been 'ranked' according to quality standards or perceived quality by users—The Consumer Quality Index. In both the United Kingdom and Germany, the outcome of care home inspections by the regulatory agencies is publicly available. This is not a straightforward issue however. The care home sector is complex and fragmented and while regulation can go some way to improve standards as can mechanisms that enhance user choice, some 'quality systems' have been criticized as only assessing the superficial elements of care home provision such as the number of locked medicine cabinets or fire extinguishers. A lack of attention paid to the quality of therapeutic care and the social environment is a long-running criticism of regulatory systems.

Conclusions

Although long-term care is currently provided to only a minority of older people in Europe, it commands considerable resources and provides care to some of the most vulnerable and dependent members of our societies (Huber et al., 2009). For this reason alone it warrants coherent and focused attention.

The authors draw two main conclusions from this chapter. The first is that the picture of institutional care in Europe is a heterogeneous and uneven one. Although in the majority of European countries dependent older people are supported to remain at home, institutional care remains the backbone of formal care in a number of Eastern European countries. There is, however, increasing interest in the role of innovative developments that sit on the boundary between care homes and care at home. These may have a particularly important role in extending the capacity of older people to remain independent and to 'age in place'.

The second and most important conclusion is that long-term care sits at the intersection of economic, demographic, and policy change across Europe. Its users are increasingly elderly and frail as community-based care has delayed the need for admission and the prevalence of dementia is an overarching feature of all care home populations. This emerging profile raises the question of how to respond to these changing needs. For example, we must consider what is the best way to invest in new ways to provide quality care to older people with multiple and complex needs, such as the development of smaller residential units for people with dementia. Long-term care also has to rise to the challenge of meeting a burgeoning matrix of quality regulations. These arise, in part, from an increased focus on resident quality of life and the promotion of key principles such as autonomy, choice, privacy, and dignity. The provision of long-term care has also been opened up to market forces, which has demanded a redefinition of the role of public authorities and the establishment of a system of regulation and inspection.

This chapter has struggled to tell a coherent story about long-term care in Europe. It is a fragmented and diverse picture at the present time characterized by significant individual country differences and by an East/West distinction-based primarily on the extent of economic development. Although the trends identified in this conclusion form part of the background fabric of care home developments in Europe over the next 10 years, much remains unknown. The impact of global recession on welfare spending, the role of the emerging markets in Eastern Europe, and the funding challenges that an ageing population brings are all factors that will have a profound effect on future care home developments. The importance of having access to coherent data gathered across the whole of Europe, rather than only parts of it, cannot be overstated. Although we have made a start in mapping the nature of care homes and care home populations in this chapter, there is a long way to go before we can be confident that we can paint a full and accurate picture of long-term care in Europe.

References

Alzheimer Europe (2006). *Dementia in Europe Yearbook 2006*. Luxembourg: Alzheimer Europe.

Boer, de A.H. (Ed) (2006). *Report on the Elderly 2006—Changes in the Lives and Living Situation of Elderly Persons in the Netherlands*. The Hague: The Netherlands Institute for Social Research.

BMG (Bundesministerium für Gesundheit) (2009). *Long-term Care in the Health Care and Social Welfare System: Expectations and Demands from the Viewpoint of Policymakers*. Document from the German Federal Ministry of Health. Available at: http://www.bmg.bund.de/cln_151/SharedDocs/Downloads/EN/Long-term-care-insurance/Sued-Korea-2009, templateId=raw,property=publicationFile.pdf/Sued-Korea-2009.pdf (accessed in May 2010).

DZA (Deutsches Zentrum für Altersfragen) (2005). *Charter of Rights for People in Need of Long-term Care and Assistance*. Berlin: Deutsches Zentrum für Altersfragen.

Eurobarometer (2007). *Health and Long-term Care in the European Union*. Special Eurobarometer 283. Survey conducted by TNS Opinion & Social upon the request of the European Commission, Directorate General Communication, Public Opinion and Media Monitoring Available at: http://ec.europa.eu/public_opinion/archives/ebs/ebs_283_en.pdf (accessed 14 April 2011).

Glendinning, C. (2009). *Combining Choice, Quality and Equity in Social Services Provision, Synthesis Report Denmark*. Luxembourg: European Commission, DG Employment, Social Affairs and Equal Opportunities.

Huber, M., Maucher, M., & Sak, B. (2008). *Study on Social and Health Services of General Interest in the European Union: Final Synthesis Report*. Brussels: DG Employment, Social Affairs and Equal Opportunities.

Huber, M., Rodrigues, R., Hoffmann, F., Gasior, K., & Marin, B. (2009). *Facts and Figures on Long-term Care—Europe and North America*. Vienna: European Centre for Social Welfare Policy and Research.

Kendall, J., Knapp, M., Forder, J., Hardy, B., Matosevic, T., & Ware, P. (2003). *The State of Residential Care Supply in England: Lessons from PSSRU's Mixed Economy of Care (Commissioning and Performance) Research Programme.* LSE Health and Social Care Discussion Paper, 6. London: London School of Economics and Political Science.

Leichsenring, K. (2004). Providing integrated health and social care for older persons—an European overview. In: K. Leichsenring & A. Alaszewski (Eds.), *Providing Integrated Health and Social Care for Older Persons* (pp. 9–52). Aldershot: Ashgate.

Leichsenring, K. (2009a). *Contracting for Quality—Germany Country Profile.* European Social Network. Working Paper prepared for the European Social Network Policy & Practice Research Project on changing relationships between financer, provider and user of older people's services.

Leichsenring, K. (2009b). *Developing and Ensuring Quality in LTC in Austria.* Vienna: European Centre for Social Welfare Policy and Research (unpublished).

Marin, B., Leichsenring, K., Rodrigues, R., & Huber, M. (2009). *Who Cares? Care Coordination and Cooperation to Enhance Quality in Elderly Care in the European Union.* Vienna: European Centre for Social Welfare Policy and Research.

Marin, B. & Zolyomi, E. (Eds.) (2010). *Women's Work and Pensions: What is Good, What is Best? Designing Gender-sensitive Arrangements.* Aldershot: Ashgate.

Matthews, F.E. & Dening, T.R. (2002). Prevalence of dementia in institutional care. *Lancet,* *360*, 225–226.

Netten, A., Darton, R., Davey, V., et al. (2005). *Understanding Public Services and Markets.* London: Kings Fund Publishing.

Nies, H., Leichsenring, K., Van der Veen, R., et al. (2010). *Quality Management and Quality Assurance in Long-term Care—European Overview Paper.* Report prepared under the FP7 Project INTERLINKS. Utrecht/Vienna: Stichting Vilans, European Centre for Social Welfare Policy and Research.

Nogueira, J. (2009). *A dependência: o apoio informal, a rede de serviços e equipamentos e os cuidados continuados integrados* [Dependent people: informal care, social services and long-term care]. Lisbon: Ministério do Trabalho e da Solidariedade Social.

Nolan, M., Davies, S., Ryan, T., & Keady, J. (2008). Relationship-centred care and the 'Senses' framework. *Journal of Dementia Care, 16,* 26–28.

OECD (2005). *Long-term Care for Older People.* Paris: OECD.

Rothgang, H. & Igl, G. (2007). Long-term care in Germany. *The Japanese Journal of Social Security Policy, 6,* 54–84.

SALAR (Swedish Association of Local Authorities and Regions) (2009). *Developments in Elderly Policy in Sweden.* Stockholm: Swedish Association of Local Authorities and Regions.

THL (National Institute for Health and Welfare) (2009). *Statistical Yearbook on Social Welfare and Health Care 2009.* Helsinki: National Institute for Health and Welfare.

Tobis, D. (2000). *Moving from Residential Institutions to Community-based Social Services in Central and Eastern Europe and the Former Soviet Union.* Washington, DC: World Bank.

Trydegård, G. (2004). *Welfare Services for the Elderly in Sweden at the Beginning of the 21st Century—Still in Line with the Nordic Welfare State Model?* Presentation at the Conference 'Social Policy as if People Matter, A Cross-National Dialogue' at Adelphi University, Garden City, New York.

Ungerson, C. & Yeandle, S. (Eds.) (2007). *Cash-for-Care in Developed Welfare States.* Basingstoke: Palgrave Macmillan.

Van Campen, C. (Ed.) (2008). *Values on a Grey Scale—Elderly Policy Monitor 2008.* The Hague: The Netherlands Institute for Social Research.

Zoidze, A., Gotsadze G., & Cameron, S. (2007). An Overview of Health in Transition Countries. *International Hospital Federation Reference Book, 2006/2007*, 29–32.

Part 3

Mental health and care

Chapter 12

Meeting mental health needs

Tom Dening

Abstract

This chapter introduces the section of the book on mental health problems, setting out the context of the high level of mental disorders among care home residents, especially dementia and depression. Moving into a care home is a major step for any person to take and it is often the last address that he or she will have in his or her life. The circumstances of the move may well be traumatic, associated with bereavement or serious illness. However, some residents may show improvements after the move, probably due to better nutrition or the effects of company. The impact of moving into a home on depression appears to be complex and incompletely understood. The final part of this chapter discusses important issues around care homes and people with intellectual difficulties (ID). More people with ID are living in relatively advanced ages, though their life expectancy is still less than the general population. They are also at risk of dementia at a younger age. It is often difficult to ensure that older people with ID are cared for in care homes appropriate to their needs.

Introduction

This chapter introduces the section which lies at the heart of this book. The following chapters discuss the mental health problems most often seen in long-term care settings. It has two main aims: to introduce the chapters about mental health problems; and to discuss two important topics that might otherwise be overlooked—the impact of moving into a care home, and residential care for older people with ID.

From earlier chapters, we have gained some measure of the importance of mental health issues for care home residents, their family supporters, and care home staff. The regulatory and legal context also makes it clear how issues around mental health, dignity, and mental capacity are crucial in assessing the quality of care and quality of residents' lives. This leads, in the next part of the book, into consideration of how treatments and services can be effectively employed to support residents with mental health problems and their physical needs.

It is important to be aware of the high levels of physical and mental health problems in the care home population and how common multiple pathology is. For example, in one UK study of 16,000 residents, over half had dementia, stroke, or other neurode-generative disease, 78% had at least one form of mental impairment, 71% were incontinent, and 76% needed help with mobility or were immobile (Bowman et al., 2004). Overall, 27% were immobile, confused, and incontinent.

It is also clear that the care home population has become more frail and disabled over time. This probably reflects the intersection of a number of factors. Certainly, the availability of better community-based care is one factor; this has enabled many more disabled older people to remain in their own homes or to return home after hospital admission, rather than going into a care home. As the number of care homes has remained relatively static despite the increasing older population, the 'dependency threshold' for entering a home has also been raised, a trend probably also accelerated by the increasing costs of residential care.

Probably, the biggest single change in the last 20 years has been the steadily increasing proportion of people with dementia in residential care; it has been estimated that around two-thirds of care home residents have dementia, even if it has not been formally diagnosed (Matthews and Dening, 2002). Although it has taken some time for this fact to be acknowledged, there are now signs that dementia is being recognized as an important issue by the care home sector. It is evident, for example as discussed in this volume by John Killick and Lynda Martin (Chapter 4) and by Dorothy Runnicles (Chapter 5), that even people with advanced dementia in care homes can express their views about the kind of care they want much more clearly than was previously believed.

In considering the care of people with dementia in care homes, several issues are especially topical, and these are considered in detail in Chapter 13. There is a growing body of research looking at behavioural problems in care home residents and how some of these, such as aggressive behaviour, can be surprisingly persistent. There has been justified concern about the use of powerful drugs, especially antipsychotic drugs, to control disturbed behaviour, in particular the extent to which their use may be a substitute for proper person-centred care, as well as the serious side-effects (Banerjee, 2009). As a result, all guidance, including that from NICE (National Collaborating Centre for Mental Health, 2007) says that psychological and social approaches to management should be used first, but it is important that we consider what this means and what the evidence is for the efficacy of various interventions that may be employed. In any case, there is a huge need to train care staff to be more aware of dementia and the challenges that are inherent in caring for people with this condition. The recent training materials from SCIE (Social Care Institute for Excellence) (http://www.scie. org.uk/publications/dementia/index.asp) are especially welcome in this regard (and the important role of training is explored in Chapter 24). Graham Stokes assesses the evidence for psychological interventions in Chapter 16.

Chapter 14 discusses the importance of depression in care homes, how it can be easily overlooked, and what can be done to treat it and also to promote good mental health in all residents. Chapter 15 concerns a small but often neglected group of people, those with severe and enduring mental illnesses. Historically, many such individuals might have languished in old long-stay mental hospitals but newer cohorts will have received more of their care in the community, for example living in group homes. It is not entirely clear what is the best model for providing care for this group in old age. As the numbers are relatively small, it is difficult to do robust research on different models of care.

We have also included contributions on the roles of primary care and specialist services in supporting care homes (Chapter 17); diversity (Chapter 18); and physical health (Chapter 19). The section closes by discussing end-of-life care (Chapter 20), an area of growing interest and importance.

Moving into residential care

A big decision

The decision to move into a care home is one of the last major decisions a person will make for themselves or someone else will make for them. For most people it will be their last address, unless they happen to move to another home or, more rarely, move to another form of accommodation. What do we know about the factors influencing people's decision to move into a care home, and what do we know about the impact of making this move both on the older person and their families?

Most of the older people wish to remain in their own homes and to live as independently as possible until death. It is only fairly reluctantly that most people will accept, first, help provided in the community and, later, the need to be in full time residential or nursing care. Residential care is widely regarded as an option of last resort. The commonest causal triggers that prompt a move into a care home are one or more of the following: bereavement; concerns about health; poor or unsuitable housing; inadequate or unsatisfactory care or a breakdown in care arrangements at home; and/or other people's concerns and anxieties for their well-being, safety, and protection (Bowers et al., 2009). The 'other people' who may be concerned include relatives, friends, and health or social care personnel. There is a risk that their concerns and their wish for a 'safe' option may sometimes override the wishes of the older person. In some cases, for example if the older person has dementia, he or she may lack capacity to make a competent choice about his or her own care, in which case a 'best interests decision' can be made.

The move to a care home often follows some form of crisis, so there is relatively little time to plan the move or to make informed choices about which home the older person might prefer. The cause of the crisis may be the death of a spouse—or other long-term carer—or an episode of serious illness requiring hospital admission so, quite apart from the stress of giving up one's home, there will probably be other losses to contend with. And, once admitted to the care home, possible opportunities for moving back to one's own home often rapidly disappear, for example if the person's house or flat is sold to fund the residential care. If a move to a care home is necessary, then one of the primary needs older people and their families have is for information; some excellent guidance is available covering many of the practical and financial issues that need to be addressed (Alzheimer Scotland, 2007; Counsel and Care, 2009). Publically available information about quality of care, including care home standards, is also published by the Care Quality Commission (previously the Commission for Social Care Inspection) (see Chapter 7). It is difficult though, faced with a crisis and short timeline to make a decision—which may be driven by concerns such as freeing up a hospital bed—for the older person and/or their relatives to avail themselves of all available information.

The biggest single predictor of care home admission appears to be dementia. For example, Bharucha et al. (2004), in a US study, found that dementia increased the risk of admission to a nursing home fivefold. In the United Kingdom, Banerjee et al. (2003) found that having a co-resident carer at home had a strongly protective effect— the risk of being institutionalized was 20 times higher in people who did *not* have a carer living with them. This must be one of the most striking demonstrations of the importance of carers anywhere in the research literature. In people without dementia, perhaps unsurprisingly, medical ill health appears to be the second biggest influential factor (Bharucha et al., 2004).

Most of the evidence about moving into care from older people themselves is in the form of qualitative accounts; see for example the *My Home Life* programme (Owen and NCHRDF, 2006) and the Joseph Rowntree study of *Older People's Vision for Long-term Care* (Bowers et al., 2009). The former provides several personal testimonies that cover the span of life in a care home (a total of 25 older people), including the move into care, and the latter involved 84 older people in discussions and focus groups, presenting a synthesis of their findings but also several illustrative quotes from residents. For various reasons it may be easier to study families and carers of older people, though caution is needed in drawing inferences from this work about older people's perspectives. Davies and Nolan (2003, 2004, 2006) studied the experience of transition into residential care from the perspective of relatives, based on 37 interviews with 48 people who had assisted a close relative to move in. They distinguished three phases embedded in the process of transition: making the best of it; making the move; and making it better, referring to the times before, during, and after the move. The chapters in the first section of this book also contribute to this evidence base.

Several key points emerge from these findings. Better outcomes are more likely if older people are not put under undue pressure to make decisions about care homes; they need accurate and relevant information to inform their choice; and they should retain control over decision-making (although their families and other people close to them will also be involved) (Owen and NCHRDF, 2006). On arrival in the home, an older person will require support and understanding from staff. This will include taking account of his or her feelings of guilt, loss, sorrow, grief, and/or anger that may be associated with the change. The opportunity simply to talk to people may be the most important element in helping new residents to settle in satisfactorily (Andersson et al., 2007). Families have a major part to play in supporting this transition, as they occupy a role intermediate between the person and the care staff, and can act as a bridge or conduit between life inside and outside the care home (Kellett, 2007). And of course, relatives and carers will be undergoing their own transitions too, often with feelings that mirror those of the person entering care, so their needs have to be considered as well (Clarke and Bright, 2006; Milne et al., 2004).

Mental health impacts

Although dementia is a progressive and irreversible condition, evidence suggests that care home admission does not hasten health-related decline, at least in the short term. In fact, as a consequence of identifying and treating hitherto unknown medical conditions and good nutrition the overall health of some demented residents may improve. Buttar et al. (2003) found that, among residents with severe cognitive impairment, 14% showed improvements in the first 6 months following admission; apparently due to better and more regular diet, treatment of physical illnesses, and antidepressant treatment. McConnell et al. (2003) found different patterns of change over 12 months depending on the degree of cognitive impairment on admission—residents with mild cognitive impairment showed initial improvement, then slow decline, moderate impairment was associated with steady decline, and severe impairment was associated with initial improvement and then stability. This may indicate that there are subgroups among new residents who are at particular risk of increased morbidity and mortality.

Furthermore, while some people with dementia are physically frail, a significant number—who tend to be admitted as a consequence of behavioural problems such as aggression or wandering—are relatively robust. Magaziner et al. (2005) found that newly admitted nursing home residents with dementia were more physically fit and had *lower* rates of mortality than residents without dementia. Although other studies (e.g. Landi et al., 1998) have found an association between severe dementia and mortality, this probably results from limited use of medical services and medication. It may also reflect a 'palliative care approach' with less aggressive treatment of people with dementia (Burton et al., 2001). There are also some concerns about prescribing for older people entering care homes. For example, a Canadian study including 20,000 residents across Ontario (Bronskill et al., 2004), found that 17% of people were started on antipsychotics within 100 days of admission, and 24% within 1 year, not having received them in the year prior to admission. A prescription was more likely in the case of men and those with dementia. By contrast, Zuckerman et al. (2005), looking at inappropriate prescribing, found that 20% plus of residents were receiving potentially inappropriate medications prior to admission, and this percentage *increased* in residents without dementia but fell slightly in residents with dementia.

Identifying depression in care homes is important as it has a potent effect on well-being (Smallbrugge et al., 2006) and social engagement (Achterberg et al., 2003). In addition, high depression scores on admission are associated with increased mortality (Sutcliffe et al., 2007). Although high rates of depression have been reported, it is not clearly established that rates are higher in care homes than in other settings. The course of depression in homes is incompletely understood, but most studies suggest the symptoms tend to persist. For example, Sutcliffe et al. (2007) found that almost half the residents with depression at admission were still depressed after 9 months; Bruce et al. (2002) found that most of the episodes of major depression lasted more than 2 months; and Scocco et al. (2006) reported high levels of depressive symptoms on admission and these increased over a 6-month period, suggesting that nursing home admission did not bring about improvement or stability for this group of people. By contrast, Payne et al. (2002) found that, although 20% of residents were depressed on admission, only 7.5% of these were still depressed 12 months later. However, the annual rate for new episodes of depression was 26%, though most new episodes resolved within 6 months or less, possibly because of the availability of adequate treatment.

In summary, our knowledge of the relationship between depression and entering residential care is incomplete. Some depressive symptoms may be relatively mild and transient and related to the factors around the move, but other manifestations of depression may be more severe, chronic, and disabling. They may be related to pre-existing depressive disorders, cognitive impairment, and the approaching end of life. Evidence about whether residents receive treatment, and the results of such treatment, is also patchy (Sutcliffe et al., 2007; Ames, 1990).

People with intellectual difficulties

Older people with ID face the same issues as other care home residents but with certain distinct features. The most important of these are discussed below.

Ageing populations of people with ID

Because of improved medical and social care, many people with lifelong developmental disorders, variously referred to as learning disabilities or ID, live longer than was the case with previous generations although their lifespan remains shorter. Although there is an ageing of the ID population alongside that of the general population, the key difference is that 'old age' is considered to begin around the age of 50 years for those with ID, with age-related problems often beginning at an even younger age (Hatzidimitriadou and Milne, 2005). It should also be borne in mind that a proportion of people with ID may have lived in institutional settings all their lives and the population within these homes will experience 'ageing in place'. Therefore, for an individual facility, one of two things may happen. Either the residents move on when they reach a certain age or level of need, or else the average age of the residents, and consequently their level of physical (and perhaps cognitive) dependency, will also increase. In practice, both of these processes may operate, but in any case, the home providers and commissioners of care need to be aware and planning for these changes in advance of their emergence. For example, Kandel et al. (2009) found that there was a significant increase in residents aged 50–59 years in residential care centres in Israel over a 7-year period (6%), with a smaller increase in numbers aged over 60 years, while the numbers aged 40–49 years remained stable.

Physical and mental health problems, including dementia

Several of the conditions that may cause ID are associated with higher levels of physical and mental health problems, including increased rates of mental disorders such as psychosis, mood disorders, and behavioural problems (see Holland, 2008, for discussion of these). However, the most frequent age-associated problem is dementia, which occurs at higher rates in relatively young people with ID of all causes, but is especially associated with Down's syndrome (Holland et al., 1998). The occurrence of Alzheimer-type dementia in people with Down's syndrome mirrors that of the normal population, except that it occurs some 30–40 years earlier in life, with typical prevalence figures of 1–2% between ages 30–39 and 40% above age 50 (Holland, 2000).

Dementia can be difficult to diagnose, since there may be functional decline alone or it may be associated with physical health problems and/or changes in personality and behaviour. The development of dementia leads to several challenges in the social care of the person with ID, and these have been explored by Wilkinson et al. (2004) in a thoughtful review of the issues. One of the main questions is where care should most appropriately be provided. Broadly, there are three options—ageing in place; in place progression; and referral out—which refer to whether the person with ID and dementia remains where they are, whether they move to a specific area in the same home, or whether they move somewhere completely different that specializes in dementia care. In practice, the third option is the most common but each poses its own difficulties not only from the point of view of the resident but also the appropriate level of skills required for staff. Tools such as dementia care mapping that aim to enhance person-centred dementia care can be used with people with ID and dementia but rarely are (Finnamore and Lord, 2007).

Carers and families

For people with ID, their main carers have often been their parents. Thus, by the time the person with ID is getting into the older age range, their parents may be very old, frail, or even deceased. Ageing parents of adults with ID often feel that they have no option but to continue caring (Eley et al., 2009) and this is obviously the cause of considerable stress in some cases. As a result, there may be little preparation for the future needs of the person with ID until some crisis befalls their parent and something has to be done. Thus, the death of a parent will often be the reason for the person with ID entering residential care, so the person will often be recently bereaved as well as facing the loss of the parent and erstwhile home. Research evidence supports this; the main reasons for older people with ID to enter residential care are rarely to do with their own needs but are more commonly a consequence of the ageing or death of their family carer(s) or else a move from another facility, often when that has closed down or been reorganized (Thompson and Wright, 2001). Although families usually wish to be involved in planning such moves, in the event they often have little influence. Moves frequently occur at short notice, and relatives seem to have limited knowledge of their rights, leaving them feeling they are dealing with a fait accompli (Bigby et al., 2010).

Out-of-area placements

Sometimes, because of a lack of suitable placements, people with ID may be placed at a distance from where they previously lived, and this may make it harder for relatives and other significant people in their lives to keep in contact with them. Out-of-area placements are more likely for those people with the highest levels of mental ill health and behavioural problems (Allen et al., 2007). Such placements are often made inconsistently (Mansell et al., 2006), and it can then be difficult for the person with ID to return to their 'home' locality. In addition, the most disabled people seem to experience the worst outcomes (Beadle-Brown et al., 2006), perhaps as there are perverse incentives for the funders of services not to review the placements or bring them to an end.

There is certainly a need to use information from out-of-area placements to plan and provide suitable residential facilities closer to home (Brown and Paterson, 2008).

Inappropriate care

Finally, for various reasons, there may be problems in providing appropriate care for older people with ID or for people with ID who have dementia. There may be a lack of relevant expertise and competencies in the care staff team. For example, if the person has remained in an ID residential setting, there may be scarcity of experience with physical illness, ageing, dementia, and end-of-life care. As well as this, the other residents may not understand what is happening when the person with ID develops dementia and they may well be upset by, or intolerant of, the associated behaviour changes (Wilkinson et al., 2004).

Or else, if the person with ID is in a mainstream care home for older people, there may be a lack of recognition of the fact that he or she may be significantly younger than the other residents. People under, say, the age of 60 residing in care homes for older people form a very isolated and often excluded group, tending to receive few visits from outside, participating in few leisure activities, and having few outings (Winkler et al., 2006). Residents with ID in old people's homes tend to be younger than other residents and to remain living in the home for longer periods. They often have difficulties in fitting into the resident community and in establishing or maintaining meaningful relationships (Bigby et al., 2008). There may also be a tendency among staff or fellow residents to attribute any problems to the intellectual difficulty rather than considering physical health, emotional needs, or the onset of dementia. Thompson and Wright (2001) concluded that many people with ID residing in homes for older people were misplaced. Although many homes claimed that they were suitable to care for people with ID, they also complained that they lacked suitable training, had inadequate staffing levels, the activities provided were unsuitable for people with ID, and people with ID did not 'fit in'.

Irrespective of the setting, there is good evidence to suggest that emphasis should be placed on improving particular aspects of care such as feeding, pain management, and end-of-life care (Ng and Li, 2003; Wilkinson et al., 2004). Furthermore, on top of the problems with care provision, people with ID may need even more help than other care home residents to access appropriate primary or specialist care when they need it.

Better care for older people with ID

Holland (2000) suggested that there are three key health and social care service requirements of older people with ID: a responsive and appropriate social care environment, access to appropriately skilled health professionals, and emotional support as their circumstances change.

Thompson and Wright (2001) argued that improving the lives of older people with ID inappropriately placed in mainstream older people's care homes requires action on several fronts. These include ensuring that services for people with ID are better equipped to meet age-related needs; preventing people from entering older people's services which are unable to offer them an appropriate level of care and quality of life; and reviewing the appropriateness and quality of placements of all people with ID in residential and nursing homes for older people. They also commented that there are financial incentives for local authorities to use older people's services rather than developing good quality provision for older people with an intellectual difficulty. Unless this is addressed, the common practice of *misplacing* people with ID in older people's homes and then *forgetting* them will continue.

For people with ID who develop dementia, several things are required (Wilkinson et al., 2004) including access to assessment and diagnosis of dementia, and treatment when it is appropriate. There needs to be proper consideration of the environment and the care to be provided within a residential facility for people with ID and dementia, involving commissioners, regulators, and providers of care. All this suggests a large agenda for training staff and providing them with the appropriate skills and knowledge. The current situation remains confused and fragmented, with a lack of clear perspective from people with ID and their supporters. A coherent, effective, and well-funded approach to service planning and provision is required to improve care for this neglected and marginalized population (Hatzidimitriadou and Milne, 2005). But, as the next few chapters make apparent, these elements are also needed to address other mental health needs too.

References

Achterberg, W., Pot, A.M., Kerkstra, A., Ooms, M., Muller, M., & Ribbe, M. (2003). The effect of depression on social engagement in newly admitted Dutch nursing home residents. *Gerontologist, 43*, 213–218.

Allen, D.G., Lowe, K., Moore, K., & Brophy, S. (2007). Predictors, costs and characteristics of out of area placement for people with intellectual disability and challenging behaviour. *Journal of Intellectual Disability Research, 51*, 409–416.

Alzheimer Scotland (2007). *A Positive Choice: Choosing Long-stay Care for a Person with Dementia.* Edinburgh: Alzheimer Scotland.

Ames, D. (1990). Depression among elderly residents of local-authority residential homes: its nature and the efficacy of intervention. *British Journal of Psychiatry, 156*, 667–675.

Andersson, I., Pettersson, E., & Sidenvall, B. (2007). Daily life after moving into a care home—experiences from older people, relatives and contact persons. *Journal of Clinical Nursing, 16*, 1712–1718.

Banerjee, S. (2009). *The Use of Antipsychotic Medication for People with Dementia: Time for Action.* London: Department of Health.

Banerjee, S., Murray, J., Foley, B., Atkins, L., Schneider, J., & Mann, A. (2003). Predictors of institutionalisation in people with dementia. *Journal of Neurology Neurosurgery & Psychiatry, 74*, 1315–1316.

Beadle-Brown, J., Mansell, J.L., Whelton, B., Hutchinson, A., & Skidmore, C. (2006). People with learning disabilities in 'out-of-area' residential placements: 2. Reasons for and effects of placement. *Journal of Intellectual Disability Research, 50*, 845–856.

Bharucha, A.J., Pandav, R., Shen, C., Dodge, H.H., & Ganguli, M. (2004). Predictors of nursing facility admission: a 12-year epidemiological study in the United States. *Journal of the American Geriatrics Society, 52*, 434–439.

Bigby, C., Bowers, B., & Webber, R. (2010). Planning and decision making about the future care of older group home residents and transition to residential aged care. *Journal of Intellectual Disability Research* [Epub ahead of print].

Bigby, C., Webber, R., Bowers, B., & McKenzie-Green, B. (2008). A survey of people with intellectual disabilities living in residential aged care facilities in Victoria. *Journal of Intellectual Disability Research, 52*, 404–414.

Bowers, H., Clark, A., Crosby, G., et al. (2009). *Older People's Vision for Long-term Care.* York: Joseph Rowntree Foundation.

Bowman, C., Whistler, J., & Ellerby, M. (2004). A national census of care home residents. *Age and Ageing, 33*, 561–566.

Bronskill, S.E., Anderson, G.M., Sykora, K., et al. (2004). Neuroleptic drug therapy in older adults newly admitted to care homes: incidence, dose, and specialist contact. *Journal of the American Geriatrics Society, 52*, 749–755.

Brown, M. & Paterson, D. (2008). Out-of-area placements in Scotland and people with learning disabilities: a preliminary population study. *Journal of Psychiatric Mental Health Nursing, 15*, 278–286.

Bruce, M.L., McAvay, G.J., Raue, P.J., et al. (2002). Major depression in elderly home health care patients. *American Journal of Psychiatry, 159*, 1367–1374.

Burton, L.C., German, P.S., Gruber-Baldini, A.L., Hebel, J.R., Zimmerman, S., & Magaziner, J. (2001). Medical care for nursing home residents: differences by dementia status. *Journal of the American Geriatrics Society, 49*, 142–147.

Buttar, A.B., Mhyre, J., Fries, B.E., & Blaum, C.S. (2003). Six-month cognitive improvement in nursing home residents with severe cognitive impairment. *Journal of Geriatric Psychiatry & Neurology, 16*, 100–108.

Clarke, A. & Bright, L. (2006). *Moving Stories: The Impact of Admission into a Care Home on Residents' Partners.* London: Relatives and Residents Association.

Counsel and Care (2009). *Care Home Handbook*, 3rd Edition. London: Counsel and Care.

Davies, S. & Nolan, M. (2003). 'Making the best of things': relatives' experiences of decisions about care-home entry. *Ageing & Society, 23*, 429–450.

Davies, S. & Nolan, M. (2004). 'Making the move': relatives' experiences of the transition to a care home. *Health & Social Care in the Community, 12*, 517–526.

Davies, S. & Nolan, M. (2006). 'Making it better': self-perceived roles of family caregivers of older people living in care homes: a qualitative study. *International Journal of Nursing Studies, 43*, 281–291.

Eley, D.S., Bowes, J., Young, L., & Hegney, D.G. (2009). Accommodation needs for carers of and adults with intellectual disability in regional Australia: their hopes for and perceptions of the future. *Rural & Remote Health, 9*, 1239. Available at: http://www.rrh.org.au. (last accessed 15 February 2011).

Finnamore, T. & Lord, S. (2007). The use of Dementia Care Mapping in people with a learning disability and dementia. *Journal of Intellectual Disabilities, 11*, 157–165.

Hatzidimitriadou, E. and Milne, A. (2005). Planning ahead: meeting the needs of older people with intellectual disabilities in the UK. *Dementia, 4*, 341–359.

Holland, A.J. (2000). Ageing and learning disability. *British Journal of Psychiatry, 176*, 26–31.

Holland, A.J. (2008). Working with older people with intellectual difficulties. In: R. Jacoby, C. Oppenheimer, T. Dening, & A. Thomas (Eds.), *Oxford Textbook of Old Age Psychiatry* (pp. 663–672). Oxford: Oxford University Press.

Holland, A.J., Hon, J., Huppert, F.A., Stevens, F., & Watson, P. (1998). Population-based study of the prevalence and presentation of dementia in adults with Down's syndrome. *British Journal of Psychiatry, 172,* 493–498.

Kandel, I., Merrick-Kenig, E., Merrick, J., & Morad, M. (2009). Increased aging in persons with intellectual disability in residential care centers in Israel 1999–2006. *Medical Science Monitor, 15,* 13–16.

Kellett, U. (2007). Seizing possibilities for positive family caregiving in nursing homes. *Journal of Clinical Nursing, 16,* 1479–1487.

Landi, F., Gambassi, G., Lapane, K.L., et al. (1998). Comorbidity and drug use in cognitively impaired elderly living in long-term care. *Dementia & Geriatric Cognitive Disorders, 9,* 347–356.

McConnell, E.S., Branch, L.G., Sloane, R.J., & Pieper, C.F. (2003). Natural history of change in physical function among long-stay nursing home residents. *Nursing Research, 52,* 119–126.

Magaziner, J., Zimmerman, S., Gruber-Baldini, A.L., et al. (2005). Mortality and adverse health events in newly admitted nursing home residents with and without dementia. *Journal of the American Geriatrics Society, 53,* 1858–1866.

Mansell, J.L., Beadle-Brown, J., Whelton, B., Hutchinson, A., & Skidmore, C. (2006). People with learning disabilities in 'out-of-area' residential placements: 1. Policy context. *Journal of Intellectual Disability Research, 50,* 837–844.

Matthews, F.E. & Dening, T. (2002). Prevalence of dementia in institutional care. *Lancet, 360,* 225–226.

Milne, A., Hatzidimitriadou, E., & Chryssanthopoulou, C. (2004). Carers of older relatives in long term care: support needs and services. *Generations Review, Journal of the British Society of Gerontology, 14,* 4–9.

National Collaborating Centre for Mental Health (2007). *Dementia: The NICE-SCIE Guideline on Supporting People with Dementia and their Carers in Health and Social Care.* London: British Psychological Society.

Ng, J. & Li, S. (2003). A survey exploring the educational needs of care practitioners in learning disability (LD) settings in relation to death, dying and people with learning disabilities. *European Journal of Cancer Care (England), 12,* 12–19.

Owen, T. & National Care Home Research & Development Forum (NCHRDF) (Eds.) (2006). *My Home Life: Quality of Life in Care Homes—A Review of the Literature.* London: Help the Aged.

Payne, J.L., Sheppard, J-M., Steinberg, M., et al. (2002). Incidence, prevalence, and outcomes of depression in residents of a long-term care facility with dementia. *International Journal of Geriatric Psychiatry, 17,* 247–253.

Scocco, P., Rapattoni, M., & Fantoni, G. (2006). Nursing home institutionalization: a source of *eustress* or *distress* for the elderly? *International Journal of Geriatric Psychiatry, 21,* 281–287.

Smallbrugge, M., Pot, A.M., Jongenelis, L., Gundy, C.M., Beekman, A.T., & Eefsting, J.A. (2006). The impact of depression and anxiety on well being, disability and use of health care services in nursing home patients. *International Journal of Geriatric Psychiatry, 21,* 325–332.

Sutcliffe, C., Burns, A., Challis, D., et al. (2007). Depressed mood, cognitive impairment, and survival in older people admitted to care homes in England. *American Journal of Geriatric Psychiatry, 15,* 708–715.

Thompson, D. & Wright, S. (2001). *Misplaced and Forgotten: People with Learning Disabilities in Residential Services for Older People.* London: Mental Health Foundation.

Wilkinson, H., Kerr, D., Cunningham, C., & Rae, C. (2004). *Home for Good? Preparing to support people with learning difficulties in residential settings when they develop dementia.* York: Joseph Rowntree Foundation.

Winkler, D., Farnworth, L., & Sloan, S. (2006). People under 60 living in aged care facilities in Victoria. *Australian Health Review, 30,* 100–108.

Zuckerman, I.H., Hernandez, J.J., Gruber-Baldini, A.L., et al. (2005). Potentially inappropriate prescribing before and after nursing home admission among patients with and without dementia. *American Journal of Geriatric Pharmacotherapy, 3,* 246–254.

Chapter 13

Dementia in care homes

Janya Freer and Vellingiri Raja Badrakalimuthu

Abstract

Dementia is extremely common in care home settings, with over half
of all residents having significant cognitive impairment. It is one of
the main reasons that cause older people to move into residential
or nursing home care. The commonest causes of dementia are
Alzheimer's disease and vascular dementia. Dementia may be
associated with other physical health problems and disabilities, as
well as delirium and depression. This chapter emphasizes how good
care planning is essential to meet the diverse needs of people with
dementia. Quality care depends on having suitably trained care staff,
suitable environments, and good support from primary care and
other services. The management of behaviour problems associated
with dementia is challenging but psychological and social measures
should be tried before medication is used.

Introduction

As noted in previous chapters, there are around 18,500 care homes with over 400,000
residents in the United Kingdom (Laing & Buisson, 2009). Approximately 2.5% of the
population over the age of 65 is supported in care homes (Knapp et al., 2007). Dementia
is the most common psychiatric disorder in these settings, although reported prevalence rates vary from 6% to 60% (Rovner et al., 1990), though more recent studies find
that over half of all residents have some degree of dementia. Among residents with a
diagnosis of dementia, 40% have other psychiatric symptoms such as depression or
delusions (Rovner et al., 1990). There will of course be significant numbers of residents with as yet undiagnosed dementia (Quinn et al., 2003). Matthews and Dening
(2002) reported that standardized prevalence is slightly higher in private nursing
homes than in council or private residential homes.

The average annual cost of a patient with dementia in a care home is around £31,000
(US $45,300) with accommodation accounting for 41% of this amount (Knapp et al.,
2007). A resident with dementia requires 229 more hours of care annually than one
without dementia, resulting in a mean annual additional cost of $3900 (£2700) per
person with dementia (O'Brien & Caro, 2001).

This chapter discusses the presentation and management of dementia in the context of care homes. The authors will discuss the complex issues arising from the high degree of comorbidity of dementia with other medical and psychiatric disorders. The authors will make recommendations to address the difficult psychosocial issues that arise along the natural course of the illness.

The syndrome of dementia and types of dementia

Dementia presents as a clinical syndrome and its prominent feature is impaired memory (Table 13.1).

Alzheimer's and cerebrovascular disease are the most common causes of dementia and have overlapping risk factors, pathology, and clinical presentation (Table 13.2). There is a twofold increased risk of dementia over a 10-year period subsequent to a stroke (Ivan et al., 2004). A diagnosis of vascular dementia rests on clinical and/or neuroimaging evidence of cerebrovascular disease with a varied onset and course such as an acute onset within 3 months of a stroke or a fluctuating or stepwise deterioration.

The two next most important causes and their clinical presentations are summarized in Table 13.3. Dementia with Lewy bodies (DLB) has a population prevalence of 0.1% in those over 65 years and increases up to 3.3% in those over 75 years of age (Rahkonen et al., 2003). This form of dementia presents with features of Parkinsonism together with marked visuospatial rather than memory dysfunction.

Frontotemporal dementia (FTD) is a presenile dementia with a median age of onset between 45 and 60 years. Although the most prominent presentation is change in character with disordered social conduct, variations include a disorder of expressive language (progressive non-fluent aphasia) and a semantic disorder (semantic aphasia).

Other less common causes of dementia include idiopathic normal pressure hydrocephalus, Huntington's disease, multiple sclerosis, prion diseases, and reversible causes such as hypothyroidism and vitamin B12 and folate deficiency.

Clinical features of dementia

Cognitive symptoms

Impaired memory (amnesia) for recent events is the most typical presentation, and often progresses to impairment in retrieval of older memories. Speech and language

Table 13.1 Dementia

---

1 Multiple cognitive deficits (which must include amnesia, but also involves impairment in speech and language, reading, writing, numerical skills, attention and concentration, orientation, praxis, visuospatial skills, and higher functions such as judgement and reasoning)
2 Functional impairment
3 Clear consciousness
4 Change from previous level
5 Long duration (>6 months)

Table 13.2 Alzheimer's dementia

1 Fulfils criteria for dementia syndrome
2 Insidious onset
3 Gradual progression
4 No focal neurological signs
5 No evidence of a systematic or brain disease sufficient to cause dementia

dysfunction (dysphasia) can present with word-finding difficulties progressing to severe defects in comprehension and expression, and eventually mutism. Inability to carry out complex motor tasks with preserved sensorimotor systems and coordination (dyspraxia) and failure to correctly interpret sensory input with preserved sensory system (agnosia) can impact on relationships and activities of daily living. Impairments in problem-solving, judgement, and reasoning, a change in personality, and disordered behaviour are indicative of frontal lobe pathology.

Non-cognitive and behavioural symptoms

Psychological and behavioural symptoms can present at any stage during the course of illness affecting between 60% and 90% of people with dementia at some point during the course of the disease. These symptoms present especially in the later stage of illness and increase the likelihood of admission to long-term care. Table 13.4 lists common non-cognitive and behavioural symptoms with their relative prevalence and examples of their manifestation.

Table 13.3 Important features of other major types of dementia

Dementia with Lewy bodies
1 Fluctuating cognition with pronounced variation in attention and alertness (daytime drowsiness/lethargy/daytime sleep >2 hours/staring in to space for long periods/episodes of disorganized speech)
2 Recurrent well formed visual hallucinations (60–70%)
3 Spontaneous features of Parkinsonism (unstable gait/reduced expression/bradykinesia)
4 REM sleep behaviour disorder
5 Severe neuroleptic sensitivity
6 Low dopamine transporter uptake in basal ganglia (SPECT/PET neuroimaging)

Frontotemporal dementia
1 Progressive behavioural disorder
2 Insidious onset
3 Affective symptoms
4 Language disorder
5 Executive dysfunction
6 Preserved spatial orientation
7 Selective frontotemporal atrophy or hypoperfusion/hypometabolism on neuroimaging

Abbreviations: SPECT, single photon emission computed tomography; PET, positron emission tomography.

Table 13.4 Common non-cognitive and behavioural symptoms of dementia

Psychotic	*Delusions* (30%) Objects have been stolen, intruders
	Misidentifications (30%) Spouse, relatives, friends misidentified
	Hallucinations (20%) Visual more common than auditory
Mood	*Depression* (25%) Presents as a symptom or a syndrome, impairs quality of life
	Euphoria (<1%) Much less common
	Anxiety (30–50%) Can be health related, secondary to diagnosis, or depression
Behavioural	*Apathy* (70%) Commonly misdiagnosed as depression
	Agitation (30%) Rummaging in drawers, repeatedly taking clothes on and off, wandering (20%)
	Aggression Physical (20%), verbal (40%)
	Sleep disturbance (45–70%)—day-night reversal
	Eating—inability to use cutlery, refusal, or binge eating
	Sexual disinhibition—with severity of illness
	Personality changes—disengagement, suspicion

Assessment and diagnosis

Although many residents of care homes will have been diagnosed as having dementia before admission to the home, other residents may not have been diagnosed or may indeed develop dementia during their period of residence. Therefore, it may be helpful to set out how the assessment of investigation of possible dementia is conducted. Certain principles will aid in overcoming challenges in assessing patients with dementia: (1) adopting a flexible approach while communicating with the patient, (2) including staff, carers, family, and general practitioner (GP) in obtaining a comprehensive collateral history, (3) reviewing health and social records, and (4) establishing the circumstances leading to the assessment and the reason why it has been requested.

NICE (National Institute of Health and Clinical Excellence) guidelines (NICE, 2006) suggest that a comprehensive assessment should include history taking ('what is the experience?', 'why at this point of time?'), mental state and cognitive examination, physical examination, appropriate investigations, and a review of medications. For a resident in a care home, this should also include a review of the care home notes and care plan, together with food and fluid charts and current medication. It will often be helpful to try to understand behaviour disorders using an ABC (Antecedent-Behaviour-Consequence) analysis of the behaviour in discussion with the care staff. Discussions with the GP and other primary care health professionals (such as district nurses) can also contribute to understanding what is happening and what the causes may be. Taken together, this information enables effective interventions to be offered, as well as providing reassurance to the resident and the staff.

Rating scales

There is a huge selection of rating scales available in the assessment of dementia, including tests of cognition, functional ability, dementia severity, and behaviour. To discuss all of these is beyond the scope of this chapter and readers are referred to Burns et al. (2004) for a more detailed selection. However, a small range of scales may be helpful for staff working in care home settings, and training can be made available in each of the following.

As regards cognitive assessments, commonly used scales include the Abbreviated Mental Test Score, which is the briefest of all screening examinations but limited in its scope; the Mini Mental State Examination (MMSE), which is widely used and captures the current level of cognitive functioning especially memory and orientation; and the Addenbrooke's Cognitive Examination-Revised (ACE-R), which measures in depth the domains of orientation and attention, memory, verbal fluency, language and visuospatial skill/perception.

An ABC behavioural analysis or visual analogue scale of the severity of the behaviour or symptom is often helpful alongside a more structured tool such as the Neuropsychiatric Inventory (NPI), which analyses the duration and severity of behavioural and psychological symptoms. Individual symptom rating can be useful to measure the onset as well as the effectiveness of behaviour therapy. The overall score on the NPI is relevant in early/atypical presentations of dementia, but may be less useful when dementia is severe.

The functional impact of the symptoms of dementia on the person can be measured using the Bristol Activities of Daily Living (BADLS). Dementia Care Mapping (DCM) is an observational tool that looks at the care of people with dementia from the viewpoint of the person with dementia. These results can assist with more structured and comprehensive development of person-centred care. DCM can be used for various purposes, including assessment, development of care by repeated cycles of mapping, identification of training needs and staff development, quality assurance, and research.

Investigations

Investigations can be difficult for patients with dementia to endure especially when they are carried out in a different environment such as a hospital or GP surgery. Basic tests include urinalysis, urine test for infection, blood glucose (especially in the presence of diabetes mellitus), renal function tests, full blood count, and thyroid function tests along with inflammatory markers such as C-reactive protein (CRP) and erythrocyte sedimentation rate (ESR). NICE guidelines recommend that where a diagnosis of dementia is being explored, neuroimaging should be offered. This should be based on a balanced clinical assessment when it is expected that neuroimaging will make a significant impact on diagnosis (in atypical presentations) or management (e.g. in identifying a new cerebrovascular event). Discussion with the GP is helpful to understand previous physical health and to guide investigations.

Differential diagnosis

Not all instances of confusion or changes in behaviour are due to dementia, so it is important to consider other possibilities, of which delirium and depression are the most important.

Delirium is a syndrome with acute onset, fluctuating disturbance of consciousness, impaired attention and concentration, problems in memory, behaviour, and sleep-wake cycle, and perceptual distortions such as visual hallucinations. Delirium is usually due to a physical illness, and these are often treatable. Infections, stroke, and medications account for more than 50% of the presentations (George et al., 1997). Delirium can exacerbate a pre-existing dementia and is a medical emergency associated with a high degree of mortality (George et al., 1997). A sudden change in presentation or deterioration of dementia must be viewed as delirium and investigated thoroughly to identify and treat biological causes.

Depression may be associated with dementia in various ways. For example, depression with psychomotor retardation may appear similar to apathy associated with dementia. Depression may also be a clinical symptom of dementia. Depression is associated with poor prognosis as it has a significant impact on quality of life. Depression improves with treatment and should be explored adequately during assessment. Clues that may suggest the presence of depression include a past history of depression, negative comments about life in general, altered facial expression, and sometimes irritability.

Physical health and dementia in care homes

The 2-year survival rate for patients with dementia admitted to nursing homes is 55% (60% for women and 39% for men). Vascular dementia, physical impairment, inactivity, dependency, and comorbid physical illness all have an adverse effect on survival (Van Dijk et al., 1992). The severity of comorbidity increases with the severity of dementia. Distressing symptoms, including dyspnoea (46.0%) and pain (39.1%), are common. The 6-month mortality rate for residents with dementia who have pneumonia is 46.7%. The same mortality rate is 44.5% for a febrile episode and 38.6% for an eating problem (Mitchell et al., 2009).

Infections

Infections of various kinds can be difficult to detect in people with dementia, and they may present in a relatively non-specific way, sometimes without a raised temperature, but instead with the person simply looking ill or becoming more muddled and confused. Sepsis is commonly caused by pneumonia, urinary tract infections, or infected skin wounds. Observational studies such as Fabiszewski et al. (1990) report that antimicrobial treatment fails to achieve a positive outcome in this frail population. Nonetheless, D'Agata and Mitchell (2008) showed that 66% of residents with dementia received antimicrobial treatment more often as they approached death. Providing adequate personal hygiene to residents of care homes is very important in preventing sepsis.

Incontinence

Urinary incontinence affects approximately half of nursing home residents. In patients with dementia it is often severe and is associated with faecal incontinence. Dementia with faecal incontinence is a common reason for nursing home placement (Johanson et al., 1997). Nursing home staff generally consider urinary incontinence to be one of the most difficult conditions to care for, and they perceive that they spend a disproportionate amount of time on the care of incontinent residents.

Habit training and prompted voiding have been shown to be effective for some incontinent nursing home residents (Schnelle et al., 1990). Highly absorbent launderable and disposable pads and undergarments are however the most common method of managing urinary incontinence in care homes.

Dehydration and loss of appetite

Patients with dementia in nursing homes may be especially vulnerable to dehydration. The cause of dehydration is multifactorial, relating to swallowing difficulty, inability to perceive or report thirst, cognitive impairment, immobility, and inappropriate medications. Dehydration may indicate substandard care, or even neglect (Himmelstein et al., 1983). Recognition of dehydration can be challenging. Physical signs of dehydration have a poor sensitivity and specificity in older people compared with laboratory tests (Weinberg et al., 1995).

Patients with dementia may suffer from poor appetite, undernutrition, and involuntary weight loss. Nutritional assessments are best made in conjunction with an interdisciplinary team including nurse, dietician, speech-language therapist, occupational therapist, and dentist. Family and caregivers may be able to give valuable insight into mealtime history and cultural or personal dietary preferences.

The overall goal for mealtimes for persons with advanced dementia is the preservation of independence and social interaction as well as to ensure adequate intake of food and fluids (Amella et al., 2008). Nutritional support, including artificial (tube) feeding, should be considered if dysphagia is thought to be a transient phenomenon, but artificial feeding should not generally be used in people with severe dementia for whom dysphagia or disinclination to eat is a manifestation of disease severity (NICE, 2006). In end-stage dementia, it has been shown that aggressive treatments, such as tube feeding, are of limited benefit (Mitchell et al., 2004).

Pain

Pain is common in residents of care homes (45–80%) and has a serious impact on quality of life and functional impairment. Pain management in patients with Alzheimer's dementia is often poor because of impaired communication leading to difficulties in its detection, and because of concerns over adverse effects and polypharmacy (Frampton, 2003). An analysis of change in behaviour is a useful way to identify pain. Liaising with pain and palliative care specialists avoid unnecessary use of psychotropics such as antipsychotics to manage behaviour driven by pain.

Mental health and dementia in care homes

Depression

Among individuals with dementia, rates of all types of depression range from 14% to 39% (Cohen et al., 1998). Depression in nursing home patients with dementia has been associated with poor nutrition, behavioural problems, non-compliance with treatment, increased nursing staff time, and excessive mortality rates (Katz and Parmelee, 1994). Use of a depression screen has been shown to increase detection and treatment in this population group (Cohen et al., 2003). However, Datto (2002) reports that residents receive suboptimal levels of antidepressant medications. It is therefore essential to monitor and treat depression among care home residents with dementia.

Psychotic and behavioural symptoms

Among residents with dementia, 46.7% have moderate and 38.8% have severe non-cognitive and behavioural symptoms that require staff attention (Brodaty et al., 2003). The presence of these symptoms predicts frequent use of restraints, antipsychotic drugs, and greater consumption of nursing time (Rovner et al., 1990). Allen et al. (2005) showed that agitated nursing home residents may exhibit a heightened level of verbal agitation, decreased verbal interaction with staff, and increased bed restraint up to 3 months prior to death. There is currently considerable concern about the use of antipsychotic drugs in care homes, and this is discussed below.

Sleep disorders

Insomnia in people with dementia impacts on quality of life and often leads to institutional care as it is obviously very stressful for family carers (McCurry and Ancoli-Israel, 2003). There is evidence to suggest that behavioural approaches can be effective in treating insomnia (Morin et al., 1994). Hypnotic medications, such as zopiclone or temazepam, should be used with caution as they may cause falls, confusion, and day-time fatigue. A condition known as REM (rapid eye movement) sleep behaviour disorder, where the person is extremely restless at night, can be part of various dementias, especially DLB and dementia associated with Parkinson's disease. A safe sleep environment is essential. There is some evidence for clonazepam to treat REM sleep behaviour disorder in patients with DLB (Paparrigopoulos, 2005).

Management of dementia in care homes

Care planning

Following the advice of Hippocrates, the aim is to cure sometimes, treat often, and comfort always. Care plans are essential for the provision of good quality of care and

Table 13.5 Care plan

Care planning (a team activity and a priority) should:
- address social relationships, sexuality, spirituality, mental health, activities, and physical health
- reflect the individual resident's abilities, needs, preferences, and biography
- include appropriate risk assessment and management
- address financial and legal issues
- include regular reviews
- allow changes to be introduced as and when required
- be undertaken by the staff who know the resident best
- involve the resident and their relatives as much as possible
- include a record that is kept in the resident's room

Source: Adapted from Cantley, C. & Wilson, R. (2002). *'Put Yourself in My Place'. Designing and Managing Care Homes for People with Dementia*. Bristol: The Policy Press.

where possible should draw in the wishes of patients and family. Table 13.5 summarizes the components of a good care plan. It should address all the aspects of the residents' life, from their health needs to their everyday and social activities, and it should reflect the fact that the home is where the person is living as well as the location of the care provided for them.

High quality management of people with dementia in care home will encompass a multidisciplinary approach to develop a care plan that includes environmental measures, psychosocial interventions, pharmacological treatments where appropriate, and support for family and other carers. For example, treatment of behavioural disorder in dementia may involve a psychiatrist (or geriatrician), GP, community mental health nurse liaising with care home staff, psychologist developing a behavioural plan, and/or a social worker integrating the family into the care plan.

Environment

Creatively designed environments should be promoted for care of people with dementia in care homes. Designing facilities to support people with a reduced level of cognitive function is practical and achievable and should be based on the principles in Table 13.6. Older people should be involved in design. There needs to be space for people to move around and a recognition that this is the place where people live their lives.

Table 13.6 Environmental design

- Compensate for disability
- Maximize independence, reinforce personal identity, and enhance self-esteem/confidence
- Demonstrate care for staff
- Be orienting and understandable
- Welcome relatives and the local community
- Control and balance stimuli

Source: Adapted from Alzheimer's Australia (2004). *Dementia Care and the Built Environment: Position Paper 3*. Melbourne: Alzheimer's Australia.

Activity scheduling

Daytime activities are an unmet need among 76% of care home residents with dementia (Hancock et al., 2006). Knowledge of the person and review of his or her activity are important in matching the person's interest with appropriate and engaging challenges. Activities should include physical, sensory, cognitive, emotional, spiritual, and social components.

Psychological therapies

These include approaches that have been designed specifically to aid people with dementia, the application of behavioural techniques to manage difficult behaviour, and the psychological, potentially therapeutic, impact of general activities. Psychological interventions are further discussed in Chapter 16 of this volume.

Therapies designed for dementia are often aimed at improving or maintaining cognitive abilities and these include reminiscence therapy, reality orientation, and cognitive stimulation therapy. Reminiscence therapy (Gibson, 1994) uses materials such as old newspapers and household items to stimulate memories and enable people to share and value their experiences. There is at least one study which reports benefits in terms of better mood. Reality orientation therapy (Spector et al., 2002) is based on the idea that a lack of orientating information prevents patients with dementia from functioning well and that reminders can improve functioning. There are studies which report an improvement in terms of mood, fewer neuropsychiatric symptoms, and a reduction in the use of psychotropic medication. Cognitive stimulation therapy uses information processing rather than factual knowledge to address problems in functioning in patients with dementia. One report describes improvement of depression but there are studies which suggest an absence of long-term benefit (Spector et al., 2003). According to NICE (2006), people with mild to moderate dementia of all types should be given the opportunity to participate in a structured group cognitive stimulation programme. There is limited evidence for individualized special instruction, which involves focused individual attention and participation in an activity, and self-maintenance therapy, which aims to help patients maintain a sense of personal identity.

A slightly different approach is taken by validation therapy (Neal and Briggs, 2002), which aims to resolve unfinished conflicts by encouraging and validating expression of feelings. This does not appear to reduce nursing time or use of psychotropic medication and restraint.

There is reasonably good evidence to recommend standard behavioural management techniques in the treatment of BPSD (behavioral and psychological symptoms of dementia) (Livingston et al., 2005). This recommendation is based on consistent and long-term benefits described in large randomized controlled trials. Behavioural management techniques that focus on individual behaviours are generally successful for neuropsychiatric symptoms, and the effects of these interventions may last for months, despite qualitative disparity. Individual and group CBT (cognitive behavioral therapy) (Kipling et al., 1999), interpersonal therapy (Miller and Reynolds, 2002), and problem-solving therapy have been shown to be effective in BPSD such as depression and anxiety as well as in managing psychiatric comorbidities associated with dementia.

As regards more general interventions, there is some evidence that music therapy and Snoezelen/multisensory stimulation are effective to contain disturbed behaviour during difficult periods and for short periods afterwards but not in the long term (Livingston et al., 2005). A review of randomized controlled trials of therapeutic activities such as games, exercise, socializing, and art suggests that they are associated with significant reduction in behavioural disturbances such as agitation (Livingston et al., 2005).

Good physical health

It is important to ensure that residents with dementia have proper access to primary care, for example that they are registered with a general practitioner and that they participate in any health screening and health promotional activities that are relevant to them. In particular, there is much to be gained from a regular review of their medicines to ensure that they are not receiving unnecessary medication and that any medication that may adversely affect their mental state is kept to a minimum.

Pharmacological treatment

Pharmacological treatment has a limited but essential place in the management of dementia. Prescribing is normally a second-line approach, based on comprehensive assessment with a robust plan for follow-up to monitor the progress of the symptoms being treated. Pharmacological intervention should be offered in the first instance only if a patient is severely distressed or if there is an immediate risk of harm to the person or others. The assessment and care-planning approach, which includes behavioural management, should be followed wherever possible (NICE, 2006).

Cognitive symptoms

Alzheimer's disease

NICE (2006) recommends using acetylcholinesterase inhibitors (donepezil, galantamine, and rivastigmine) to treat moderate Alzheimer's dementia. However, there is no evidence to suggest that the beneficial effect from acetylcholinesterase inhibitors is restricted to moderately severe Alzheimer's dementia (Burns and O'Brien, 2006). Carers often report an increase in motivation, and alertness leading to an improvement in activities of daily living. They may also reduce behavioural and psychological symptoms of dementia. The commonest adverse effects of acetylcholinesterase inhibitors include nausea, vomiting, diarrhoea, and cramps, but there could be other serious effects such as bronchospasm or cardiac problems. These drugs are often discontinued in patients with severe dementia in care homes.

Another available drug is memantine, which has a different mode of action. Although NICE guidelines (2006) do not support prescribing memantine, several studies have reported it to be effective in severe dementia (Burns and O'Brien, 2006), so it may be considered for treating disturbed behaviour such as agitation or aggression if other measures have failed.

Non-Alzheimer's dementia

Acetylcholinesterase inhibitors show small benefit in the treatment of mild to moderate vascular dementia. In patients with DLB, rivastigmine is effective in reducing behavioural and psychological symptoms, and, in particular, for hallucinations although there is no significant impact on cognitive functioning (Burns and O'Brien, 2006).

Acetylcholinesterase inhibitors are generally initiated by specialists (psychiatrists, geriatricians, neurologists) with shared care protocols between primary and secondary care for follow-up.

Non-cognitive and behavioural symptoms

Treating the non-cognitive and behavioural symptoms of dementia is challenging. Treatment approaches should emphasize psychosocial interventions. Pharmacological management is reserved for the most severe and most disabling presentations where there is major risk to the patient, other residents or carers, or where there is a profound impact on quality of life.

Acetylcholinesterase inhibitors have been shown to be effective in treating depression, dysphoria, anxiety, and apathy. They may also reduce aggression and agitation (Gauthier et al., 2002) though not all studies have found this (Howard et al., 2007). In one study, memantine added to donepezil improved agitation, aggression, irritability, lability, and appetite (Gauthier et al., 2005). As these medications may help cognitive symptoms and are safer than antipsychotics, they can be tried subsequent to or along with psychosocial interventions.

Despite concern about prescribing of antipsychotics to people with dementia, about 30–40% of people with dementia in care homes receive these drugs (Alldred et al., 2007). Antipsychotic treatment of dementia is associated with reduced well-being and quality of life (Ballard et al., 2001a) and may even accelerate cognitive decline and death (McShane et al., 1997). Antipsychotics can be withdrawn in up to one-half of patients with no adverse effects on behaviour and functioning (Schmidt et al., 1998), and alternative strategies are effective in reducing agitation in people with dementia (Ballard et al., 2002). Hence, it is prudent to reserve antipsychotics as a last resort and to discontinue them once the clinical need for antipsychotics remits. Antidepressant medications such as citalopram (Pollock et al., 2007) and trazodone have been reported to be as effective as risperidone in treating agitation. There is limited evidence that carbamazepine reduces agitation (Tariot et al., 1998).

In summary, medications for non-cognitive symptoms have a role, but normally only as short-term adjuncts to psychosocial interventions provided in the care home. In all cases, the use of psychotropics should be closely monitored, and the benefits weighed carefully against the potential disadvantages and side-effects.

Quality of life

Objective 11 of the National Dementia Strategy (Department of Health, 2009) aims to provide high quality services within care homes and states that quality care should be based on managing transitions, maintaining identity, creating community, sharing decision-making, improving health and healthcare, supporting good end-of-life care, keeping the workforce fit for purpose, and promoting a positive culture. The standard of care provided to people with dementia is often poor and there is a consensus that it should be improved (Ballard et al., 2001b). Examining needs among care home residents,

Hancock et al. (2006) reported that although environmental and physical health needs are usually met, sensory or physical disability needs, mental health needs, and social needs are often unmet, leading to psychological problems and lower quality of life.

Role of staff

Ballard et al. (2001a,b) reported that over the 6-hour daytime period of observation in their study, only 50 minutes (14%) were spent talking (or communicating in other ways) with staff or other residents. A study on attitudes toward dementia and dementia care held by nursing staff in non-EMI care homes showed that a person-centred approach was associated with better recognition of cognitive impairment independent of training and experience (Macdonald and Woods, 2005). The importance of person-centred care that underpins good practice in dementia care is highlighted in NICE guidelines (2006). Adequate training of staff in care homes is a vital element in successful provision of good quality of life to patients with dementia (National Care Forum Older People and Dementia Care Committee, 2007). Table 13.7 lists the elements that contribute to successful training.

Role of primary and specialist care

GP guidelines for the management of dementia (NSW Health, 2003) suggest that GPs have a role in informing residents, carers, and families about what to expect following the diagnosis of dementia and initiation of a management plan. The guidelines also recommend that GPs regularly review patients with dementia for optimal control of comorbidities. Residents with dementia in care homes rely on care home staff who have a close working relationship with primary healthcare practitioners. It is essential that residents in care homes have the same access to specialist care as those living in the community.

Role of residents and carers

Including residents and carers in dialogue about their needs and how these can be achieved is central to an individually tailored care plan and to ensuring adequate quality of life. Relatives are equally important in discussions about care plans as they are often

Table 13.7 Aids to successful education of care home staff

- Flexibility
- Involving all staff
- Identifying and responding to training needs
- Tailoring to individual home
- Practical between-session tasks
- Developing pride in care home staff
- Support of managers and other professionals
- Minimum extra work for staff

Source: Adapted from Siddiqi, N., Young, J., Cheater, F., et al. (2008). Educating staff working in long-term care about delirium: the Trojan horse for improving quality of care? *Journal of Psychosomatic Research*, 65, 261–266, Copyright 2008, with permission from Elsevier.

distressed about the person with dementia. Relatives should be monitored for their well-being and should be encouraged to continue their active involvement in the care of their loved ones. Visits from family and friends provide assistance both with the psychosocial and identity preserving aspects of care, and help to develop trust between residents and staff in care home.

End-of-life care

NICE (2006) recommends that patients with dementia have access to palliative care services. In an important American study, Mitchell et al. (2005) reported that 71% of residents with advanced dementia died within 6 months of admission, yet only 11% were referred for palliative care. In the last 3 months of life, a high proportion of residents undergo at least one burdensome intervention such as hospitalization, emergency room visit, parenteral therapy, or tube feeding. Cardiopulmonary resuscitation (CPR) is three times less likely to be successful in a person with dementia than in one who is cognitively intact, so it is important to consider the likely outcome when developing a care plan.

Only a minority of residents discuss end-of-life care with families and even fewer provide any advance care planning. Family members are not well prepared for their role as surrogate decision makers; they often have limited understanding of dementia progression, and may be uncomfortable and ambivalent in their role. Healthcare professionals should provide support to equip families with information about palliative care and end-of-life issues. Residents and carers should be empowered to make decisions that would ensure dignity in the process of dying.

Conclusion

In this chapter, we have looked at the significant impact dementia can have on the physical, psychological, and social well-being of residents in care homes. It is important that staff in care homes are trained and supported in identifying and managing patients with dementia through closer ties between care homes, primary, and specialist services. Providing a good quality of life for residents should be a priority and this can only be achieved through active and reciprocal communication between residents and the staff in a care home.

References

Alldred, D., Petty, D., & Bowie, P. (2007). Antipsychotic prescribing patterns in care homes and relationship with dementia. *Psychiatric Bulletin, 31*, 329–332.

Allen, R., Burgio, L., & Fisher, S. (2005). Behavioural characteristics of agitated nursing home residents with dementia at the end of life. *Gerontologist, 45*, 86–91.

Alzheimer's Australia (2004). *Dementia Care and the Built Environment: Position Paper 3.* Melbourne: Alzheimer's Australia.

Amella, E.J., Grant, P.J., & Mulloy, C. (2008). Eating behaviour in persons with moderate to late-stage dementia: assessments and interventions. *Journal of the American Psychiatric Nurses Association, 13*, 360–367.

Ballard, C.G., O'Brien, J., James, I., et al. (2001a). *Dementia: Management of Behavioural and Psychological Symptoms*. Oxford: Oxford University Press.

Ballard, C., Fossey, J., Chithramohan, R., et al. (2001b). Quality of care in private sector and NHS facilities for people with dementia: cross sectional survey. *BMJ, 323*, 426–427.

Ballard, C.G., O'Brien, J.T., Reichelt, K., et al. (2002). Aromatherapy as a safe and effective treatment for the management of agitation in severe dementia: the results of a double-blind, placebo-controlled trial with Melissa. *Journal of Clinical Psychiatry, 63*, 553–558.

Brodaty, H., Draper, B., & Low, L. (2003). Behavioural and psychological symptoms of dementia: a seven-tiered model of service delivery. *Medical Journal of Australia, 178*, 231–234.

Burns, A., Lawlor, B., & Craig, S. (2004). *Assessment Scales in Old Age Psychiatry*, 2nd Edition. London: Informa Healthcare.

Burns, A. & O'Brien, J. (2006). Clinical practice with anti-dementia drugs: a consensus statement from British Association for Psychopharmacology. *Journal of Psychopharmacology, 20*, 732–755.

Cantley, C. & Wilson, R. (2002). *'Put Yourself in My Place'. Designing and Managing Care Homes for People with Dementia*. Bristol: The Policy Press.

Cohen, C.I., Hyland, K., & Magai, C. (1998). Depression among African American nursing home patients with dementia. *American Journal of Geriatric Psychiatry, 6*, 162–175.

Cohen, C.L., Hyland, K., & Kimhy, D. (2003). The utility of mandatory depression screening of dementia patients in nursing homes. *American Journal of Psychiatry, 160*, 2012–2017.

D'Agata, E. & Mitchell, S. (2008). Patterns of antimicrobial use among nursing home residents with advanced dementia. *Archives of Internal Medicine, 168*, 357–362.

Datto, C.J. (2002). Specificity of antidepressant prescribing in the nursing home setting. In: *Proceedings of the 15th Annual Meeting of the American Association of Geriatric Psychiatry*. Bethesda, MD: AAGP.

Department of Health (2009). *Living Well with Dementia—the National Dementia Strategy. Joint Commissioning Framework for Dementia*. London: Department of Health.

Fabiszewski, K.J., Volicer, B., & Volicer, L. (1990). Effect of antibiotic treatment on outcome of fevers in institutionalized Alzheimer patients. *JAMA, 263*, 3168–3172.

Frampton, M. (2003). Experience assessment and management of pain in people with dementia. *Age and Ageing, 32*, 248–251.

Gauthier, S., Feldman, H., Hecker, J., et al. (2002). Efficacy of donepezil on behavioural symptoms in patients with moderate to severe Alzheimer's disease. *International Psychogeriatrics, 14*, 389–404.

Gauthier, S., Wirth, Y., & Mobius, H. (2005). Effects of memantine on behavioural symptoms in Alzheimer's disease patients: an analysis of the Neuropsychiatric Inventory (NPI) data of two randomised, controlled studies. *International Journal of Geriatric Psychiatry, 20*, 459–464.

George, J., Bleasdale, S., & Singleton, S. (1997). Causes and prognosis of delirium in elderly patients admitted to a district general hospital. *Age and Ageing, 26*, 423–427.

Gibson, F. (1994). What can reminiscence contribute to people with dementia? In: J. Bornat (Ed.), *Reminiscence Reviewed: Evaluations, Achievements, Perspectives* (pp. 46–60). Buckingham: Open University Press.

Hancock, G.A., Woods, R., Challis, D., & Orrell, M. (2006). The needs of older people with dementia in residential care. *International Journal of Geriatric Psychiatry, 21*, 43–49.

Himmelstein, D.U., Jones, A.A., & Woolhandler, S. (1983). Hypernatraemic dehydration in nursing home patients: an indicator of neglect. *Journal of American Geriatric Society*, *31*, 466.

Howard, R., Juszczak, E., Ballard, C.G., et al. (2007). Donepezil for the treatment of agitation in Alzheimer's disease. *New England Journal of Medicine*, *357*, 1382–1392.

Ivan, C., Seshadri, S., Berser, A., et al. (2004). Dementia after stroke. The Framingham study. *Stroke*, *35*, 1264–1268.

Johanson, J., Irizarry, F., & Doughty, A. (1997). Risk factors for fecal incontinence in a nursing home population. *Journal of Clinical Gastroenterology*, *24*, 156–160.

Katz, I.R. & Parmelee, P.A. (1994). Depression in elderly patients in residential care settings. In: L.S. Schneider & C.F. Reynolds III (Eds.), *Diagnosis and Treatment of Depression in Late Life: Results of the NIH Consensus Development Conference* (pp. 463–490). Washington, DC: American Psychiatric Press.

Kipling, T., Bailey, M., & Charlesworth, G. (1999). The feasibility of a cognitive behavioural therapy group for men with a mild/moderate cognitive impairment. *Behavioural and Cognitive Psychotherapy*, *27*, 189–193.

Knapp, M., Prince, M., Albanese, E., et al. (2007). *Dementia UK: A Report into the Prevalence and Cost of Dementia.* Prepared by the Personnel Social Services Research Unit at the London School of Economics and Institute of Psychiatry at King's College London for the Alzheimer's Society. London: Alzheimer's Society.

Laing & Buisson (2009). *Care of Elderly People: UK Market Survey 2008.* London: Laing & Buisson.

Livingston, G., Johnston, K., Katona, C., et al. (2005). Systematic review of psychological approaches to the management of neuropsychiatric symptoms of dementia. *American Journal of Psychiatry*, *162*, 1996–2021.

Macdonald, A. & Woods, R. (2005). Attitudes to dementia and dementia care held by nursing staff in U.K. 'non-EMI' care homes: what difference do they make? *International Psychogeriatrics*, *17*, 383–391.

Matthews, F.E. & Dening, T. (2002). Prevalence of dementia in institutional care. *Lancet*, *360*, 225–226.

McCurry, S.M. & Ancoli-Israel, S. (2003). Sleep dysfunction in Alzheimer's disease and other dementias. *Current Treatment Options in Neurology*, *5*, 261–272.

McShane, R., Keene, J., Gedling, K., et al. (1997). Do neuroleptic drugs hasten cognitive decline in dementia? Prospective study with necropsy follow-up. *BMJ*, *314*, 211–212.

Miller, M. & Reynolds, C. (2002). Interpersonal psychotherapy. In: J. Hepple, P. Pearce, & G. Wilkinson (Eds.), *Psychological Therapies with Older People: Developing Treatments for Effective Practice* (pp. 103–127). Hove: Brunner-Routledge.

Mitchell, S.L., Kiely, D.K., & Hamel, M.B. (2004). Dying with advanced dementia in the nursing home. *Archives of Internal Medicine*, *164*, 321–326.

Mitchell, S.L., Teno, J.M., Miller, S.C., & Mor, V.A. (2005). A national study for the location of death for the older person with dementia. *Journal of American Geriatric Society*, *53*, 299–305.

Mitchell, S.L., Teno, J.M., Kiely, D.K., et al. (2009). The clinical course of advanced dementia. *The New England Journal of Medicine*, *361*, 1529–1538.

Morin, C.M., Culbert, J.P., & Schwartz, S.M. (1994). Nonpharmacological interventions for insomnia. *American Journal of Psychiatry*, *151*, 1172–1180.

National Care Forum Older People and Dementia Care Committee (2007). *Key Principles of Person-centred Dementia Care.* London: Social Care Institute for Excellence.

Neal, M. & Briggs, M. (2002). Validation Therapy for Dementia. *Cochrane Library*, issue 3. Oxford: Update Software.

NICE (2006). *Dementia: Supporting People with Dementia and their Carers in Health and Social Care*. London: NICE Clinical Guideline 42.

NSW Health (2003). *Care of Patients with Dementia in General Practice: Guidelines*. North Sydney: NSW Department of Health.

O'Brien, J. & Caro, J. (2001). Alzheimer's dementia and other dementia in nursing homes: levels of management and cost. *International Psychogeriatrics*, *13*, 347–358.

Paparrigopoulos, T.J. (2005). REM sleep behaviour disorder: clinical profiles and pathophysiology. *International Reviews of Psychiatry*, *17*, 293–300.

Pollock, G., Mulsant, B., Rosen, J., et al. (2007). A double-blind comparison of citalopram and risperidone for the treatment of behavioural and psychotic symptoms associated with dementia. *American Journal of Geriatric Psychiatry*, *11*, 942–952.

Quinn, M., Johnson, M., Andress, E., & McGinnis, P. (2003). Health characteristics of elderly residents in personal care homes: dementia, possible early dementia and no dementia. *Journal of Gerontological Nursing*, *29*, 16–23.

Rahkonen, T., Eloniemi-Sulkava, U., Rissanen, S., et al. (2003). Dementia with Lewy bodies according to consensus criteria in a geneal population aged 75 years or older. *Journal of Neurology, Neurosurgey & Psychiatry*, *74*, 720–724.

Rovner, B., German, P., Broadhead, J., et al. (1990). The prevalence and management of dementia and other psychiatric disorder in nursing homes. *International Psychogeriatrics*, *2*, 13–24.

Schmidt, I., Claesson, C.B., Westerholm, B., et al. (1998). The impact of regular multidisciplinary team interventions on psychotropic prescribing in Swedish nursing homes. *Journal of the American Geriatric Society*, *46*, 77–82.

Schnelle, J.F., Newman, D.R., & Fogarty, T. (1990). Management of patient continence in long-term care facilities. *Gerontologist*, *30*, 373–376.

Siddiqi, N., Young, J., Cheater, F., et al. (2008). Educating staff working in long-term care about delirium: the Trojan horse for improving quality of care? *Journal of Psychosomatic Research*, *65*, 261–266.

Spector, A., Orrell, M., Davies, S., et al. (2002). Reality Orientation for Dementia. *Cochrane Library*, issue 3. Oxford: Update Software.

Spector, A., Thorgrimsen, L., Woods, B., et al. (2003). Efficacy of an evidence-based cognitive stimulation therapy programme for people with dementia: a randomised controlled trial. *British Journal of Psychiatry*, *183*, 248–254.

Tariot, P., Erb, R., Podgorski, C.A., et al. (1998). Efficacy and tolerability of carbamazepine for agitation and aggression in dementia. *American Journal of Psychiatry*, *155*, 54–61.

Van Dijk, P., Van De Sande, H., Dippel, D., & Habbema, J. (1992). The nature of excess mortality in nursing home patients with dementia. *Journal of Gerontology*, *47*, M28–M34.

Weinberg, A., Minaker, K., Coble, Y., et al. (1995). Dehydration: evaluation and management in older adults. *JAMA*, *274*, 1552–1556.

Chapter 14

Depression in care homes

Briony Dow, Xiaoping Lin, Jean Tinney,
Betty Haralambous, and David Ames

Abstract

Despite increased detection and treatment of depression in recent
years, depression remains a significant problem for older people living
in care homes. Prevalence remains high and the few longitudinal
studies that have been conducted show high persistence of depression
over time. Care staff still lack knowledge and understanding of
depression with many seeing depression as a normal phenomenon
for older people. Depression is therefore often not detected or
treated. This lack of detection and treatment may have serious
consequences as depression does not often spontaneously remit in
care home residents and is a significant risk factor for mortality.
Detection is the first step in initiating assessment and treatment
for depression. Further research is needed to investigate those
treatment approaches that appear promising, particularly
multifaceted and psychosocial approaches. There is also a need for
more longitudinal studies to inform us about incidence, persistence,
and outcomes of depression.

Introduction

The term 'depression' refers to both a mood state or symptom and to a syndrome ('disorder') comprising a collection of symptoms that often occur together in a recognizable
pattern. The core feature of depression is a low mood often characterised as low, down,
miserable, sad, or blue. Other common depressive symptoms are listed in the next paragraph. In research studies and in clinical practice diagnoses of depressive disorders are
made using internationally agreed criteria such as those of the World Health Organization's
International Classification of Diseases, Tenth Revision (ICD-10) or the American
Psychiatric Association's Diagnostic and Statistical Manual, Fourth Edition (DSM-IV).

The ICD-10 defines a depressive episode as present when 4 or more of the following
10 symptoms are present most of the day, most days for at least 2 weeks in the absence
of another disorder (e.g. hypothyroidism, schizophrenia, dementia, etc.) that could

better account for the symptoms: low mood, loss of interest and enjoyment, disturbed sleep, decreased or increased weight or appetite, loss of energy, psychomotor slowing, poor concentration, feelings of guilt or self-reproach, recurrent thoughts of death or suicide, and loss of confidence (World Health Organization, 2004). In the DSM-IV, five of nine of the above symptoms (excluding loss of confidence) must be present for the same 2-week time period for a diagnosis of major depressive disorder to be confirmed (American Psychiatric Association, 1994). Both systems require that the symptoms cause clinically significant stress or impairment in social, occupational, or other important areas of functioning.

Milder forms of depression are common, and often occur with other illnesses or following bereavement. These are sometimes referred to as minor depression, dysthymic disorder (if present chronically for 2 years), or 'depressive symptoms'.

This chapter outlines knowledge about prevalence, causes, detection and screening, treatment, and outcomes of depression in care homes. The conclusion includes a summary of key messages for future action.

Prevalence and incidence

Prevalence of depression in care homes is high, ranging from 4% to 25% for major depressive disorder and 29% to 82% for minor depression or the presence of depressive symptoms (Seitz et al., 2010). A recent review by Seitz and colleagues examined 74 studies on prevalence of psychiatric disorders in nursing homes, including 26 on depression. Dementia, depression, and anxiety were the most common psychiatric disorders among older people in long-term care. A range of instruments were used to assess depression in the 26 studies cited, making it difficult to determine prevalence more precisely than the wide ranges quoted above. The Geriatric Depression Scale (GDS) was used in 12 studies but three different versions with a range of cut-off points were used (Seitz et al., 2010).

In most countries, prevalence of depression in care homes is substantially higher than among community-dwelling older people, particularly in the case of major depression. Junginger and colleagues found 21% of their sample living in nursing homes in the United States had major depression compared with 10% of community-dwelling older people (Junginger et al., 1993). Similarly, a British study found a 9.3% prevalence of *major* depression in community-dwelling older people, compared with 27.1% in nursing homes (McDougall et al., 2007).

The incidence (number of new cases arising over a defined period of time) of depression appears to be approximately 5–6% for new cases of both major and minor depression over a 6- to 12-month period (Parmelee et al., 1992a, 1992b; Smalbrugge et al., 2006). Progression from minor to major depression may be higher. One study found that 16.2% of people with minor depression progressed to major depression over 1 year (Parmelee et al., 1992a, 1992b).

Causes

A number of factors contribute to depression in care homes, but no single factor can be considered the sole cause of depressive symptoms in most residents. Nor does any single factor (or combination of factors) have the same effect on different individual residents. Factors such as the types of care homes; the education and training levels of staff; the personality, attitudes, and coping strategies of residents themselves; resident health status (psychological health, physical disability/comorbidity, and levels of function and dependence), social support, and length of time in care all have the potential to influence symptom expression.

Physical and mental health

Physical disability is strongly associated with depression. Medical comorbidities and functional impairment have emerged as important risk factors in a number of studies. Persistent pain has also been identified as a major factor affecting both mood and quality of life. Medications for a number of comorbid conditions (e.g. antihypertensive/cardiac drugs; treatment for Parkinson's disease, and certain antibiotics) may cause or worsen depression.

Medical conditions associated with depression include those whose symptoms may overlap with those of depression, and indicate a strong correlation between dementia and depression (Hyer et al., 2005). This correlation is reported in a number of studies, though it is difficult to determine cause and effect. A history of previous depression is one of the best predictors of depression in long-term care (Payne et al., 2002), and better cognitive functioning increases levels of risk of depression when associated with loss of physical function and capacity to live independently. Parkinson's disease and heart disease are risk factors for depression, although medication for these conditions may be implicated. Other studies have noted relationships between depression and impairment of hearing or vision.

Individual personality, social history, attitudes, and coping strategies

Loss, a major factor in admission into care homes, is strongly associated with depression—personal loss includes grief over the death of loved ones, loss of home, pets, social support, and close friends; loss of function and control over the body; loss of independence and autonomy; and loss of the familiar (Hyer et al., 2005). An important factor is the loss of control over one's own destiny. Personal coping styles and attitudes are important in explaining why some people are more negatively affected by loss and the presence of death. Cataldo (1994) found 'non-hardiness and health-limiting death attitudes' to be reliable predictors, and staff in another study identified social withdrawal (related to despair, loss, grief, loneliness, and isolation) as a key indicator of depression. Lack of assertiveness can lower defences against institutional risk factors. Higher education levels also correlate with greater likelihood of being depressed in long-term care, especially when associated with loss of mobility, function, and independence.

Care home environments

Institutional factors that may contribute to depression include: loss of privacy and frustration over shared rooms, noise, institutional furniture and odours, lack of stimulating social programmes, lack of close relationships, high turnover rate of staff with little training and many cultural and educational differences, and other frustrations of living in close quarters with strangers under an institutional regime (Hyer et al., 2005). The medicalized environment of long-term care settings and lack of alternative approaches to care have also been identified as risk factors, as has the constant presence of death (Cataldo, 1994).

Length of time in care

Evidence suggests that the influence of length of time in care is different for cognitively impaired residents, and more likely to be negative for those without cognitive impairment. Many residents admitted with dementia already have undiagnosed depression, which is likely to improve if diagnosed and treated (Payne et al., 2002). For residents with better cognitive function, the risk of becoming depressed increases with length of stay and an increased sense of hopelessness over health status and lack of autonomy (Hyer et al., 2005).

Detection

Despite high prevalence, depression is still underdetected in care homes (Davidson et al., 2006). The GDS, the Cornell Scale for Depression in Dementia (CSDD), and in the United States, the mood subscale of the Minimum Data Set (MDS) are the most frequently used tools for screening and detection.

Screening and detection instruments

The GDS has been widely used in care homes and several shorter versions have been developed, the most popular being the 15-item version, generally preferred over the original as it is quicker to complete (6 minutes vs. 12 minutes) and has good psychometric properties (McCurren, 2002). A five-item version of the GDS is also effective as a screening tool for depression in cognitively intact older adults (Rinaldi et al., 2003). As the GDS relies on self-report, there is debate as to whether it is suitable for use with people with mild to moderate dementia. A recent study comparing the GDS-15 with DSM-IV-TR criteria in people with and without dementia found adequate specificity and sensitivity, suggesting that it may be appropriate for use in these populations (Lach et al., 2010).

The CSDD has been extensively evaluated for use in care homes. The CSDD covers five areas and takes approximately 30 minutes to complete: 20 minutes with a carer (or other informant) and 10 minutes with the older person. It is reliable, valid, and sensitive and can differentiate the entire range of severity, including mild to no depression (Alexopoulos et al., 1988). Its limitations are that it takes 30 minutes to complete, requires trained personnel, does not correlate well with a psychiatrist's assessment, and is not always accurate in people with advanced dementia (De Bellis and Williams, 2008). Despite these limitations, De Bellis and Williams concluded that it is the most comprehensive depression screening tool for older people with and without dementia, making it suitable for use in aged care homes. The main advantage of the tool is its use of multiple sources of information. Routine use of the CSDD in care homes could improve doctor, nurse, and personal carer communication as personal care staff can be informants in the assessment of depression (Koritsas et al., 2006). Poor communication between professionals has been identified as a barrier to identification of depression in care homes.

Seven items from the mandated MDS from the Resident Assessment Instrument in the United States have been validated for use as a depression-screening tool known as the MDS Depression Rating Scale (DRS) (Burrows et al., 2000). In the original study, the DRS compared favourably with the GDS-15 and the DRS has adequate sensitivity and specificity and can be reliably administered via self-report to residents with a Mini Mental State Examination (MMSE) score ≥12 (Ruckdeschel et al., 2004). However, other studies have found poor correlation between the DRS and the GDS-15 (Jones et al., 2004; McCurren, 2002). This is probably due to the use of different information sources, as the GDS relies on self-report and the DRS is observational. It may also be that the tools are measuring different elements of depression.

A single screening question 'Do you feel that your life is empty?' was trialled as a screening tool for depression in care homes in London and compared with the CSDD. A yes response indicated that the resident was twice as likely to have depression and a no response meant that there was a 75% chance that the resident did not have depression. Half of the study sample (n = 209) scored less than 15 on the MMSE, but there was no difference in sensitivity or specificity for the screening question for different levels of cognitive impairment. Watson et al. (2009) trialled five strategies for depression screening in residential aged care. The best strategy was a two-item version of the Patient Health Questionnaire (PHQ-2) with a sensitivity of 0.80 and specificity of 0.75 as it was brief and easy to administer.

Underdetection

Nurses and personal care staff should be well placed to detect depression because of their close involvement with residents, but they are generally not good at recognizing the symptoms of depression (Ayalon et al., 2008). There is a poor relationship between resident and nurse CSDD ratings. Brühl and colleagues (2007) found the GDS detected 50% more depression than did nurses. Nurses recognized depression in only 55% of residents diagnosed via a psychiatric interview using DSM-IV criteria; furthermore they detected depression in 40% of residents not diagnosed as depressed. In the study by Watson et al. (2009), mentioned above, measures completed by care staff (modified version of the CSDD and a one-item screen) failed to detect depression adequately. In the United Kingdom, Bagley et al. (2000) found that only 15–27% of 308 newly admitted residents with depression were identified as depressed by staff. They concluded that more education was needed, as less than 2% of staff in their study had received in-service training on depression in older people. Ayalon et al. (2008) found that paraprofessional staff working in care homes were more likely to view depression as a normal phenomenon, had less accurate beliefs about signs and symptoms, and were less familiar with the effectiveness of treatments for depression than nurses, social workers, and activity staff. Education should be targeted to meet the needs of this group, as they provide the bulk of the care to residents.

Education

A number of studies have investigated the impact of education on detection and treatment of depression in care homes. In an American study investigating nursing home physicians' beliefs about how well they can detect and treat depression, excellent training (vs. good, fair, poor, or none) and the use of screening tools were associated with better recognition and treatment skills, and practice guideline awareness was associated with greater self-reported treatment competency (Banazak et al. 1999). A single education session for general practitioners (GPs) on late-life depression was associated with improved GP recognition of depression in nursing home residents in an Australian study (Davidson et al., 2006). In another Australian study, staff education was one component of a successful multifactorial intervention for improving detection and treatment of depression in care homes (Llewellyn-Jones et al., 1999). The Netherlands nursing home staff randomized to a 4-hour training session on recognition of depression through observation of activities of daily living (ADLs) (using the Behaviour Rating Scale for Psychogeriatric Inpatients) were better able to recognize depression than those in the control group. The ability to recognize residents who were not depressed did not differ between groups. The use of video-based training improves nursing staff's ability to detect mood symptoms in nursing home residents. Having a mandated screening tool also improves recognition and initiation of treatment for depression in care homes.

Treatment and management

Assessment is an essential prerequisite to treatment. Assessment may identify factors that could cause or contribute to depression, such as drug reaction, medical illness, pain, or environmental factors. Addressing such issues may alleviate depressive symptoms.

Treatment approaches

The main approaches in treatment of depression anywhere at any age can be divided into biological (e.g. antidepressants and electroconvulsive therapy [ECT]), psychological (e.g. cognitive behaviour therapy [CBT]), and social (e.g. recreational activities). Treatments may be used singly or in combination depending on circumstances.

Antidepressants are the most common treatment for depression in care home residents (Brown et al., 2002), and research suggests that they are effective and should be included in the first-line treatment for residents with major depression (American Geriatrics Society and American Association for Geriatric Psychiatry, 2003). The choice of medication should be based on possible side-effects, interactions with other medications, and the resident's other illnesses. Antidepressants should be started at a low dose and be increased slowly (American Geriatrics Society and American Association for Geriatric Psychiatry, 2003; Kallenbach and Rigler, 2006). ECT is usually administered in hospital and is reserved for severe depression, but because it works quickly it should be considered as the first-line treatment for residents with high risk of suicide (Kallenbach and Rigler, 2006).

A number of psychological approaches can treat depression in care homes. These include behaviour therapy, cognitive therapy, CBT (Hyer et al., 2008), and life review approaches. Social interventions include various types of recreational activities (Snowden et al., 2003), for example therapeutic biking programmes. Most of the studies cited above reported significant beneficial effects and some review papers have concluded that psychosocial approaches are effective in treating depression, in particular minor depression, in care home residents (Hyer et al., 2005; Snowden et al., 2003). Consistently, it is suggested that non-pharmacological methods should be considered as first-line treatment for residents with minor depression (American Geriatrics Society and American Association for Geriatric Psychiatry, 2003). It is important to note that many of these approaches were delivered in a group format. Group therapy is a more practical and cost-effective strategy as individual psycho-therapy is not readily available due to a shortage of psychotherapists (Snowden et al., 2003).

There is also some evidence that other approaches, such as staff training, changes in health service model (Snowden et al., 2003), and care home environment might also be effective in reducing residents' depressive symptoms.

It seems likely that a combination of medical and psychosocial approaches would be the ideal method to manage depression in care homes (American Geriatrics Society and American Association for Geriatric Psychiatry, 2003). Although further studies assessing the utility of such combined approaches are required, in recent years there has been increasing interest in multifaceted approaches to the treatment of depressed residents (Hyer et al., 2008; Jordan et al., 2009; Llewellyn-Jones et al., 1999). For example, the multifaceted shared care intervention of Llewellyn-Jones et al. (1999) included: (a) multidisciplinary consultation and collaboration to remove barriers to care, (b) training of general practitioners and carers in detection and management of depression, (c) depression-related health education and activity programmes for residents, such as gentle exercise classes and volunteer programmes to help frail and isolated residents. These studies have reported significant improvement in residents' depression and suggest that integrating multiple modalities should be an important direction.

As discussed, it can be difficult to identify depressed residents. It is also challenging to treat them effectively. Some antidepressants, such as selective serotonin reuptake inhibitors (SSRIs), may have limited effect in residents with dementia. In addition, these residents may not be able to participate in psychotherapy because of their limited cognitive function (Kallenbach and Rigler, 2006).

There are some important methodological limitations in current treatment studies. These include: small sample sizes, variable inclusion criteria (Hyer et al., 2005; Snowden et al., 2003), short treatment duration (Hyer et al., 2005), few randomized controlled trials, and differing outcome measures. However, these studies, as a group, provide strong evidence that depression is treatable in nursing home residents (Hyer et al., 2005).

Issues in treatment of depression

In spite of the evidence that depression is treatable in care home residents, it is under-treated in this group (Hyer et al., 2005;). About 50%, or even up to 75% of residents with depression receive no treatment at all (George et al., 2007; Rovner et al., 1991).

Although there is evidence that the initiation of treatment for depression has improved in recent years, it is often inadequate or inappropriate. First, there is a reliance on antidepressants and very few residents receive other treatments (George et al., 2007). Second, many residents receiving antidepressants are on doses too low to be effective (Brown et al., 2002; Draper et al., 2001). Antidepressant use is rarely reviewed by physicians (O'Connor et al., 2010). Given these problems, it is not surprising that only a minority of residents on antidepressants show improvements in symptoms (Draper et al., 2001). The findings of under treatment and inadequate treatment of depression in care home residents have major implications for the management of depression in these environments. Many researchers have suggested that the management should go beyond first level problems, such as identification and initial treatment, to include second level problems, such as strategies for partial responders and non-responders, and ongoing management through the maintenance phases (Draper et al., 2001).

Outcome and prognosis

There is a two-way relationship between depression and risk factors for depression. Depression in care homes is linked to poor physical health, decreased physical and cognitive abilities, pain, and poor nutrition. Depressed residents also have lower levels of social engagement, more behavioural and vocal disturbance (Brodaty et al., 2001), poorer quality of life, and increased use of healthcare services (Smalbrugge et al., 2006).

The most alarming outcome of depression is that it is a significant risk factor for mortality in care home residents. Rovner et al. (1991) found that the likelihood of death at 1 year was increased by 59% for residents with major depression as compared with those with only depressive symptoms or no depression. Ashby et al. (1991) followed 973 care home residents for 8 to 16 months and found that depression was associated with increased mortality; depressed residents were three times more likely to die than those without depression or dementia. In a study by Parmelee et al. (1992a, 1992b) of 898 nursing home and congregate apartment residents, the mortality rates were 33% for residents with major depression, 28% for residents with minor depression, and 16% for non-depressed residents after 18 months. This result indicates a systematic and significant increase in mortality with increasing severity of depression.

These studies indicate that depression is related to increased mortality in care home residents. However, there is controversy about how depression exerts its effect. While some studies found that depression was an independent risk factor for mortality in care home residents (Rovner et al. 1991), others found no significant relationship between depression and mortality when age, sex, physical health, functional impairment, cognitive status, and history of depression were taken into account (Parmelee et al., 1992a, 1992b). The different results in these studies might be due to methodological differences, such as the definition of depression, the sampling strategies, and the sample sizes, and more studies are needed for a clearer understanding of the relationship between depression and mortality in care home residents.

Much depression in care homes is chronic, with persistence rates ranging from 44% to 63%. Sutcliffe et al. (2007) followed 308 newly admitted UK care home residents for 9 months. Of the residents who were depressed at baseline, 44% were still depressed after 5 and 9 months. Similarly, Barca et al. (2010) reported a persistence rate of 45% after 12 months. Smalbrugge et al. (2006) followed 350 Dutch nursing home residents for 6 months and reported a persistence rate of 63%. Weyerer et al. (1995) followed 120 newly admitted residents (60 from German residential homes and 60 from UK homes) for 8 months. The prevalence of depression was high in both cities at admission (35% in Mannheim and 48% in London) and did not change significantly over 8 months. Most importantly, the study found that in both places, depression at baseline was the best predictor for depression 3 months and 8 months later, but sex, age, social isolation, ADLs, and cognitive impairment at the time of admission were not significantly associated with depression 3 and 8 months later.

The persistence rate seems to be lower for depressed residents with dementia. Payne et al. (2002) followed 201 residents with cognitive impairment. They found that at 6 months, only 15% of the depressed patients were still depressed, and at 12 months only 7.5% were depressed. The study suggested that the decline in depression over the year after admission likely reflects appropriate diagnosis and treatment of depression in care homes.

Depression is probably a risk factor for suicide in care home residents. A study in Finland found that 12 nursing home residents died by committing suicide in a 12-month period, accounting for 0.9% of all suicides in Finland in that year. Nine (75%) of them were diagnosed with a depressive syndrome, although only three (33%) were recognized by staff as having depressive symptoms before their death (Suominen et al., 2003).

It is important to point out that there are as yet relatively few outcome studies of depression in care homes and most of those studies have short follow-up periods (Llewellyn-Jones and Snowdon, 2007). More longitudinal studies are needed for a better understanding of the outcomes of depression in care homes.

Conclusion

Despite increased detection and treatment of depression in recent years, depression remains a significant problem for older people living in care homes. Prevalence remains high and the few longitudinal studies that have been conducted show high persistence of depression over time. Care staff still lack knowledge and understanding of depression, with many seeing depression as a normal phenomenon for older people (Ayalon et al., 2008). Depression is therefore often not detected or treated. This lack of detection and treatment may have serious consequences, as depression does not often remit spontaneously in care home residents (Barca et al., 2010; Smalbrugge et al., 2006) and is a significant risk factor for mortality (Ashby et al., 1991; Rovner et al., 1991) and suicide (Suominen et al., 2003). Detection is the first step in initiating assessment and treatment for depression.

Further research is needed to investigate those treatment approaches that appear promising, particularly multifaceted (Llewellyn-Jones et al., 1999) and psychosocial approaches (Hyer et al., 2005; Snowden et al., 2003). There is also a need for more longitudinal studies to inform us about incidence, persistence, and outcomes of depression.

There is a strong need for education of care staff (particularly personal carers) to ensure they recognize the signs and symptoms of depression and understand that it is a serious and treatable condition. Screening for depression should be mandatory in all care homes and linked to a process for referral and initiation of assessment and treatment. Finally, care homes should address environmental factors associated with depression, such as lack of privacy, and institute interventions known to benefit people with depression, such as recreational activities, for all residents.

References

Alexopoulos, G.S., Abrams, R.C., Young, R.C., & Shamoian, C.A. (1988). Cornell Scale for depression in dementia. *Biological Psychiatry*, *23*, 271–284.

American Geriatrics Society and American Association for Geriatric Psychiatry (2003). Consensus statement on improving the quality of mental health care in U.S. nursing homes: management of depression and behavioral symptoms associated with dementia. *Journal of the American Geriatrics Society*, *51*, 1287–1298.

American Psychiatric Association (1994). *DSM-IV: Diagnostic and Statistical Manual of Mental Disorders*. Washington, DC: American Psychiatric Association.

Ashby, D., Ames, D., West, C.R., MacDonald, A., Graham, N., & Mann, A.H. (1991). Psychiatric morbidity as predictor of mortality for residents of local authority homes for the elderly. *International Journal of Geriatric Psychiatry*, *6*, 567–575.

Ayalon, L., Arean, P., & Bornfeld, H. (2008). Correlates of knowledge and beliefs about depression among long-term care staff. *International Journal of Geriatric Psychiatry*, *23*, 356–363.

Bagley, H., Cordingley, L., Burns, A., et al. (2000). Recognition of depression by staff in nursing and residential homes. *Journal of Clinical Nursing*, *9*, 445–450.

Banazak, D.A., Mullan, P.B., Gardiner, J.C., & Rajagopalan, S. (1999). Practice guidelines and late-life depression assessment in long-term care. *Journal of General Internal Medicine*, *14*, 438–440.

Barca, M.L., Engedal, K., Laks, J., & Selbaek, G. (2010). A 12 months follow-up study of depression among nursing-home patients in Norway. *Journal of Affective Disorders*, *120*, 141–148.

Brodaty, H., Draper, B., Saab, D., et al. (2001). Psychosis, depression and behavioural disturbances in Sydney nursing home residents: prevalence and predictors. *International Journal of Geriatric Psychiatry*, *16*, 504–512.

Brown, M.N., Lapane, K.L., & Luisi, A.F. (2002). The management of depression in older nursing home residents. *Journal of the American Geriatrics Society*, *50*, 69–76.

Brühl, K.G., Hendrika, J.L., & Martien, T.M. (2007). Nurses' and nursing assistants' recognition of depression in elderly who depend on long-term care. *Journal of the American Medical Directors Association*, *8*, 441–445.

Burrows, A., Morris, J., Simon, S., Hirdes, J., & Phillips, C. (2000). Development of a minimum data set-based depression rating scale for use in nursing homes. *Age and Ageing*, *29*, 165–172.

Cataldo, J.K. (1994). Hardiness and death attitudes: predictors of depression in the institutionalized elderly. *Archives of Psychiatric Nursing*, *8*, 326–332.

Davidson, S., Koritsas, S., O'Connnor, D.W., & Clarke, D. (2006). The feasibility of a GP led screening intervention for depression among nursing home residents. *International Journal of Geriatric Psychiatry, 21*, 1026–1030.

De Bellis, A. & Williams, J. (2008). The Cornell Scale for depression in dementia in the context of the Australian aged care funding instrument: a literature review. *Contemporary Nurse, 30*, 20–31.

Draper, B., Brodaty, H., Low, L.-F., et al. (2001). Use of psychotropics in Sydney nursing homes: associations with depression, psychosis, and behavioral disturbances. *International Psychogeriatrics, 13*, 107–120.

George, K., Davison, T.E., McCabe, M., Mellor, D., & Moore, K. (2007). Treatment of depression in low-level residential care facilities for the elderly. *International Psychogeriatrics, 19*, 1153–1160.

Hyer, L., Carpenter, B., Bishmann, D., & Wu, H.-S. (2005). Depression in long-term care. *Clinical Psychology: Science and Practice, 12*, 280–299.

Hyer, L., Yeager, C.A., Hilton, N., & Sacks, A. (2008). Group, individual, and staff therapy: an efficient and effective cognitive behavioral therapy in long-term care. *American Journal of Alzheimer's Disease and Other Dementias, 23*, 528–539.

Jones, R., Koehler, M., Hirdes, J., et al. (2004). Measuring depression in nursing home residents with the MDS and GDS. *The Gerontologist, 44*, 55–56.

Jongenelis, K., Pot, A.M., Eisses, A.M.H., et al. (2005). Diagnostic accuracy of the original 30-item and shortened versions of the Geriatric Depression Scale in nursing home patients. *International Journal of Geriatric Psychiatry, 20*, 1067–1074.

Jordan, F., Byrne, G., & Bushell, A. (2009). *Improving Mental Health in Aged Care Facilities: A Feasibility Study*. Lutwyche, Queensland: in partnership with GPpartners, Deakin University, *beyondblue*, University of Queensland and Carers Queensland (funded by the Australian Government Department of Health and Ageing).

Junginger, J., Phelan, E., Cherry, K., & Levy, J. (1993). Prevalence of psychopathology in elderly persons in nursing homes and in the community. *Hospital and Community Psychiatry, 44*, 381–383.

Kallenbach, L.E. & Rigler, S.K. (2006). Identification and management of depression in nursing facility residents. *Journal of the American Medical Directors Association, 7*, 448–455.

Koritsas, S., Davidson, S., Clarke, D., & O'Connor, D. (2006). Diagnosing and treating depressions in nursing home residents: challenges for GPs. *Australian Journal of Primary Health, 12*, 104–108.

Lach, H., Chang, Y., & Edwards, D. (2010). Can older adults with dementia accurately report dementia using brief forms? *Journal of Gerontological Nursing, 36*, 30–37.

Llewellyn-Jones, R.H., Baikie, K.A., Smithers, H., Cohen, J., Snowdon, J., & Tennant, C.C. (1999). Multifaceted shared care intervention for late life depression in residential care: randomised controlled trial. *British Medical Journal, 319*, 676–682.

Llewellyn-Jones, R.H. & Snowdon, J. (2007). Depression in nursing homes: ensuring adequate treatment. *CNS Drugs, 21*, 627–640.

McCurren, C. (2002). Assessment for depression among nursing home elders: evaluation of the MDS mood assessment. *Geriatric Nursing, 23*, 103–108.

McDougall, F.A., Matthews, F.E., Kvaal, K., Dewey, M.E., & Brayne, C. (2007). Prevalence and symptomatology of depression in older people living in institutions in England and Wales. *Age and Ageing, 36*, 562–568.

Meeks, S., Shah, S.N., & Ramsey, S.K. (2009). The pleasant events schedule—nursing home version: a useful tool for behavioral interventions in long-term care. *Aging & Mental Health, 13,* 445–455.

O'Connor, D.W., Griffith, J., & McSweeney, K. (2010). Changes to psychotropic medications in the six months after admission to nursing homes in Melbourne, Australia. *International Psychogeriatrics, 22,* 1149–1153.

Parmelee, P.A., Katz, I.R., & Lawton, M.P. (1992a). Depression and mortality among institutionalized aged. *Journal of Gerontology, 47,* 3–10.

Parmelee, P.A., Katz, I.R., & Lawton, M.P. (1992b). Incidence of depression in long-term care settings. *Journal of Gerontology, 47,* M189–M196.

Payne, J.L., Sheppard, J.-M.E., Steinberg, M., et al. (2002). Incidence, prevalence, and outcomes of depression in residents of a long-term care facility with dementia. *International Journal of Geriatric Psychiatry, 17,* 247–253.

Rinaldi, P., Mecocci, P., Benedetti, C., et al. (2003). Validation of the five-item geriatric depression scale in elderly subjects in three different settings. *Journal of the American Geriatrics Society, 51,* 694–698.

Rovner, B.W., German, P.S., Brant, L.J., Clark, R., Burton, L., & Folstein, M.F. (1991). Depression and mortality in nursing homes. *Journal of American Medical Association, 265,* 993–996.

Ruckdeschel, K., Thompson, R., Datto, C.J., Streim, J.E., & Katz, I.R. (2004). Using the minimum data set 2.0 mood disturbance items as a self-report screening instrument for depression in nursing home residents. *American Journal of Geriatric Psychiatry, 12,* 43–49.

Seitz, D., Purandare, N., & Conn, D. (2010). Prevalence of psychiatric disorders among older adults in long-term care homes: a systematic review. *International Psychogeriatrics, 22,* 1025–1039.

Smalbrugge, M., Jongenelis, L., Pot, A.M., Eefsting, J.A., Ribbe, M.W., & Beekman, A.T. (2006). Incidence and outcome of depressive symptoms in nursing home patients in the Netherlands. *American Journal of Geriatric Psychiatry, 14,* 1069–1076.

Smalbrugge, M., Pot, A.M., Jongenelis, L., Gundy, C.M., Beekman, A.T.F., & Eefsting, J.A. (2006). The impact of depression and anxiety on well being, disability and use of health care services in nursing home patients. *International Journal of Geriatric Psychiatry, 21,* 325–332.

Snowden, M., Sato, K., & Roy-Byrne, P. (2003). Assessment and treatment of nursing home residents with depression or behavioral symptoms associated with dementia: a review of the literature. *Journal of the American Geriatrics Society, 51,* 1305–1317.

Suominen, K., Henriksson, M., Isometsä, E., Conwell, Y., Heilä, H., & Lönnqvist, J. (2003). Nursing home suicides—a psychological autopsy study. *International Journal of Geriatric Psychiatry, 18,* 1095–1101.

Sutcliffe, C., Burns, A., Challis, D., et al. (2007). Depressed mood, cognitive impairment, and survival in older people admitted to care homes in England. *American Journal of Geriatric Psychiatry, 15,* 708–715.

Watson, L.C., Zimmerman, S., Cohen, L.W., & Dominik, R. (2009). Practical depression screening in residential care/assisted living: five methods compared with gold standard diagnoses. *American Journal of Geriatric Psychiatry, 17,* 556–564.

Weyerer, S., Häfner, H., Mann, A.H., Ames, D., & Graham, N. (1995). Prevalence and course of depression among elderly residential home admissions in Mannheim and Camden London. *International Psychogeriatrics, 7,* 479–493.

World Health Organisation (2004). *International Classification of Diseases: 10th Revision.* Geneva: World Health Organisation.

Chapter 15

Functional mental illness

Catherine Hatfield and Tom Dening

Abstract

The term 'functional' mental illness applies to mental disorders other than dementia, and includes severe mental illness such as schizophrenia and bipolar mood disorder. Symptoms of these disorders frequently persist into old age or, less frequently, begin in old age. Older people with long-term functional mental illness are often neglected in research with, and services for, older people. There are limited epidemiological data about the number of people with lifelong mental disorders or their needs profile. Often they have experienced social isolation and disadvantage throughout their lives, for example losing contact with relatives. In old age, they are more likely to experience various difficulties, including cognitive impairment, poor physical health, psychiatric comorbidity, side-effects from treatment, and social exclusion. Various models of residential care for the most disabled exist, though there is no single ideal form of provision. The chapter discusses how needs may be assessed and met, with support from primary care and specialist mental health services.

Definitions

This chapter addresses the needs of people with long-term mental illness other than dementia and depression. These comprise mainly patients with schizophrenia and bipolar affective disorder but, as will become evident, this is a very mixed group.

The so-called 'functional' mental illnesses are those where no organic basis for the symptoms has been found such as an identifiable lesion in the brain or a hormonal abnormality. This label has classically been applied to mood and anxiety disorders and to schizophrenia. With advances in technology it has become apparent that many so-called functional mental illnesses are associated with changes in brain structure and/or function such as increased ventricle size in schizophrenia (Johnstone et al., 1976; Shenton et al., 2001). Thus, this distinction is becoming obsolete but it continues to be in common use. Functional mental illnesses have been regarded as the province of psychiatrists, whereas organic brain disorders may be treated by neurologists or geriatricians. The International Classification of Diseases, Tenth Revision (ICD-10) continues to use the term organic disorder although the term functional has been discarded.

Natural history

Schizophrenia

Schizophrenia is a mental illness characterized by hallucinations and delusions. A hallucination is a perception in the absence of a stimulus and can occur in any sensory modality but auditory hallucinations are the most common. Sufferers typically hear voices speaking to them or about them or commenting on their actions.

A delusion is a fixed abnormal idea out of keeping with the individual's social and cultural background. Common themes include a belief that the person is being pursued or that others are plotting against him or her (persecutory delusion) or that things in the environment such as newspaper articles, television broadcasts, or the gestures of passers-by hold special significance for the person (referential delusion). The person may believe that he or she is being controlled by some external agency (delusion of passivity) or that his or her thoughts can be read by others (thought interference). In addition, the person's thoughts and speech may become disorganized and difficult to understand. These experiences are referred to as the positive symptoms of schizophrenia, and they are most apparent during acute episodes.

The negative symptoms are less well known and less obvious but can be the most disabling features of the illness in the long term. The person becomes apathetic and loses interest and motivation sometimes to the extent of neglecting basic hygiene. Emotional responses are reduced (blunted or flattened affect) or inappropriate to the situation (incongruous affect).

The peak age of the onset of schizophrenia is 15–25 for men and 20–40 for women. Nonetheless, 25% have an onset between 40 and 60 (late-onset schizophrenia) or over age 60 years (very late-onset schizophrenia) (Harris and Jeste, 1988; Castle and Murray, 1993). There has been considerable debate over whether late-onset schizophrenia is the same as the early-onset illness or a distinct disorder. Women greatly predominate in the late-onset illness. A female to male ratio of between 9 and 4 to 1 has been observed among those with onset over age 40. A family history of schizophrenia is less common and there is an association with sensory impairment and social isolation. In terms of clinical presentation, persecutory delusions are common, there tend to be less severe negative symptoms, and the illness is more responsive to lower doses of antipsychotic medication (Vahia et al., 2010).

The course of the illness is very variable. Some patients have one isolated episode of psychosis from which they make a full recovery (20%). Another 30% have recurrent episodes but make a full recovery in between. About 40% have recurrent episodes and never regain their premorbid function and a minority (10%) are resistant to treatment and continue to experience disabling positive and negative symptoms and require extensive support (Harding et al., 1987; De Sisto et al., 1995). Those with the poorest prognosis are most likely to be admitted to long-term institutional care.

Bipolar affective disorder

Bipolar affective disorder (commonly known as manic depression) is characterized by extremes of mood. Patients experience episodes of depression with loss of pleasure, low energy, poor sleep, and appetite together with hopeless, worthless, and guilty thoughts; and episodes of mania with elevated mood, overtalkativeness, less need for sleep, very high energy levels, and excessive self-confidence. In this state they may spend excessively or take unaccustomed risks. In either state they may experience psychotic symptoms of delusions or hallucinations.

Four or more mood episodes occurring in 1 year are referred to as rapid cycling and this is harder to treat, with worse outcomes.

Again, bipolar disorder commonly has its onset in adolescence or early adult life. There is however a further peak in old age which is associated with more organic aetiology, particularly vascular lesions.

Other mental disorders

This includes a range of other mental health problems, including anxiety disorders, obsessive-compulsive disorder, addictions, and personality disorders. There are also individuals who may have more than one diagnosis. Among older people in long-term care, there will be some in whom no clear diagnosis can be made, for example because there are no available informants and the earlier history of the problem cannot be traced. This mixed group of 'other' diagnoses constitutes approximately 10% of the population with long-term functional illness, though such a figure is likely to be imprecise.

Epidemiology

There are no national data for the numbers of older people with functional mental illness living in institutional settings in the United Kingdom.

The adult psychiatric morbidity survey last undertaken in 2007 included data for people aged 16–74 years, but was restricted to those living in private households and excluded the 4% of people aged over 65 years living in care homes.

A previous survey looked at the extent of psychiatric morbidity in those living in institutions but was restricted to the 16–64 age group (Meltzer et al., 2003). That survey found 33,200 adults permanently resident in accommodation for people with mental health problems. One-third of residents were in NHS hospitals, while about two-thirds were in residential care facilities. About two-thirds of adults interviewed suffered from schizophrenia, delusional, and schizoaffective disorders, 8% suffered from neurotic disorders, and 8% suffered from affective psychoses (mainly bipolar affective disorder).

Smaller community surveys have given prevalence rates of 0.1–0.5% (Copeland et al., 1998; Castle and Murray, 1993; McNulty et al., 2003). Regional prevalence figures will be affected by the historical structure of services, in particular the presence of large old mental hospitals in some areas. These prevalence rates are much lower than the 1% lifetime prevalence usually quoted for schizophrenia overall (Perälä et al., 2007). The difference might be accounted for by excess mortality or by incomplete ascertainment due to refusal to participate.

Social exclusion

People with schizophrenia are less likely to marry and have children than the general population. About two-fifths never marry and a further quarter are divorced. Two-fifths do not have children (Cohen and Talavera, 2000). They are also less likely to have been in employment and their lives may be disrupted by substantial periods of hospitalization. All of these factors lead to them having substantially reduced social networks (Abdallah et al., 2009). Of those contacts that they do have most are based on provision of sustenance or support (59% vs. 15% for age-matched peers) and few are intimate, confiding relationships (44% vs. 67%) (Cohen et al., 1996). This lack of financial and social resources predisposes people with enduring mental illness to care home admission.

On measures of social skills they are significantly impaired in accepting and initiating contact with others, group participation, and making friendships (Bartels et al., 1997a,b). Social withdrawal may be a mechanism to cope with distressing psychotic symptoms such as persecutory delusional beliefs or thought interference or may result from reduced capacity to enjoy friendships due to negative symptoms.

Despite these deficits older people with enduring mental illness do identify social needs as important. Auslander and Jeste (2002) examined the self-reported needs of a sample of 72 people (41–80 years). Around half of them lived independently and the remainder (47%) lived in an assisted care facility. The study excluded people with dementia or with a comorbid alcohol or substance abuse problem. The main priorities they identified were around social relationships (developing and sustaining friendships), managing their illness, and improvements in mood, physical health, and memory.

Routes to care home admission

Hospital discharge

In the early part of the twentieth century, people with long-term functional mental illness in the United Kingdom were cared for in large county asylums. From the 1960s onwards, this model of care was questioned as the disadvantages of long-term institutionalization became clear and bed numbers were gradually reduced with a shift of focus to care in the community. Older people with chronic psychosis were among the last to benefit from this approach. In addition to the impairments associated with their illness they were further handicapped by their long hospital stay and by having no independent living skills. Nonetheless studies in particular from the TAPS (team for the assessment of psychiatric services) group studying a cohort of people discharged from Friern Barnet Hospital in London have found some positive outcomes. Only 71 out of 130 were alive 3 years later (not significantly different from those remaining in hospital). Of those, half had returned to hospital but those remaining in the community had more social contacts and were more satisfied than those in hospital (Trieman et al., 1999; Leff and Trieman, 2000; Trieman and Leff, 2002).

Between 1954 and 1996, 110,000 psychiatric hospital beds were closed and only 13,000 community placements replaced them (Lelliott et al., 1996). With the closure of long-stay institutions, it is clear that some people with mental illness have been diverted to the prison or homeless populations (Crane and Warnes, 2000).

Admission from the community

Less is known about admission to institutions for older people with functional mental illness who had previously been dwelling in the community. Andrews et al., (2009) studied admissions to nursing homes over a 10-year period in New Hampshire, USA. They found a much younger age of entry to a nursing home among those with a diagnosis of schizophrenia (a mean age of 65 compared with 80 for those with no mental illness). The rates of admission started to diverge significantly between the ages of 40 and 65, where nursing home admission risk was 3.9 times greater than for peers with no mental illness. The reasons for this are not known but one could speculate that loss or burnout of the primary carer, who might be the parent for those diagnosed at a young age (usually young men) or the spouse for women with a later onset, may contribute. The percentage of people with mental illness living with their families varies between countries depending on cultural expectations and on provision of alternative resources. In the United States, approximately 40% of white people with severe mental illness lived with their families, increasing to 60–80% for those from ethnic minorities (Lefley and Hatfield, 1999). The majority of these were living with their parents. Increasing burden of negative symptoms, cognitive impairment, or physical frailty may also be determinants of care home admission.

Providing care for long-term mental illness

Suitable accommodation

From the 1970s and 1980s onwards, with the decline of long-stay wards within NHS hospitals, other types of provision have arisen to fill the void. Hostels and care homes run by private sector and voluntary organizations vary from those with 24-hour staffing by qualified staff to those with daytime cover only from a smaller number of staff without specialist qualifications. Group homes are unstaffed facilities where small groups of residents with chronic mental illness live together supported by visits from staff. A more recent model of care is where each individual has his or her own flat or bedsit but within a unit where there is a staff member present and often some communal facilities. There is evidence that this form of support is preferred by patients (Tanzman, 1993). Patterns of provision may be driven less by need and more by historical precedent. Some patients previously resident in long-stay hospital wards were 'trans-institutionalized' rather than deinstitutionalized as they were moved into nursing homes which differed very little from the wards from which they had come.

As people with enduring mental illness become older, physical disabilities may mean that their needs can no longer be met in their previous setting. Because their numbers are small, those with functional illness are often placed in settings designed mainly for people with severe dementia that may be poorly placed to meet their needs. Opportunities for social interaction and participation in particular are likely to be severely limited and freedoms curtailed. These problems might be overcome by better staff education and individual care planning and risk assessment.

Two examples of different types of home are described in the two vignettes.

Vignette: home A

The home was purpose built to accommodate the residents of two old wards in the Victorian mental hospital. It was provided by a housing association that already provided several group homes in the town but this was their first experience for older people in a residential setting. The home consisted of four flats each with six residents. It was centrally located, so residents could access the town centre. There was generous communal space and provision for activities, such as art therapy. A consultant psychiatrist visited every 6 weeks to review residents and their care plans.

As it was a specialist home for older people providing nursing care for mental health problems, the establishment included a registered mental nurse with each shift. However, recruitment always proved difficult and this aim was not always achieved. The home was popular with its residents, many of whom had high levels of persisting psychotic symptoms. As time went on, levels of physical need increased but the home was able to transfer very frail residents to mainstream nursing homes. Few residents required readmission to psychiatric hospital care. Several were on high doses of medication and it proved difficult to reduce these to safer levels.

Over time, the environment deteriorated, especially when the open plan staircase had to be boxed in after an incident. The difficulty of recruiting staff took its toll and the host organization wished to move away from providing this type of unit. Numbers of referrals, and hence of residents fell, and the home was eventually closed after almost 20 years.

Vignette: home B

A newly built extra care housing scheme consisting of 46 self-contained two-bedroom apartments, each with their own kitchen, bathroom, and living room. There are communal facilities including a restaurant and rooms for activities such as exercise classes and social events which are open to residents and to the wider community. The complex is owned by a housing association that also provides another extra care scheme, three care homes and four sheltered housing schemes. It is situated in a suburb of the city with local amenities such as small shops, a post office, a general practitioner (GP) surgery, and a chapel. There are care staff on site 24 hours a day 7 days a week who are able to provide assistance with personal care, cleaning, meals, and medication according to individual need. The residents have individual tenancy agreements with the housing association. The costs of additional care and support are charged on top of rent and service charges depending on usage and residents may refuse additional care or choose a different provider. Couples can move in together if one has needs which meet the criteria. There is an emphasis on promoting independence and autonomy and on involvement of service users. The scheme is not a specialist mental health placement but is open to all older people with care needs. Nonetheless, it has been successful in meeting the needs of a number of older people with functional mental illness who had previously experienced multiple hospital admissions and were unable to live independently. The community mental health team provide specialist support to residents and care staff as required.

Meeting residents' needs

There are significant challenges in caring for patients with long-term functional mental illness in a care home setting. The number of people with these diagnoses is small compared with those with dementia and their needs differ substantially from those of dementia patients. There will be fewer staff with experience or expertise in caring for this client group and less access to training or resources. These individuals will often have no family members or friends to act as advocates or supporters.

The symptoms and experiences of people with long-term mental illness may combine to make it harder to provide good care in a residential setting. For example, people with psychotic mental illness may have persecutory delusions about staff and this may make it very hard to establish any trusting relationships. This group of people will have a long experience of healthcare services, much of which may be negative. They may have suffered invasive treatments, lack of autonomy, negative attitudes, and discrimination. Such experience can lead to a profound mistrust of healthcare professionals. In addition, negative symptoms can make the person difficult to motivate, for example to attend to their personal hygiene or to join in group activities. The chronicity of symptoms means that any change resulting from an intervention may take a long time to see. Lack of insight is very common meaning that the person may deny that they have any illness or are in need of care or treatment. This can lead to difficult decisions about whether they have capacity to refuse and whether or when to intervene in a person's best interests.

As well as these challenges, there are other problems that are quite frequent in older people with functional disorders—cognitive impairment, psychiatric comorbidity, poor physical health, and issues around medication and other treatment—and these are discussed in the following sections. Taken as a whole, these characteristics mean that caring for this client group can be a very unrewarding experience, especially if the nature of their illnesses and their experiences is poorly understood. This needs to be acknowledged and provision made for staff support and supervision.

Support from mental health services

There has been much debate about who should provide services to older people with functional mental illness. People growing older with functional mental illnesses may perceive a great injustice in being discharged from services they have previously been able to access due to an arbitrary age cut-off of 65 years. Older people's mental health services are often more poorly resourced than rehabilitation services for younger adults and focused around dementia rather than functional illness. Access to services such as crisis resolution and home treatment teams for acute relapses or assertive outreach teams may be restricted to working age adults.

On the other hand, older people's services may be better placed to meet the needs of those with physical frailty or cognitive impairment whatever their age. In the United Kingdom, a recent Royal College of Psychiatrists report (Benbow et al., 2009) has recommended that transfer should be based on need rather than chronological age and that there should be agreed protocols in place.

In addition to age discrimination, people living in care homes receive poorer care from mental health services. They are often prevented from accessing day hospitals or community groups because of an assumption that their needs are being met within the care home. Community mental health teams may also be reluctant to provide input to clients in care homes for the same reason.

Complications of long-term mental illness

Cognitive impairment

Cognitive impairment has long been recognized as a component of the clinical syndrome of schizophrenia. Memory and executive functioning seem to be the most prominently impaired (Heinrichs and Zakzanis, 1998).

There is evidence that cognitive deficits are present at first episode and indeed even predate the onset of illness (Jones et al., 1994), but whether these deficits remain static throughout life or continue to deteriorate over time remains controversial (Rund, 1998; Kurtz, 2005). Cross-sectional studies of mostly younger community-dwelling patients with schizophrenia showed no differences in performance with age (Heaton et al., 1994; Eyler Zorilla et al., 2000), although they were grossly impaired compared with normal subjects. By contrast, studies of older institutionalized patients have shown deterioration over 2.5 years (Harvey et al., 1999; Friedman et al., 2001). Studies of long-term institutionalized patients may be confounded by the effects of institutionalization itself, use of long-term psychotropic medication, and selection for those with a poorer prognosis but they may better reflect the care home population (Auslander et al., 2001). Cognitive impairment is a better predictor of adaptive function than psychotic symptoms and thus patients with more severe cognitive impairment are more likely to be placed in care homes (Velligan et al., 1997).

Psychiatric comorbidity

Older people with functional mental illness are not more likely to have the neuropathological brain abnormalities of Alzheimer's disease than the general population (Arnold et al., 1998) but given the high prevalence of dementia in older age groups the conditions can co-occur. It can be very difficult to distinguish the cognitive impairments associated with schizophrenia from a new onset of dementia. Short-term memory loss, word finding difficulties, and disorientation are more associated with Alzheimer's disease, whereas frontal executive deficits are more associated with schizophrenia. The time course of cognitive decline should also be helpful in making the distinction.

Schizophrenia is frequently accompanied by mood problems: approximately 60% of people with schizophrenia suffer a major depression during the course of their illness and around a quarter experience depression following an acute schizophrenic episode (Martin et al., 1985). Depression is associated with poorer outcomes, including increased rates of relapse, longer duration of inpatient care, poorer response to drug treatments, chronic course, and suicide (Siris 2001). The diagnostic term schizoaffective disorder is sometimes applied to people who show evidence of both psychosis and mood disorders.

There is also a relationship between mood disorders and cognitive impairment, especially when the mood disorder has its onset in the second half of life. Such patients often show more evidence of organic brain changes, especially diffuse cerebrovascular disease and neuropsychological impairments.

With changing patterns of alcohol and drug use in recent years, there will indubitably be more older people with a history of illegal drug use in future decades and this may have implications for health services in general, as well as for the care home sector (Sajatovic et al., 2006).

Physical health

People with schizophrenia have a twofold to fourfold increased mortality rate compared with the general population and on average their life expectancy is reduced by 10–15 years (Brown et al., 2000). Much of this excess mortality is accounted for by suicides in earlier life but there is also an excess of deaths from natural causes.

There is an increased risk of death from cardiovascular and respiratory disease, infections, and type 2 diabetes (Jeste et al., 1996; Harris and Barraclough, 1998). This is likely to be multifactorial relating to lifestyle factors, side-effects of medication, and reduced access to healthcare. People with schizophrenia are more likely than the general population to have lifestyle risk factors for cardiovascular disease. They were found to be more likely to smoke, less likely to exercise, and more likely to have high fat, low fibre diets even when the study population was controlled for socioeconomic status (McCreadie and Scottish Schizophrenia Lifestyle Group, 2003; Osborn et al., 2008).

Side-effects of antipsychotic medication may also contribute to increased morbidity and mortality. The cardiovascular side-effects of antipsychotic medication include lengthening of the QT interval on electrocardiography which may contribute to arrhythmia and sudden cardiac death. The newer atypical antipsychotic medications are significantly associated with weight gain, raised cholesterol levels, and the development of type 2 diabetes. Conventional antipsychotic medications significantly elevate prolactin levels, which interferes with sexual functioning and reduces bone density increasing the risk of osteoporosis.

People with schizophrenia are less likely to receive treatment for physical health problems (Kilbourn et al., 2008; Vahia et al., 2008). Data from the Patient Outcomes Research Team (PORT) study in the United States (Dixon et al., 2000) showed that 30% of patients reporting a physical health condition were not receiving treatment. Patients may lack the motivation to attend appointments or cognitive deficits or delusional ideas may make it hard for them to comply with treatment plans. It is also likely that negative attitudes of care providers towards those with chronic mental illness play a role. In one study, GPs were less likely to offer screening for cardiovascular risk factors to people with schizophrenia than to those with asthma or another diagnosis (Roberts et al., 2007).

Medication

Older patients require lower doses of medication due to physiological changes associated with ageing. For example, there is an increase in the proportion of body fat with ageing, which increases the volume of distribution of lipid soluble drugs and prolongs their action, glomerular filtration rate decreases reducing clearance of renally excreted drugs such as lithium, and liver metabolism may also be reduced leading to increased plasma concentration of drugs such as benzodiazepines.

Older people are also more susceptible to side-effects from medication. Tardive dyskinesia (TD) is a particular problem with older typical antipsychotic medications such as haloperidol. TD describes involuntary movements, usually of the mouth and face but sometimes involving the limbs and trunk, which are associated with long-term use of antipsychotics. TD is often irreversible even after stopping medication and although patients are usually not aware of the movements they are obvious to others and can be stigmatizing. Studies of older hospitalized patients have shown rates of TD of over 60% (Quinn et al., 2001). Other common side-effects are those related to anticholinergic actions such as delirium, constipation, and urinary retention. All of these can be more severe in elderly people due to the interaction with physiological ageing, for example prostatic hypertrophy in older men causes them to have a higher risk of urinary retention. Orthostatic hypotension is more likely to lead to falls in older people.

Newer atypical antipsychotic medications carry less risk of TD but increased risk of weight gain, diabetes, and derangements of lipid metabolism. Earlier claims that atypical antipsychotics were more effective for negative symptoms have not been proven.

Clozapine is the only antipsychotic medication shown to have greater efficacy in treatment resistant schizophrenia (Kane et al., 1988) and has negligible risks of TD but its use is tightly controlled due to rare but serious adverse effects including agranulocytosis, cardiomyopathy, and seizures. Common adverse effects include sedation and postural hypotension. There is very little evidence to guide its use in older patients. One randomized controlled trial (RCT) comparing it with chlorpromazine in patients over 55 years found no differences between the two drugs (Howanitz et al., 1999).

Non-pharmacological treatments

There is now considerable evidence of benefit from cognitive behavioural therapy (CBT) in younger patients with schizophrenia (Tai and Turkington 2009). It is recommended for improving persistent psychotic symptoms and increasing insight and treatment adherence. Techniques include identifying and challenging irrational ideas, generating alternative explanations for symptoms, and testing out these explanations in behavioural experiments. This can be delivered in 1:1 sessions with a psychologist or in a group. Other psychological therapies such as social skills training and cognitive remediation have also been shown to be valuable in younger adults. Skills training is usually done in a group and may include learning about verbal and non-verbal communication and rules of social interaction using role-play and exercises.

There is very little research evidence for the use of psychological treatments of this kind in older people with long-term mental illness but one RCT of a combined social skills training and CBT intervention in 76 outpatients aged between 42 and 74 years found increased participation in social activities and greater insight (Granholm et al., 2005, 2008). In clinical practice these interventions are not widely available to older people. There has been considerable interest in psychological approaches to treatment in care homes (Vahia and Cohen, 2007), but most of this interest has been limited to people with dementia and challenging behaviour rather than those with functional illnesses.

Conclusions

Older people with enduring functional mental illness represent a vulnerable, marginalized group in society. They are liable to a double discrimination on grounds of age and mental illness and they are likely to receive poor quality care despite having profound needs. It is not clear what model of long-term care may be most suitable for this group of people. There may be a balance to be struck between some individuals whose needs may be best met in ordinary care homes and those who may require some more specialized accommodation. For this group, imaginative solutions, such as small supported group homes, may be the best option.

In caring for this group of people, there is a need for specialist training and support for staff to enable them to understand the wide-ranging impact of psychotic mental illness on patients' lives and tailor care plans to their individual needs. Again, how this is best met in practice remains unclear, but good support from both primary care and from specialist mental health services is likely to be important. Residents need access to good physical and mental health care, especially given their high risk of physical ill health, psychiatric comorbidity, and drug side-effects. Many of these harms might be avoided or reduced by screening, health promotion, and early treatment. As well as this, much better provision of psychosocial interventions needs to be extended to older people, together with more systematic study of what is effective.

References

Abdallah, C., Cohen, C.I., Sanchez-Almira, M., Reyes, P., & Ramirez, P. (2009). Community integration and associated factors among older adults with schizophrenia. *Psychiatric Services, 60,* 1642–1648.

Andrews, A.O., Bartels, S.J., Xie, H., & Peacock, W.J. (2009). Increased risk of nursing home admission among middle aged and older adults with schizophrenia. *American Journal of Geriatric Psychiatry, 17,* 697–705.

Arnold, S.E., Trojanowski, J.Q., Gur, R.E., Blackwell, P., Han, L.Y., & Choi, C. (1998). Absence of neurodegeneration and neural injury in the cerebral cortex in a sample of elderly patients with schizophrenia. *Archives of General Psychiatry, 55,* 225–232.

Auslander, L.A. & Jeste, D.V. (2002). Perceptions of problems and needs for service among middle-aged and elderly outpatients with schizophrenia and related psychotic disorders. *Community Mental Health Journal, 38,* 391–401.

Auslander, L.A., Lindamer, L.L., Delapena, J., et al. (2001). A comparison of community-dwelling older schizophrenia patients by residential status. *Acta Psychiatrica Scandinavica, 103,* 380–386.

Bartels, S.J., Mueser, K.T., & Miles, K.M. (1997a). A comparative study of elderly patients with schizophrenia and bipolar disorder in nursing homes and the community. *Schizophrenia Research, 27,* 181–190.

Bartels, S.J., Mueser, K.T., & Miles, K.M. (1997b). Functional impairments in elderly patients with schizophrenia and major affective disorders living in the community: social skills, living skills and behaviour problems. *Behaviour Therapy, 28,* 43–63.

Benbow, S.M., Ramakrishnan, A.N., Sibisi, C., et al. (2009). *Links not Boundaries: Service Transitions for People Growing Older with Enduring or Relapsing Mental Illness.* College report CR153. London: Royal College of Psychiatrists.

Brown, S., Inskip, H., & Barraclough, B. (2000). Causes of the excess mortality of schizophrenia. *British Journal of Psychiatry, 177*, 212–217.

Castle, D.J. & Murray, R.M. (1993). The epidemiology of late-onset schizophrenia. *Schizophrenia Bulletin, 19*, 691–700.

Cohen, C.I. & Talavera, N. (2000). Functional impairment in older schizophrenic persons: towards a conceptual model. *American Journal of Geriatric Psychiatry, 8*, 237–244.

Cohen, C.I., Talavera, N., & Hartung, R. (1996). Depression among older persons with schizophrenia who live in the community. *Psychiatric Services, 47*, 601–607.

Copeland, J.R., Dewey, M.E., Scott, A., et al. (1998). Schizophrenia and delusional disorder in older age: community prevalence, incidence, comorbidity, and outcome. *Schizophrenia Bulletin, 24*, 153–161.

Crane, M. & Warnes, A. (2000). Evictions and prolonged homelessness. *Housing Studies, 15*, 757–773.

De Sisto, M., Harding, C.M., McCormick, R.V., et al. (1995). The Maine and Vermont three decade studies of serious mental illness I: matched comparison of cross sectional outcome. *British Journal of Psychiatry, 167*, 331–342.

Dixon, L., Weiden, P., Delahanty, J., et al. (2000). Prevalence and correlates of diabetes in national schizophrenia samples. *Schizophrenia Bulletin, 26*, 903–912.

Eyler Zorrilla, L.T., Heaton, R.K., McAdams, L.A., Zisook, S., Harris, M.J., & Jeste, D.V. (2000). Cross-sectional study of older outpatients with schizophrenia and healthy comparison subjects: no differences in age-related cognitive decline. *American Journal of Psychiatry, 157*, 1324–1326.

Friedman, J.I., Harvey, P.D., Coleman, T., et al. (2001). Six-year follow-up study of cognitive and functional status across the lifespan in schizophrenia: a comparison with Alzheimer's disease and normal aging. *American Journal of Psychiatry, 158*, 1441–1448.

Granholm, E., McQuaid, J.R., McClure, F.S., et al. (2005). A randomized, controlled trial of cognitive behavioral social skills training for middle-aged and older outpatients with chronic schizophrenia. *American Journal of Psychiatry, 162*, 520–529.

Granholm, E., McQuaid, J.R., Link, P.C., Fish, S., Patterson, T., & Jeste, D.V. (2008). Neuropsychological predictors of functional outcome in Cognitive Behavioral Social Skills Training for older people with schizophrenia. *Schizophrenia Research, 100*, 133–143.

Harding, C.M., Brooks, G.W., Ashikaga, T., Strauss, J.S., & Breier, A. (1987). The Vermont longitudinal study of persons with severe mental illness. II: Long-term outcome of subjects who retrospectively met DSM-III criteria for schizophrenia. *American Journal of Psychiatry, 144*, 727–735.

Harvey, P.D., Silverman, J.M., Mohs, R.C., et al. (1999). Cognitive decline in late-life schizophrenia: a longitudinal study of geriatric chronically hospitalized patients. *Biological Psychiatry, 45*, 32–40.

Harris, E.C. & Barraclough, B. (1998). Excess mortality of mental disorder. *British Journal of Psychiatry, 173*, 11–53.

Harris, M.J. & Jeste, D.V. (1988). Late-onset schizophrenia: an overview. *Schizophrenia Bulletin, 14*, 39–55.

Heaton, R., Paulsen, J.S., McAdams, L.A., et al. (1994). Neuropsychological deficits in schizophrenics. Relationship to age, chronicity, and dementia. *Archives of General Psychiatry, 51*, 469–476.

Heinrichs, R.W. & Zakzanis, K.K. (1998). Neurocognitive deficit in schizophrenia: a quantitative review of the evidence. *Neuropsychology, 12*, 426–445.

Howanitz, E., Pardo, M., Smelson, D.A., et al. (1999). The efficacy and safety of clozapine versus chlorpromazine in geriatric schizophrenia. *Journal of Clinical Psychiatry*, *60*, 41–44.

Jeste, D.V., Gladsjo, J.A., Lindamer, L.A., & Lacro, J.P. (1996). Medical comorbidity in schizophrenia. *Schizophrenia Bulletin*, *22*, 413–430.

Johnstone, E.C., Crow, T.J., Frith, C.D., Husband, J., & Kreel, L. (1976). Cerebral ventricular size and cognitive impairment in chronic schizophrenia. *Lancet*, *2*, 924–926.

Jones, P., Rodgers, B., Murray, R., & Marmot, M. (1994). Child development risk factors for adult schizophrenia in the British 1946 birth cohort. *Lancet*, *344*, 1398–1402.

Kane, J.M., Honigfeld, G., Singer, J., & Meltzer, H. (1988). Clozapine treatment in treatment resistant schizophrenics. *Psychopharmacology Bulletin*, *24*, 62–67.

Kilbourne, A.M., Welsh, D., McCarthy, J.F., Post, E.P., & Blow, F.C. (2008). Quality of care for cardiovascular disease-related conditions in patients with and without mental disorders. *Journal of General Internal Medicine*, *23*, 1628–1633.

Kurtz, M.M. (2005). Neurocognitive impairment across the lifespan in schizophrenia: an update. *Schizophrenia Research*, *74*, 15–26.

Leff, J. & Trieman, N. (2000). Long-stay patients discharged from psychiatric hospitals. Social and clinical outcomes after five years in the community. The TAPS Project 46. *British Journal of Psychiatry*, *176*, 217–223.

Lefley, H.P. & Hatfield, A.B. (1999). Helping parental caregivers and mental health consumers cope with parental aging and loss. *Psychiatric Services*, *50*, 369–375.

Lelliott, P., Audini, B., Knapp, M., & Chisholm, D. (1996). The mental health residential care study: classification of facilities and description of residents. *British Journal of Psychiatry*, *169*, 139–147.

Martin, R.L., Cloninger, C.R., Guze, S.B., & Clayton, P.J. (1985). Frequency and differential diagnosis of depressive syndromes in schizophrenia. *Journal of Clinical Psychiatry*, *46*, 9–13.

McCreadie, R.G. & Scottish Schizophrenia Lifestyle Group (2003). Diet, smoking and cardiovascular risk in people with schizophrenia: descriptive study. *British Journal of Psychiatry*, *183*, 534–539.

McNulty, S.V., Duncan, L., Semple, M., Jackson, G.A., & Pelosi, A.J. (2003). Care needs of elderly people with schizophrenia. Assessment of an epidemiologically defined cohort in Scotland. *British Journal of Psychiatry*, *182*, 241–247.

Meltzer, H., Gill, B., Hinds, K., & Petticrew, M. (2003). The prevalence of psychiatric morbidity among adults living in institutions. *International Review of Psychiatry*, *15*, 129–133.

Osborn, D.P., Wright, C.A., Levy, G., King, M.B., Deo, R., & Nazareth, I. (2008). Relative risk of diabetes, dyslipidaemia, hypertension and the metabolic syndrome in people with severe mental illnesses: systematic review and metaanalysis. *BMC Psychiatry*, *8*, 84.

Perälä, J., Suvisaari, J., Saarni, S., et al. (2007). Lifetime prevalence of psychotic and bipolar I disorders in a general population. *Archives of General Psychiatry*, *64*, 19–28.

Quinn, J., Meagher, D., Murphy, P., Kinsella, A., Mullaney, J., & Waddington, J.L. (2001). Vulnerability to involuntary movements over a lifetime trajectory of schizophrenia approaches 100%, in association with executive (frontal) dysfunction. *Schizophrenia Research*, *49*, 79–87.

Roberts, L., Roalfe, A., Wilson, S., & Lester, H. (2007). Physical health care of patients with schizophrenia in primary care: a comparative study. *Family Practice*, *24*, 34–40.

Rund, B.R. (1998). A review of longitudinal studies of cognitive functions in schizophrenia patients. *Schizophrenia Bulletin*, *24*, 425–435.

Sajatovic, M., Blow, F.C., & Ignacio, R.V. (2006). Psychiatric co-morbidity in older adults with bipolar disorder. *International Journal of Geriatric Psychiatry, 21*, 582–587.

Shenton, M.E., Dickey, C.C., Frumin, M., & McCarley, R.W. (2001). A review of MRI findings in schizophrenia. *Schizophrenia Research, 49*, 1–52.

Siris, G. (2001). Depression in schizophrenia: perspective in the era of 'atypical' antipsychotics. *American Journal of Psychiatry, 158*, 1528–1529.

Tai, S. & Turkington, D. (2009). The evolution of cognitive behaviour therapy for schizophrenia: current practice and recent development. *Schizophrenia Bulletin, 35*, 865–873.

Tanzman, B. (1993). An overview of surveys of mental health consumers' preferences for housing and support services. *Hospital and Community Psychiatry, 44*, 450–455.

Trieman, N. & Leff, J. (2002). Long term outcome of long-stay psychiatric in-patients considered unsuitable to live in the community: TAPS Project 44. *British Journal of Psychiatry, 181*, 428–432.

Trieman, N., Leff, J., & Glover, G. (1999). Outcome of long stay psychiatric patients resettled in the community: prospective cohort study. *BMJ, 319*, 13–16.

Vahia, I.V. & Cohen, C.I. (2007). Psychosocial interventions and successful aging: new paradigms for improving outcome for older schizophrenia patients? *American Journal of Geriatric Psychiatry, 15*, 987–990.

Vahia, I.V., Diwan, S., Bankole, A.O., et al. (2008). Adequacy of medical treatment among older persons with schizophrenia. *Psychiatric Services, 59*, 853–859.

Vahia, I.V., Palmer, B.W., Depp, C., et al. (2010). Is late-onset schizophrenia a subtype of schizophrenia? *Acta Psychiatrica Scandinavica, 122*, 414–426.

Velligan, D.I., Mahurin, R.K., Diamond, P.L., Hazleton, B.C., Eckert, S.L., & Miller, A.L. (1997). The functional significance of symptomatology and cognitive function in schizophrenia. *Schizophrenia Research, 25*, 21–31.

Chapter 16

Psychosocial interventions in care homes

Graham Stokes

Abstract

This chapter considers the range of mental health needs to be found in care homes embracing both dementia and the psychological consequences of adjustment. The content addresses the need to restore resident function, promote well-being, and enhance quality of life through the provision of care homes that are therapeutic and have recovery of the person at the heart of what they do. The evidence for the success of psychosocial interventions is appraised, as is the contribution of narrative psychology whereby storytelling enables carers to understand their residents better and helps them to resolve distress and challenges. It is argued that the successful delivery of psychosocial interventions involves not only the relationship between carers and 'cared for' but also the need for systems of care to support therapeutic interventions. As such, organizational changes designed to deliver job satisfaction, staff support, and learning opportunities may be critical psychosocial interventions.

Introduction

This chapter addresses the efficacy of psychosocial interventions to meet the mental health needs of care home residents, most of whom are aged people living with dementia, using the term mental health to cover the emotional and behavioural consequences of dementia, as well as consequential and coexisting psychological disorders of depression and anxiety.

Dementia

A significant number of people living with dementia, probably a third to a half, live in care homes (Froggat and Parker, 2010). Research has suggested that the prevalence of dementia in care homes is over 60% and possibly as high as 75% (Matthews and

Dening, 2002; Macdonald et al., 2002) with many residents living with advanced dementia, some with complex challenging needs. Consequently, care homes have an important role to play in the provision of health and social care for people with dementia. Yet this state of affairs has not been planned for, either through commissioning services or through workforce planning and hence a number of challenges exist that inhibit the delivery of quality dementia care. The workforce is fluid in terms of retention and while staff may be caring most lack specific knowledge and expertise regarding psychosocial interventions. Yet without doubt it is care workers and nurses, not visiting professionals such as psychologists who are in the best position to deliver psychosocial interventions for the benefit of those in their care. A UK Parliamentary report (All-Party Parliamentary Group, 2009) recommended that psychological interventions and staff training in dementia care should be prioritized.

Psychosocial interventions

In the beginning, psychosocial approaches to dementia care were 'symptom-specific' and mechanistic (e.g. reality orientation [RO]) regarding people living with dementia as a homogeneous group with uniform needs and failings. Nowadays, psychological interventions are embedded within and pay heed to the individual needs of people with dementia. Consequently, we embrace a person with a psychology that is dimmed by dementia but not destroyed; a person with a unique life history that exerts influence over how he or she lives in a world that is rendered more complex and mysterious as time passes.

Acknowledging the presence of a person with dementia means striving to support and improve his or her well-being and quality of life though evidence-based psychosocial interventions even though to date evidence of efficacy remains meagre (Livingston et al., 2005). It is possible though that measures of success may be flawed as psychosocial gains may be transient, fading as soon as the support or intervention is withdrawn. Yet this cannot debase what has been achieved, for lasting maintenance of a positive emotional state may not be the appropriate goal. As dementia progresses and people are denied the capacity to retain experience, the 'here and now' is the therapeutic ground we ultimately occupy.

Interventions within care homes that meet people's psychological needs, affirm personhood, promote emotional well-being, and uphold social value constitute what is called person-centred care (Brooker, 2007).

Psychosocial interventions to understand and resolve behaviours that challenge

Behaviours that challenge carers have traditionally been understood in terms of symptoms of disease. Sometimes referred to as 'behavioural and psychological symptoms of dementia' (Finkel, 2003), behaviours such as repetitive questioning, walking with risk and nuisance, aggression, agitation, confusion, and screaming are invariably regarded as symptomatic of neurological disease. Consequently, therapeutic nihilism has historically prevailed with the attendant result that too often care homes strive to 'manage' residents' behaviour as best they can and hard-pressed general practitioners or remote psychiatrists viewing the care setting as the 'patient' resort to prescribing antipsychotic medication (Ballard and Margallo-Lana, 2001). Alldred et al. (2007) established a point prevalence antipsychotic prescribing rate of 32% for care home residents with dementia. Although the safety and efficacy of antipsychotics is controversial, Ballard and Aarsland (2010) conclude that the benefits of short-term antipsychotic use are modest while ongoing treatment benefits are limited.

Nowadays, many investigators contend that behaviours seen as challenging have multiple aetiologies and are amenable to psychosocial interventions (Osborne et al., 2010). Stokes (1996; 2000) argues that behaviours that challenge are often attempts to communicate unmet need and in most instances viewing these behaviours as symptoms of pathology is evidence of diagnostic overshadowing. A person who walks away from a chair, loses his or her way, and is said to be wandering is clearly affected by impaired recall and communication, but these cognitive decrements are not the reasons why the person decided to leave where he or she was sitting.

Behavioural (ABC) analysis (Stokes, 2000) establishes the environmental context—'the setting event'—of a behaviour (i.e. *where*, *when*, and *what* happened before, during, and immediately after the behavioural sequence) and determines whether a pattern and triggers exist. In turn, functional analysis attempts to identify the possible reasons *why* a person acts in that way in that specific setting at that particular time in the company of those people.

Case study 1

Mr G was unpredictably violent. Behavioural analysis identified 47 violent assaults (B = behaviour) in 9 days and a consistent pattern. On 96% of occasions, Mr G was violent while he was receiving intimate personal care, nearly always if those actions were to do with his toileting (A = antecedents).

It was equally clear that the actions of the staff were not maintaining his violence for their responses were varied and unpredictable (C = consequences). Sometimes they persisted in their actions to care for him, at other times they would walk away, recoil, or scold him. On the odd occasion they would attempt to restrain him.

Behavioural analysis provided the foundation for the functional analysis. Mr G had been a teacher. His wife disclosed that her husband was a reserved, conservative, and stubborn man. Keeping up appearances was all important to him. His passion was the solitary pursuit of gardening. Yet in his teaching what motivated him more than anything was seeing students learn. Unfortunately, his standards were high and his manner was frequently misunderstood. As a result people rarely warmed to him.

Mr G was clearly not a man who was going to prosper living in a care home. A proud and insular man, he was never going to be comfortable receiving intimate care that to him would constitute an inexplicable invasion of his privacy.

Behavioural and functional analysis had revealed both an understanding of Mr G's behaviour and a possible solution.

Mr G's need for hygiene could only be met with assistance. This would, however, violate his need for privacy and self-respect and result in a violent reaction. Yet, if carers addressed his need to be left alone they would fail to meet Mr G's need for hygiene. Consequently, a care plan was required that would permit staff to reconcile Mr G's need to be assisted to the toilet with his need to be free of unwelcome attention.

The sensory garden provided the hope of achieving change. Every 2 hours, Mr G was approached but the word 'toilet' was never mentioned. Instead, the topic to be talked about was the garden, not simply in terms of 'would you like to visit the garden' but the care plan embraced the pleasure he had derived from helping his students learn. In the process, the disempowerment so commonly observed in the lives of people with dementia living in care homes was reversed.

Acknowledging his position as a teacher, Mr G was placed in a position of authority and his advice sought—do the roses need pruning, were they weeds or flowers, does the lawn need mowing, or the bugs exterminating? His status had been blended with his joy of gardening.

Mr G understood a fair amount, even though he said little. Without saying a word Mr G would rise from his chair and as he was assisted along the corridor towards the garden he was repeatedly reminded where they were heading. The route ensured he would walk past two communal toilets. On reaching the toilet he was asked whether he wanted to use the toilet before going into the garden. For an enthusiastic gardener of his generation this would be customary practice. He could be outside for hours and would not want to be caught short and have to walk back through his house wearing muddy boots because he desperately needed the toilet.

On nearly all occasions, Mr G would use the toilet and his dressing skills were sufficiently well preserved to enable him to do so independently.

After using the toilet he was reminded that they were heading off to the garden and how grateful they were for his help. Once in the garden, Mr G gazed at the flowers and foliage with obvious delight.

Two hours later he was approached again and a fresh episode would unfold. So severe was his dementia that Mr G could not remember that what was unfolding had occurred 2 hours earlier.

To evidence-base the effectiveness of the revised care plan the frequency of violent incidents continued to be recorded. In 2 weeks Mr G was violent on just six occasions.

Functional analysis considers the contribution of neurobiological factors, life history, 'unobservable antecedent private events', which may include thoughts, beliefs, and the meaning of the behaviour (Samson and McDonnell, 1990), and the interrelationships with the 'setting event'. Hypotheses that are generated about the function of a person's behaviour lead to case-specific interventions.

However, what is commonly heard from staff working in care homes is 'we haven't got time to . . .' Consequently, behavioural and functional analysis does not need to be a planned intervention but instead provides the conceptual framework when thinking about behaviour in dementia. Encouraging carers to think about 'what, when, where, and why' rather than being seduced by the simplicity of the erroneous analysis, 'it's because (s)he has dementia' enables care homes to become therapeutic care settings.

Case study 2

Mrs D was 'unmanageable' at night. She would not stay in her bedroom to sleep and if she was returned she would become agitated and destructive. Out of her room she would return to the lounge or enter the bedrooms of other residents and get into bed alongside them.

The colour scheme of Mrs D's bedroom was purple and mauve. Deep purple duvet, curtains, and carpet set against mauve wallpaper. A review of her life history revealed that Mrs D had been a devout Roman Catholic and in the Catholic faith the colour purple is associated with death, grief, and mourning. It was hypothesized that Mrs D's behaviour was revealing an engrained morbid dread of the colour purple and its distressing association with death and mourning. When away from her room she was psychologically comfortable, however when confronted with her bedroom and its colour scheme she was consumed by foreboding and sought sanctuary elsewhere. Thus, it was not where she was heading, but where she was leaving that was significant. If the analysis was right and her room constituted a traumatic 'setting event' then the solution lay in a simple exchange of bedrooms.

One evening Mrs D moved into a bedroom that was colour coordinated light and dark green and she slept throughout the night. Never again did Mrs D try to leave her room. Informal behavioural and functional analysis had resolved Mrs D's distressed behaviour.

There is a growing evidence-based support for the concept of needs-related behaviours that challenge (Downs et al., 2008), as well as accumulating narrative-based evidence to illustrate that such behaviours are often driven by enduring psychological need (Stokes, 2008). Recently, a UK dementia care clinical guideline stated that 'Health and social care staff should identify the specific needs of people with dementia . . . understanding behaviour that challenges as a communication of unmet need' (National Institute for Health and Clinical Excellence, 2006).

Following analysis functional displacement is an intervention that consists of providing the person with functionally equivalent but more socially appropriate ways of meeting their needs (Moniz-Cook et al., 2003). However, for functional displacement to work the alternative action must be functionally equivalent to the challenging behaviour not just socially appropriate; the new behaviour cannot be more 'effortful'; and in dementia care, because profound learning impairments inhibit the acquisition of new information, the functionally equivalent alternative must be either a feature of the interaction between caregivers and the person with dementia, thereby allowing the behaviour to be maintained by the carer, or the functionally equivalent response must at the very least be the most obvious option available (Stokes, 2008).

Simulated presence therapy (SPT) was first described by Woods and Ashley (1995). Recording the voice of a significant attachment figure simulates their presence and may help to reduce distress-related aggression and agitation. A number of studies have shown that SPT can successfully alleviate 'problem behaviours' (Byatt and Cheston, 1999), although SPT does not work for all people (Peak and Cheston, 2002).

Activity therapy

A subjective indicator of good practice in care homes is the provision of recreational and social activities.

Physical exercise sessions requiring gentle movement and task attention have reported improvements in both fitness and cognitive function (Hopman-Rock et al., 1999).

To address the severity of dementia accommodated in care homes, passive and multisensory stimulation interventions have been used to improve the quality of life for people with advanced dementia. Music, aromatherapy, massage, and pet therapy have all been advocated, and the benefits of music have been shown (Goddaer and Abraham, 1994). In a comparison of three types of activity—music, puzzle exercises, and recreational activities, such as drawing and painting—it was found that music elicited the greatest degree of enjoyment, pleasure, and engagement (Lord and Garner, 1993), although there is no evidence of lasting benefits for either music or multisensory stimulation (Livingston et al., 2005).

Although there is evidence to support the use of aromatherapy, responses seem to be individual. A recent review identified 11 prospective randomized controlled trials (RCTs) of aromatherapy in people with dementia (Nguyen and Paton, 2008) and found that the data supporting efficacy were meagre with both negative and positive effects being reported. The same review also draws attention to the potential toxicity of the oils and the need to be vigilant for side-effects.

Multisensory rooms (sometimes referred to as a Snoezelen) have subdued lighting and comprise relaxing music, visual stimulation from optic fibres, kaleidoscopes, and lava lamps, tactile stimulation, and at times aromatherapy. Now found in many care homes, their use has been associated with mood improvement and a reduction in behavioural disturbance (Baker et al., 1997). A study in nursing homes evaluated an 18-month programme of individualized exposure to multisensory stimulation integrated into a resident's 24-hour plan of care and showed an improvement in depression, a reduction in apathy, and less disturbed behaviour (Van Weert et al., 2005). However, what can contaminate evaluations of multisensory stimulation is that such interventions can be affected by non-specific effects such as the presence of the carer who engages with the person in a way that is invariably intimate, patient, and encouraging.

Recently, interest has been shown in brief social and activity encounters when caring for people with advanced dementia, what Sheard (2008) calls 'butterfly moments'. Communication between residents with dementia and care workers can be very limited again because carers feel they have little time. However, 'butterfly moments' involve carers engaging with residents for no more than a minute or two before moving onto a similarly brief purposeful interaction with other residents. Such brief interactions are not to be dismissed as superficial, delivered in this way because that is all time allows. The methodology is predicated on the awareness that if a person's capacity to remember is measured in minutes, then why not provide engagement that corresponds with this restricted memory span? Furthermore, while episodic memory is fragile and degrades rapidly, emotional benefits may not be similarly brief for the psychological and physiological correlates of well-being may well persist for longer than the memory of why a person should feel calm and content. Clearly, the benefit for the culture of care is that brief encounters are less likely to fall prey to the press of time that care staff experience and which often conspires against the introduction and maintenance of time-consuming recreational activities.

Cognitive stimulation therapy

Cognitive stimulation therapy (CST) is an intervention that has a strong evidence base and draws on the practice of the once-popular group RO. CST has a similar social format but also includes non-cognitive and cognitive exercises, reminiscence, and multisensory stimulation. In a controlled trial of a 14-session programme for older people with mild to moderate dementia, CST resulted in significant improvements on two measures of cognition, with associated improvements in quality of life although if therapy gains are to be maintained CST needs to be continued on a regular basis (Spector et al., 2003). Studies have also suggested that CST may enhance the effects of acetylcholinesterase inhibitors though expectations must be tailored to the findings that there is little evidence that CST positively affects day-to-day behaviour and performance (Woods and Clare, 2008) and CST is unlikely to benefit people with severe dementia.

Reality orientation

Reality orientation was in many ways the first psychological intervention to enter dementia care (Folsom, 1968). Practised within the framework of either structured, time-limited groups or as part of daily discourse (24-hour RO), it began to fall into disrepute during the 1980s as it became apparent that not only was it no 'miraculous cure' but it also did not attempt to understand the personal experience of dementia. Reports of its limitations and adverse effects led some to question whether there was a place for RO in contemporary dementia care (Woods, 1994).

Although 'group RO' has evolved into CST, there remains a role for 24-hour RO. Orienting people to their environment offers valued support and common sense dictates the need to use environmental cues, natural as well as the cues offered by signage and directional information (e.g. while a toilet sign may alert a resident to the fact that he or she is in the proximity of a toilet, seeing armchairs and a settee are the natural cues that tell someone this is where he or she can sit and rest), as well as verbal orientation to help people find their way.

However, RO is a prosthetic therapy that can never resolve the underlying inability to learn and in advanced dementia the prosthetic value of cues may never be acquired. For this reason, the results of RO in counteracting the more disabling consequences of disorientation have been generally disappointing. However, one study found that while orientation designs improved way-finding and helped foster independence the most significant development was the way in which staff became enthusiastic and adopted a positive outlook (Bignall, 1996).

Nowadays, 24-hour verbal orientation is also one of the means by which the fears of a person living with dementia can be acknowledged, the accuracy of their observations affirmed, and empathic support offered (Stokes, 2000).

If 24-hour RO remains part of the therapeutic care offered to people struggling with disorientation, it has little or no role to play in a carer's response to confusion. Confusion can be defined as the living or reporting of a reality that is different to our own (Stokes, 2000) and exposing people with dementia to RO is unlikely to result in involvement in present-day reality. Instead, carers engage in reality confrontation. The focus of attention therefore needs to be not on a person's factual errors but the feelings that flow from what constitutes his or her personal truth—a world of small children to be found, jobs to go to, a home to return to, and parents and partners to find.

Validation

While it would be wrong to dismiss RO as the mechanistic communication of information, validation therapy (VT) disputes the need to orientate and argues that we accept 'whatever reality they are in, in order to ease distress...' (Morton and Bleathman, 1991). Happening in small groups or as an aspect of individual caring relationships, VT does not concern itself with factual errors, but acknowledges that the emotion underlying a person's words and actions is true and real, and this is the material for therapeutic intervention. However, we need to distinguish VT from validation.

VT has been described as theoretically incoherent and unconvincing, offering little to our understanding of dementia (Goudie and Stokes, 1989). A Cochrane review identified only three studies of group VT that warranted inclusion in the review and the results from these studies were inconclusive (Neal and Barton-Wright, 2007).

Validation is neither a theory nor therapy but is an essential aspect of relating to people living with dementia and is the acceptance of the reality and 'personal truth' of another's experience (Kitwood, 1996).

Case study 3

A woman with dementia struggled with her inability to remember. She found difficulty storing experiences that were ongoing or recent. Her memory for what she intended to do often let her down. Her problems at work accumulated. With failing insight her behaviour was erratic and eventually intolerable. After months on sick leave she retired on the grounds of ill-health.

Aged 51 years, divorced and living alone when she awakes on the first morning of her retirement where does she go? To work. To her yesterday has not happened. She cannot recall the gifts, tearful embraces, and fond farewells. From our perspective she is confused. Yet she does not believe she has a job, she *knows* it. As months pass her family are ever more exasperated as they are telephoned again and again by neighbours telling them their mother has left her house to go to work.

As Ribot's law slowly and remorselessly exercises its effect, more and more experiences from her recent past disappear into the abyss of lost memories. She is now more inclined on waking to search for her young children who need to be taken to school. As before she does not believe she is a mother, she knows it. Her desperate searching is founded on complete conviction.

As she ventures outside the risks and nuisance become ever greater and Mrs M is admitted to a care home where she continues to search and plead to go home to her children. But now living behind a baffled door she screams out 'help' and bangs on the windows and if carers approach she lashes out. Worsening symptoms of pathology or distress beyond our comprehension.

Despite VT's theoretical failings, Feil's methods of engagement helped practitioners to appreciate the benefits of validation when caring for people living with confusion. Feil combined a respect for the subjective world of the confused person with a concern for their emotional welfare by maintaining that whatever the facts are their emotions possess their own validity. Feelings that cannot be disregarded as if they are not real. Stokes (2000) describes validation in practice.

SPECAL (Specialized Early Care for Alzheimer's) is a controversial psychosocial intervention that aims to resolve distress by actively creating a state of confusion (James, 2008). Carers systematically support the re-experience of historical memories and make 'a present of the past'. Having identified a significant theme from a person's history that is absorbing and emotionally comfortable carers collude in order to maintain this aspect of person's life that while being at odds with the present is nevertheless familiar and reassuring.

Reminiscence therapy and life story work

The use of reminiscence with people living with dementia is of potential benefit. It not only taps into a well of distant memory that may resonate with feeling, and also, with the destruction of recent memories, the past may be all that remains and hence all that can be acknowledged. For carers it helps them to get to know their residents better.

Music, photographs, archive recordings, household paraphernalia, and foods are used to evoke memories as well as offering the opportunity for social engagement. Life story books enable carers to learn about the people they care for while memory boxes are found in many care homes adjacent to residents' bedrooms as a personalized orientation cue and a stimulus to personally relevant conversation; although a risk is that the boxes end up being no more than wall furniture with little evidence of engagement. Woods and Clare (2008) describe the use of life story work in the development of meaningful individualized care plans.

Although higher levels of well-being during reminiscence have been reported (Brooker and Duce, 2000), it has been suggested that reminiscence is not truly a therapy (Woods and Clare, 2008) but is best regarded as a diversionary activity (Thornton and Brotchie, 1987). Without doubt, while the practice of reminiscence is to be found in most care settings, as is the use of 'nostalgia' interior designs in care homes for people with dementia, research is needed regarding the outcomes of the different types of reminiscence activity. One outcome of life story work can be the understanding and resolution of challenging behaviours (Stokes, 2008).

Case study 4

Sylvia's determination to walk was risky and a nuisance. Not only might she fall, Sylvia would walk over to people, and having reached them bend over and softly say, 'I'm so, so sorry. Terrible, terrible' and then walk on. This would happen over and over again.

The content of what Sylvia had to say also bore no relationship to reality for she had nothing to apologize for, nor had anything terrible happened. She was a woman with dementia living on a unit who had harmed or offended no one.

Life story work with Sylvia's family revealed that 27 years earlier Sylvia had lost her youngest son during the Troubles in Northern Ireland when he was just 17 years old. Sylvia was devastated, but only fleetingly. To the astonishment of her family 'Mum never grieved'. She would not talk about her son's death. Nor would she talk about him. He had literally ceased to exist. His photographs and possessions were stored in the cellar for safekeeping and she never ventured into his bedroom again.

Sylvia had survived the shock of her son's death by repressing her feelings. Now she was dementing and there was only the past, and confusion reigned. As a result she endured unremitting anguish. Years previously Sylvia had invoked the psychological defence of repression to contain the magnitude of her grief, and now her mind employed projection. She projected onto others her own feelings and fears so it was not she who was overwhelmed by sorrow, but others. This is why she comforted others.

Life story work would be a risky endeavour, for reminiscing about her son might cue Sylvia to become even more aware of her loss and thus become more agitated and desperate to defend herself, but logic is not a characteristic of confusion and so the hope was that if memories of him as a child could occupy her she would gain pleasure and most importantly peace of mind. With pleasurable memories absorbing her attention she would no longer be preoccupied with his death. And in the absence of unbearable recollections there would be no intolerable upset and she would no longer be driven to console others.

Her children told the staff all they could remember about their brother's life. From what they learned they compiled a life story book. To bring it alive they asked for photos and any other memorabilia that could be pasted into the book. Carers would sit next to Sylvia, as would her family, and talk to her about her youngest child. And it worked. It was not so much the reminiscing of others that was uplifting, it was what she could see, touch, and caress. Always engrossed, time would pass without incident. Life story work had not helped to manage Sylvia's wandering, it had resolved it.

Psychological sequelae

People with dementia are experiencing many transitions in care homes. Not simply a need to adjust to the progressive loss of cognitive function but also the need to adapt to discontinuity and the loss of familiarity following admission, which may require in turn adjustment to the death of a caring partner who had been old themselves. As many aged people living with dementia have comorbidity, they may also be coming to terms with frailty and disability. For all, the process of adjustment is hindered by cognitive impairment and loss of insight. For many, consequent depression and adjustment anxiety is to be expected. Yet in the majority of instances depression is unacknowledged and the screening for depression considered by many to be an indicator of high quality dementia care rarely takes place (Feil et al., 2007). Instead, as the person becomes passive and withdrawn or on the other hand repeatedly calls out, paces from room to room, wrings his or her hands or sleeps poorly, these signs of psychological maladjustment are misinterpreted as symptoms of neurological degeneration and consequently a culture of 'management' rather than 'recovery' descends. Consequently, a challenge facing care homes is how to create a therapeutic culture of openness to a person's experience of living with dementia.

Knight (2004) noted that therapists often feel that older people are unlikely to benefit from psychological interventions even though this is not necessarily so. Laidlaw (2001) reported the effectiveness of cognitive behaviour therapy (CBT) in treating late life depression, while Scholey and Woods (2003) demonstrated the applicability of CBT in early stage dementia. However, psychologists and therapists have traditionally shied away from therapy with older people which probably contributes to the finding that the majority of older people with psychological needs do not receive adequate mental health services. This applies even more if aged people live in institutional care as many care homes, to the detriment of carers and 'cared for', have evolved into 'isolated wards in the community'.

Instead of relying on visiting specialists to deliver psychosocial interventions, the need for therapeutic interventions may be best addressed by reference to the care setting. Yet transforming care cultures wherein one set of individuals attends to another set of individuals in a perfunctory, superficial way with little regard for their humanity and psychology rarely happens by chance, while Georgiades and Phillimore (1975) warned us of the fate of the lone 'hero innovator'. If a therapeutic culture is to be introduced wherein the person is recovered in the eyes of others and his or her emotional world is acknowledged, intervening at the level of the care home must include skills and attitude-based training, staff support, leadership development, mentoring, and service evaluation.

Without systemic change psychosocial interventions rarely happen and change may require a concerted effort to remove the belief that dementia robs a person of not only his or her cognitive ability but also their identity and human worth for only then will there be an organizational commitment to address feelings of separation, helplessness, and hopelessness. Feelings that are not predicated on an ability to remember, reflect, or anticipate, but sentiments that exist and recur in discrete episodes of the 'here and now', each instance divorced from any underpinning narrative.

Chenoweth et al. (2009) trained care home staff in person-centred care and dementia care mapping (Brooker, 2005) with a resultant lowering of resident agitation. Nolan et al. (2008) suggest that educational initiatives need to be embedded within the organizational culture of a care setting. Using an intervention that embraced staff training in psychosocial care and systemic consultation to tackle 'whole home issues', Fossey et al. (2006) reported a reduction in the number of residents taking antipsychotics with no increase in agitation and aggressive behaviour.

Although such ways of systemic working are not always considered to be psychosocial interventions in their own right, there is much to be gained by viewing them as such (Brooker, 2008) for we underestimate the power of institutional inertia at our peril.

Job satisfaction and staff support are critical variables when promoting quality care, achieving resident satisfaction and delivering service innovation and job dissatisfaction can often implicate and embrace systemic issues beyond the care home. In Western societies, income is a commanding cultural signifier and when you can earn more stacking shelves in a supermarket than you can earn working in a care home then the perception is that society does not value care work. Consequently, cultural forces can undermine job satisfaction and the ensuing quality of care observed despite leadership within a care home valuing staff and attempting to stimulate a strong sense of accomplishment.

Similarly staff stress and burnout may not only pertain to the work setting but may also involve carers bringing personal 'problems' and stresses from home to work. The consequence is that if staff feel unsupported and are made to feel they as people do not matter and their life struggles are not appreciated they may ameliorate their distress by adopting distancing coping strategies (Woods, 2008), which in turn result in task-oriented care delivery that runs contrary to the implementation of empathy-centred psychosocial interventions.

Although the influence of the social environment is paramount, transitions to living well in a care home are also eased by interior design. Care homes that are designed to be 'homely' and where there is not a slavish commitment to communal care (wherein people sit in lounges simply because the physical space exists) helps facilitate psychological adjustment. A resident's room that resonates with his or her identity embraces familiarity and a sense of belonging that will help salve a troubled psychology.

Case study 5

Penny hated being in the lounge. Severely disabled by vascular dementia she would call out unintelligibly, curse the person sitting next to her, and glare at those who passed too close. But the people against whom she vented her anger were doing no more than being in her presence. These were people with dementia; people with whom she knew she shared nothing in common. Without self-awareness, Penny saw them as distasteful and repugnant.

Her transition to living in a care home would be helped if her life was centred on her own room. Enriched with personal touches and the nostalgic trivia of her life, Penny's room embraced familiarity and continuity. Penny's family brought in ornaments, photographs, and all sorts of knickknacks. Her dressing table was simply that, *her* dressing table with hairbrush, perfume, and jewellery. She adored musicals and so a portable TV, CD player, and a library of videos and albums now adorned the unit by the window. Above her bed was a collage made by her granddaughter. Family, past and present now smiled down on Penny. The room was truly Penny's home.

Penny was now a contented lady. Safe and comfortable among her familiar things, undisturbed by the people who had once tormented her, she had no reason to be agitated. Instead she sat quietly for hours watching her films, listening to music, or simply gazing around at the story of her life.

The promotion of care practices that preserve dignity, acknowledge individuality, and encourage autonomy in making decisions and choices counter the powerlessness and helplessness that are rife in care homes and which contribute to depression (Boyle, 2005).

Finally, systemic psychosocial interventions need to not only engage residents but there is also a need to support caring families as well. Although, in theory, families are regarded as integral to the functioning of a care home, in practice there is a risk that they become marginalized because the tasks inherent in running a busy care home get in the way (Bauer, 2006). Yet when supporting people with profound dementia it is hard to see how care settings that aspire to engage with residents on an affective level and build meaningful relationships can scale such heights unless families collaborate in drawing up care plans, are involved in life story work and participate in the meaningful provision of social activities. Involvement with families also brings us a step closer to breaking down institutionalized care practices. However, engagement is unlikely to happen if families continue to believe that living in a care home is tantamount to failure. For if this is how they are perceived then the understandable and more likely outcome, founded on feelings of guilt and shame, is avoidance. Only when care homes are seen as providing both care and quality of life solutions at a time of greatest vulnerability and complex need will families be psychologically open to a true partnership.

Conclusion

While there is enthusiasm for psychosocial non-pharmacological interventions to support and restore levels of well-being, caution is required. There must be realism as to what can be achieved, especially when dementia is characterized by severe cognitive impairment and frailty, and the temptation to believe that simply because interventions resonate with the term 'psychosocial' that success is all but inevitable must be resisted. For if history is to be our guide, without systemic change, transformational developments in care quality are unlikely to happen.

References

Alldred, D.P., Petty, D.R., Bowie, P., Zermansky, A.G., & Raynor, D.K. (2007). Antipsychotic prescribing patterns in care homes and relationship with dementia. *Psychiatric Bulletin*, *31*, 329–332.

All-Party Parliamentary Group (2009). *Always a Last Resort: Inquiry into the Prescription of Antipsychotic Drugs to People with Dementia Living in Care Homes*. London: Alzheimer's Society.

Baker, R., Dowling, Z., Wareing, L.A., Dawson, J., & Assey, J. (1997). Snoezelen: its long-term and short-term effects on older people with dementia. *British Journal of Occupational Therapy*, *60*(5), 213–218.

Ballard, C. & Margallo-Lana, M.L. (2001). The relationship between anti-psychotic treatment and quality of life for patients with dementia living in residential and nursing home care facilities. *Journal of Clinical Psychiatry*, *65*(11), 23–28.

Ballard, C. & Aarsland, D. (2010). Pharmacological management of neuropsychiatric symptoms in people with dementia. In: J.C. Hughes, M. Lloyd-Williams, & G.A. Sachs (Eds.), *Supportive Care for the Person with Dementia*. Oxford: Oxford University Press, 105–115.

Bauer, M. (2006). Collaboration and control: nurses' constructions of the role of family in nursing home care. *Journal of Advanced Nursing*, *54*, 45–52.

Bignall, A. (1996). Look and learn: designs on the care environment. *Journal of Dementia Care*, *4*, 12–13.

Boyle, G. (2005). The role of autonomy in explaining mental ill health and depression among older people in long-term care settings. *Ageing and Society*, *25*, 731–748.

Brooker, D. (2005). Dementia care mapping: a review of the research literature. *The Gerontologist*, *45*, 11–18.

Brooker, D. (2007). *Person-centred Dementia Care: Making Services Better*. London: Jessica Kingsley Publishers.

Brooker, D. (2008). Interventions at the care team level. In: R. Woods & L. Clare (Eds.), *Handbook of the Clinical Psychology of Ageing*, 2nd Edition. Chichester: John Wiley, 595–611.

Brooker, D. & Duce, L. (2000). Wellbeing and activity in dementia: a comparison of group reminiscence therapy, structured goal-directed activity and unstructured time. *Aging & Mental Health*, *4*(4), 287–296.

Byatt, S. & Cheston, R. (1999). Taped memories: a source of emotional security. *Journal of Dementia Care*, *7*, 28–32.

Chenoweth, L., King, M.T., Jeon, Y.H., et al. (2009). Caring for Aged Dementia Care Resident Study (CADRES) of person-centred care, dementia-care mapping, and usual care in dementia: a cluster-randomised trial. *Lancet Neurology*, *8*, 317–325.

Downs, M., Clare, L., & Anderson, E. (2008). Dementia as a biopsychosocial condition: implications for practice and research. In: R. Woods & L. Clare (Eds.), *Handbook of the Clinical Psychology of Ageing*, 2nd Edition. Chichester: John Wiley, 145–159.

Feil, D.G., MacLean, C., & Sultzer, D. (2007). Quality indicators for the care of dementia in vulnerable elders. *Journal of the American Geriatric Society*, *55*, 293–301.

Finkel, S. (2003). Behavioural and psychological symptoms of dementia. *Clinical Geriatric Medicine*, *19*, 799–824.

Folsom, J.C. (1968). Reality orientation therapy for the elderly mental patient. *Journal of Geriatric Psychiatry, 1,* 291–207.

Fossey, J., Ballard, C., Juszczak, E., et al. (2006). Effect of enhanced psychosocial care on antipsychotic use in nursing home residents with severe dementia: cluster randomised trial. *BMJ, 332,* 756–758.

Froggatt, K. & Parker, D. (2010). Care homes and long-term care for people with dementia. In: J.C. Hughes, M. Lloyd-Williams, & G.A. Sachs (Eds.), *Supportive Care for the Person with Dementia.* Oxford: Oxford University Press, 181–188.

Georgiades, N. & Phillimore, L. (1975). The myth of the hero innovator and alternative strategies for organisational change. In: C. Kiernan & P. Woodford (Eds.), *Behaviour Modification for the Severely Retarded.* New York: Associated Scientific Publishers, 313–319.

Goddaer, J. & Abraham, I.L. (1994). Effects of relaxing music on agitation during meals among nursing home residents with severe cognitive impairment. *Archives of Psychiatric Nursing, 8*(3), 150–158.

Goudie, F. & Stokes, G. (1989). Understanding confusion. *Nursing Times, 85,* 35–37.

Hopman-Rock, M., Staats, P.G.M., Tak, E.C.P.M., & Droes, R.M. (1999). The effects of a psychomotor activation programme for use in groups of cognitively impaired people in homes for the elderly. *International Journal of Geriatric Psychiatry, 14,* 633–642.

James, O. (2008). *Contented Dementia.* London: Ebury Press.

Kitwood, T. (1996). A dialectical framework for dementia. In: R. Woods (Ed.), *Handbook of the Clinical Psychology of Ageing.* Chichester: John Wiley, 267–282.

Knight, B. (2004). *Psychotherapy with Older Adults,* 3rd Edition. Thousand Oaks, CA: Sage.

Laidlaw, K. (2001). An empirical review of cognitive therapy for late life depression: does research evidence suggest adaptations are necessary for cognitive therapy with older adults? *Clinical Psychology and Psychotherapy, 8,* 1–14.

Livingston, G., Johnston, K., Paton J., & Lyketsos, C. (2005). Systematic review of psychological approaches to the management of neuropsychiatric symptoms of dementia. *The American Journal of Psychiatry, 162,* 1996–2021.

Lord, T.R. & Garner, J.E. (1993). Effects of music on Alzheimer's patients. *Perceptual & Motor Skills, 76,* 451–445.

Macdonald, A.J., Carpenter, G.I., Box, O., Roberts, A., & Sahu, S. (2002). Dementia and use of psychotropic medication in non-'Elderly Mentally Infirm' nursing homes in South East England. *Age and Ageing, 31,* 58–64.

Matthews, F. & Dening, T. (2002). Prevalence of dementia in institutional care. *Lancet, 360*(9328), 225–226.

Moniz-Cook, E., Stokes, G., & Agar, S. (2003). Difficult behaviour and dementia in nursing homes: five cases of psychosocial intervention. *Clinical Psychology and Psychotherapy, 10,* 197–208.

Morton, I. & Bleathman, C. (1991). The effectiveness of validation therapy in dementia—a pilot study. *International Journal of Geriatric Psychiatry, 6,* 327–330.

National Institute for Health and Clinical Excellence—Social Care Institute for Excellence (2006). *Dementia: Supporting People with Dementia and their Carers in Health and Social Care.* London: HMSO.

Neal, M. & Barton-Wright, P. (2007). *Validation Therapy for Dementia (Cochrane Review). The Cochrane Library, 2.* Chichester: John Wiley.

Nguyen, Q. & Paton, C. (2008). The use of aromatherapy to treat behavioural problems in dementia. *International Journal of Geriatric Psychiatry, 23,* 337–346.

Nolan, M., Davies, S., Brown, J., et al. (2008). The role of education and training in achieving change in care homes: a literature review. *Journal of Research in Nursing*, *13*(5), 411–433.

Osborne, H., Simpson, J., & Stokes, G. (2010). The relationship between pre-morbid personality and challenging behaviour in people with dementia: a systematic review. *Aging & Mental Health*, *14*, 503–515.

Peak, J.S. & Cheston, R.I.L. (2002). Using simulated presence therapy with people with dementia. *Aging & Mental Health*, *6*, 77–81.

Samson, D.M. & McDonnell, A.A. (1990). Functional analysis and challenging behaviours. *Behavioural Psychotherapy*, *18*, 259–272.

Scholey, K.A, & Woods, B.T. (2003). A series of brief cognitive interventions with people experiencing both dementia and depression: a description of techniques and common themes. *Clinical Psychology and Psychotherapy*, *10*, 175–185.

Sheard, D. (2008). *Enabling*. London: Alzheimer's Society.

Spector, A., Thorgrimsen, L., Woods, R., et al. (2003). Effectiveness of an evidence-based cognitive stimulation therapy programme for people with dementia: randomised controlled trial. *British Journal of Psychiatry*, *183*, 248–254.

Stokes, G. (1996). Challenging behaviour in dementia: a psychological approach. In: R. Woods (Ed.), *Handbook of the Clinical Psychology of Ageing*. Chichester: John Wiley, 601–628.

Stokes, G. (2000). *Challenging Behaviour in Dementia: A Person-centred Approach*. Bicester: Winslow Press.

Stokes, G. (2008). *And Still the Music Plays: Stories of People with Dementia*. London: Hawker Publications.

Thornton, S. & Brotchie, J. (1987). Reminiscence: a critical review of the empirical literature. *British Journal of Clinical Psychology*, *26*, 93–111.

Van Weert, J.C.M., Van Dulmen, A.M., Spreeuwenberg, P.M.M., Ribbe, M.W., & Bensing, J.M. (2005). Behavioural and mood effects of Snoezelen integrated into 24-hour dementia care. *Journal of American Geriatric Society*, *53*, 24–33.

Woods, P. & Ashley, J. (1995). Simulated presence therapy: using selected memories to manage problem behaviours in Alzheimer's disease patients. *Geriatric Nursing*, *16*, 9–14.

Woods, R. (1994). Reality orientation. *Journal of Dementia Care*, *2*, 24–25.

Woods, R. (2008). Residential care. In: R. Woods & L. Clare (Eds.), *Handbook of the Clinical Psychology of Ageing*, 2nd Edition. Chichester: John Wiley, 289–309.

Woods, R. & Clare, L. (2008). Psychological interventions with people with dementia. In: R. Woods & L. Clare (Eds.), *Handbook of the Clinical Psychology of Ageing*, 2nd Edition. Chichester: John Wiley, 523–548.

Chapter 17

Support to care homes

Amanda Thompsell

Abstract

Care home residents suffer high levels of physical and mental health problems, and there is concern that their needs are often not well met by primary and/or specialist healthcare. General practitioners (GPs) may provide medical services through the ordinary general medical service (GMS) contract or there may be incentivized through contracts with homes or locally enhanced services. Various models of specialist support services have developed recently. These include community pharmacists and specialist mental health and/or nursing support. The latter may take several forms, from specialist outreach clinics to designated care home support teams, of which several examples are provided. In general, care home support teams have been found to be reasonably effective in managing behavioural problems, management of medications, and reduction of need for other specialist care, such as hospital admissions. Despite their likely cost-effectiveness, however, they are often vulnerable to being lost in times of economic stringency.

Background

The elderly population in care homes is a large one—in 2010, 435,000 people aged 65 years or older were living in care homes in England (Wild et al., 2010)—and this figure is set to rise as the population ages. Furthermore, the care home population has progressively changed and now consists of older residents (aged 80 years upwards), many with complex physical and mental comorbidity. Bowman et al. (2004), reviewing 15,483 residents, found that 41% had two or more diagnoses and 27% were confused, incontinent, and immobile. Residents have a wide range of healthcare needs including pain relief and nutrition (Cowan et al., 2003a,b) and mental health problems (Bowman et al., 2004). Care home residents are also often on more medications, and require more frequent reviews, than other patients of the same age (National Prescribing Centre, 2000). This population is very frail. Generally, they leave only to go into hospital or as a result of death. The median length of stay in a care home is 24 months and only 18 months in nursing care homes. As many residents in nursing care homes have advanced, incurable, and progressive diseases, they also will have end-of-life needs.

Care homes now are also seen as central to the planning of good end-of-life care, currently a particular focus in the United Kingdom and elsewhere. The recent National Dementia Strategy and End of Life Strategy have both focused on the importance of delivering good end-of-life care to the person in his or her preferred place of care. Few care home residents wish to die in hospital in unfamiliar surroundings being cared for by staff who do not know them. It therefore is essential to be able to give good end-of-life care in care homes. The Gold Standards Framework (Badger et al., 2009) provides a suitable model, aiming to meet the preferences of residents and also to reduce costly hospital admissions. The Framework promotes a shift in staff attitude from seeing someone dying in the home as a failure to one of normality. It is a nurse-led model but input from physicians is an integral component.

Care homes therefore have great need of skilled medical intervention but, by and large, this need is not met by any specialist provision. GPs have primary responsibility for medical care, but often they lack specialist training in the health and social needs of older people. Geriatricians have tended to become disengaged from care homes (Steves et al., 2009). Residential care homes which do not have nursing staff are also dependent on district nurses. District nurses spend a significant amount of time in care homes, usually ranging from 4 to 6 hours per week (Goodman et al., 2003). The work that they do is often defined by what the care home staff do not undertake, or are not allowed to, for the resident (Perry et al., 2003).

With no central planning for the delivery of services into care homes, it is unsurprising that there is extensive variation in the medical services received by various homes (Glendinning et al., 2002). Although the experience will vary by locality, there is evidence that, overall, care home residents get a poor deal when it comes to medical services. Fahey et al. (2003) compared the quality of care offered by nurses for elderly residents in care homes with that given to a control population in the community in Bristol. Care home residents were less likely to have their blood pressure measured and more likely to be placed on antipsychotics before any specific diagnosis had been confirmed to validate this prescription. Fahey et al. found care was inadequate across all quality markers. This inadequate management of long-term conditions is likely to be linked to greater morbidity and possibly more hospital admissions.

There are, then, substantial medical needs in care homes and the current arrangements fall short in meeting these needs. This state of affairs has been noted with concern by various bodies such as the Care Homes Residents and Relatives Association (Bright, 2008) and also now by the Care Quality Commission (2010), in its audit of medical and specialist input into care homes. It is timely then to review what these arrangements are and how they might be improved.

GP provision to care homes

Medical input under the GMS contract

Currently, there are several models of medical support to care homes but the most common is for medical input to be provided by GPs under the terms of their GMS contracts—the general contract under which the GP provides services to the community at large. Residents are served individually by their own GP rather than the home being served exclusively by a single GP practice.

Although the GMS contract does take some account of the complex needs of care home residents in its scheme for rewarding GPs, the higher capitation does not adequately reimburse GPs for the extra time needed to meet fully the medical needs of the residents. A typical workload would be around four GP visits a year for a resident in a care home without nursing or six visits a year for a resident in a care home with nursing. For a home of 60 residents, this equates to 240 visits a year for a home without nursing or 360 visits a year for a home with nursing.

Groom et al. (2000) reviewed the impact of nursing home residents on general practitioners' workload over a year, studying 540 patients in 9 different practices in Nottingham, pairing nursing home residents with controls in the community. They found that nursing home residents had more face-to-face visits and interventions than controls in the community. The cost to the GP of the input to residents in care homes was £18.70 per patient per month which was £10.50 (128%) more than for the controls. However, substantial savings could be made in the costs of GP provision if more than one patient can be seen in the same visit. Groom et al. (2000) demonstrated a potential saving of 27% if one extra patient was seen and 44% if four extra patients were seen, on the same visit.

GPs are generally organized to see patients at their surgeries and find it more difficult to operate at care homes. Generally, their electronic records are held at the surgery and are often not accessible at the care homes, so residents may be seen without relevant clinical information to hand. Arranging referrals is also more difficult and time-consuming from the care home. Inevitably, some GPs will have more experience or enthusiasm for this type of work and this too can lead to worrying variations in the quality of care provided.

If the GMS contract has shortcomings from the viewpoint of the GP, this is equally true from the care home perspective. The GMS contract does not cover enhanced or supplementary services or require (or reward) any particular level of liaison with the home. For example, GPs are not obliged to make entries in the nursing notes, undertake regular 'reviews', or attend multidisciplinary team meetings in care homes. Of course many GPs do these things out of a sense of professionalism, but as services come under increasing strain, it is more likely that the basic GMS contract will be strictly adhered to, and therefore it may be unrealistic to rely on the goodwill and professionalism of GPs in undertaking these extra activities—or to support new initiatives such as good end-of-life care.

When the GP visits only infrequently the staff are less likely to develop a trusting relationship with that GP and may become less confident in supporting residents to stay in the home rather than go to hospital. Communication between the staff members, a vital element of good quality care, is also made more difficult if the GP is not often present. The Department of Health recently issued an alert about medication errors in care homes, and it is easy to see how having to deal with perhaps 15 or more GPs can increase the risks of prescribing or dispensing errors.

So, while many GPs deliver care well beyond their contractual obligations, if we are to look after frail individuals in care homes the level of medical input will need to be greater, more targeted, and better trained.

Other models for providing GP input to care homes

Although the most common model for providing medical input is through the GMS contract, several other models exist, each having particular benefits and disadvantages and these are considered below. Later in the chapter we will consider non-GP-based models.

GMS contract to a care home where the GP has a special interest

This model is more applicable to smaller homes as it depends on the availability of the individual GP. His or her colleagues need to cover when he or she is away, which may sometimes lead to delays while the covering GPs wait for their colleague to return. This model may not work so well in the future, as the current trend is for care homes to be larger, around 60 places is thought to be the minimum size for economic viability.

Private contracts between the care homes and the GP

This model usually applies to larger homes and involves the payment to the GP of a so-called retainer fee. This is controversial, with critics pointing out that residents should enjoy the same access to health services as the rest of the population. For example, the Health Select Committee Inquiry into Elder Abuse (House of Commons Health Committee, 2004) concluded that 'such fees are paid so that residential homes are assured of a service by the local GP. We recommend that the practice of the payment of retainer fees is abolished as every patient registered with a GP should have a right to a service from the GP without the payment of additional retainer fees'. In response, the Government made a distinction between the rights of the individual to access a GP and any business arrangement that the home may come to with the GP to provide management support.

One large care group recently reported that 12% of its homes paid retainers, ranging from £895 to £24,000 per annum, with a median of £7,000. This variation suggests that fees are calculated in a largely arbitrary manner. The English Community Care Association (2008) opposed this practice, arguing that there is often no difference between the care provided under the GMS contract and that under the private contract. In some cases, however, an enhanced package of care is specified, including regular reviews and routine visits to the home, with the GPs keeping a clinical record in the home. Nevertheless, there remains little clarity and consistency about what services justify the payment of a retainer and how much it should cost.

Such contracts are often poorly monitored and it may be that self-funding residents are paying for care from a GP to which they are already entitled. Retainers are negotiated directly between the home and the GP practice, so it is hard for health commissioners to monitor them. Finally, care homes who cannot afford to pay retainer fees may be disadvantaged if other local homes do so, and as a result it may be difficult to find GPs to provide a service for them.

Local enhanced service agreement between commissioners and GPs for individual care homes

In Lambeth, South London, where I work, a local enhanced service (LES) has been developed for GPs to provide services beyond the GMS contract to care homes with nursing. The contracts were awarded after competitive tendering and specify regular attendance in the home for clinical reviews, medication reviews, and multidisciplinary team meetings, and support for the Gold Standards Framework for end-of-life care.

Payment under the contract for the LES depends on the number of beds in the home. The contract is monitored partly by the care home manager as well as the primary care trusts (PCTs). Compulsory attendance at training is built into the contract. Monitoring also includes auditing, for example, of the number of visits made in the year, number of residents with documented annual reviews, and number of residents dying within the care home if that was their wish.

Although this system involves additional cost, it appears to provide a number of substantial benefits. For example, it places the residents in the care home under the same GP with obvious advantages for clinical continuity, although some residents may want to keep their previous GP. The benefits for GPs are improved relationships with staff, better working conditions with fewer requests for acute visits, and more job satisfaction. From my observations, increased availability of the GPs has helped staff to become more confident in managing clinical situations.

For PCTs, a LES contract allows a more proactive approach and continuity of care by improving chronic disease management and medication reviews. It aims to reduce hospital admissions by enhancing staff confidence and to reduce the numbers of drugs prescribed and drug errors. Regular medication reviews may also produce significant cost savings (see section 'Pharmacy input into care homes').

As the LES can be awarded on an annual basis it allows for regular reviews of its effectiveness and adaptation to any new clinical priorities.

Local enhanced service agreement with one GP practice and several care homes

In this model, the PCT commissions a particular GP practice to provide an enhanced service to several care homes. The considerations here are similar to a one-home LES, but these arrangements on a larger scale could provide additional administrative efficiencies especially for the PCT.

Dedicated primary care service

Here the PCT commissions a multidisciplinary team to support care homes (as discussed below in 'Specialist Support to Care Homes' on p. 227) and the team's functions might include providing full primary care so that the team includes a salaried GP to provide medical care to the residents. The difficulty is ensuring cover for the GP's absence and he/she could only be responsible for a limited number of homes.

The care home's responsibility for ensuring good medical care

The most crucial factor for delivering high quality medical care to residents is good cooperation between the GP and the management of the care home. If there is an enhanced agreement with the GPs it is essential that responsibility for managing this contract is shared with the home. Having a fully briefed supernumerary member of staff available for the GP's visits is a good way of ensuring this. Not only does it avoid confusion and make the best use of the GP's time but it also provides a good opportunity for learning.

The care home should provide a private space for the GP and staff to discuss the residents and appropriate facilities where the GP can see the resident and examine them in private. Finally, the care home should also provide the GP with up-to-date information and measurements, such as residents' weight and blood pressure.

Ideally, there should be an electronic link with the GP surgery for access to clinical records.

Defining good GP support to care home residents

If an enhanced contract with a GP or GP practice is being considered by PCT commissioners or by a care home, the following issues should be considered:

- that the GP actually likes to work with elderly residents;
- that the GP has or is considered able to develop a good working relationship with and mutual respect for the care home staff;
- that the GP is knowledgeable about the physical and mental conditions that he/she will meet in a care home;
- that the GP is knowledgeable about end-of-life care and the Mental Capacity Act;
- that the GP proposes a regular programme of review of the health status of the residents;
- that the GP will perform a new residents check on admission or near to admission;
- that the GP will perform regular medication reviews;
- that the GP will show respect for residents by conducting consultations in a private space;
- that the GP will make time available to talk to concerned relatives; and
- that the GP will hold regular meetings with care home staff to discuss the residents.

Pharmacy input into care homes

There has been justifiable concern about the quality of medicines management in care homes, including prescribing, dispensing, monitoring, and administration of drugs. In 2004, the National Care Standards Commission (NCSC), and following that the Commission for Social Care Inspection (NCSC's successor), published reports which showed that nearly half the care homes were failing to meet the National Minimum standards set by the Department of Health for the safe management of medicines. Other studies have reported similar findings, for example, the Care Home Use of Medicines Study (CHUMS) (Barber et al., 2009), which found high levels of poor medication management. The report found that, in any 1 month, 7 out of 10 care home residents experienced at least one medication error, some with potential for 'serious harm'. As a result, the Department of Health ordered an urgent safety review and instructed PCTs to work with GPs, pharmacists, and social care providers to review the safety of local prescribing, dispensing, administration, and monitoring arrangements in care homes. This alert, which was issued for 'immediate action' via the NHS Central Alerting System, demonstrates the increasing Government concern over medicines management in residential and nursing care homes for older people.

There is evidence to show that medication reviews can be effective, and several studies of pharmacist-conducted reviews have shown that many prescribed medications could be reduced or stopped altogether (Furniss et al., 2000). However, the availability of such support is variable. PCTs can choose to commission a LES to care homes from community-based pharmacists, but not all PCTs elect to do so.

Several approaches may improve the monitoring of medication. Firstly, there is the education of the care staff. If staff are informed of the adverse consequences of night sedation and they know that their home tends to use these drugs relatively often, they can reflect on this. After such reflection I have found on re-auditing a reduction from 25% down to zero. The same also can apply to antipsychotics. Reporting systems for care staff to indicate to primary/secondary care that the person is on a particular medication can also reduce the time between reviews thereby stopping the medication earlier.

Some PCTs have developed locally enhanced services for their GPs, as described above, which includes ensuring that medication is regularly reviewed and that they liaise with pharmacists about medicines.

Other PCTs have clinically trained pharmacists to review and monitor the use of medicines prescribed in care homes. This varies from looking at inhaler technique to ensure that respiratory diseases are being effectively treated, to auditing prescribed antipsychotic drugs or completing full clinical medication reviews.

Finally, there is the alternative of a multidisciplinary team tasked with reviewing medication, probably as part of a wider support service to care homes. This can be an effective way of ensuring a holistic approach to deciding the most appropriate therapeutic approach—it may not always be medication that is needed. The South East London Care Homes Support Team (CHST) where I have worked (described further in Box 17.2), has used the statutory nursing assessment and regular audits to review those on antipsychotics and sedatives and make recommendations to the GPs and homes based on assessment of the need for the medication. This proactive approach has meant that fewer than 7% of residents with dementia in non-specialist care homes with nursing in our locality were on antipsychotics, compared with up to 48% quoted elsewhere (Fossey et al., 2006). Work presented to the British Geriatrics Society (Burns, 2010) found that regular medication reviews in care homes supported by a geriatrician resulted in an estimated savings on direct medication costs alone of £168,000 per year in Leeds.

Specialist support therefore provides a good alternative for promoting and ensuring good medication practice. This raises the question of how far it should be seen as the way forward for medical provision in care homes generally.

Specialist support to care homes

In recent years, interest has grown in the possibilities of improving care in care homes by the use of specialist teams. It is difficult, however, to establish the true current extent of this type of service as it is often not separately identified or funded, despite a growing consensus that it can be valuable.

The British Geriatrics Society (Gladman et al., 2009) estimated that only 18% of PCTs funded the involvement of a specialist geriatrician in care homes despite evidence that assessment by a geriatrician prior to admission can often identify unmet medical needs. Indeed, in some cases care home admission might have been avoided, thus saving money.

The interim report by the National Audit Office (2009), Improving Dementia Services in England, included a survey of old age psychiatrists. In this, 87% of respondents said that they did work with care homes although 64% were not specifically commissioned to do so. Old age psychiatrists thought that care homes were important for implementation of the National Dementia Strategy but with low likelihood of achievement. The recent report on antipsychotic use in care homes (Banerjee, 2009) may also require more future engagement of old age psychiatrists with care homes.

Despite a lack of ring-fenced funding, there has been a long history of partnership and innovation in supporting care homes although, as has been pointed out before (Goodman et al., 2003), teams supporting care homes rarely survive longer than 5 years as often they are the first services to be cut in times of economic stringency. The current picture is difficult to describe as existing teams often merge or morph into something different. Much of the rest of this chapter will consider input into care homes by specialist services, especially the role of care home support teams, but there are also various examples of partnership working, including initiatives such as:

- designating some care homes as teaching care homes or centres of learning. Seconding care home staff to wards or local hospices to increase their knowledge has also been felt to be helpful, as has student nurse placements in care homes;

- developing training to support care homes based on the needs identified by the care homes themselves or as stipulated by the commissioners. This training may be linked with positive financial incentives such as attendance at training and increased payments for the beds from the Local Authority dependent on the extent to which the homes participate;

- specialist interventions, such as using dementia care mapping to help improve practice in care homes, or the SOFI (Short Observation Framework for Inspection) tool as used by the Care Quality Commission (2008) in their inspections.

Studies have considered the positive results and challenges for health professionals in supporting care staff. Research by Proctor et al. (1998, 1999) and Lyne et al. (2006) showed reduced depression scores and increased activity levels for residents after health professionals introduced care planning training and support for care staff. Lyne et al. also pointed out how collaborative working improved staff confidence and morale. However, the major barriers encountered were generally the lack of available staff and the time taken to implement the interventions.

There is unfortunately a lack of studies based on the views of the residents themselves about what ways they would like to see their healthcare improved and this is clearly an area that should be addressed. Another tension that arises in these medically based initiatives lies between the wish to improve the residents' healthcare without medicalizing their environment, as it is their home.

Innovative secondary services models of support to care homes

As we have seen there are many ways in which specialist services may engage with care homes, but these may be grouped into certain broad categories.

Outreach clinics

In this approach, secondary services (usually mental health teams) engage directly with the homes by running regular clinics. These clinics are usually held once or twice a month, usually by community psychiatric nurses (CPNs) or specialist registrars. Referrals are as far as possible seen at these clinics.

This model has some advantages over the GP referral/expert consultation model as it is less reliant on GPs to identify problems and secondary services gain a better understanding of the dynamics of the home and how their treatment might work in that particular setting. Staff can be encouraged to refer problems for they might not have consulted a GP and there is an opportunity for specialist and care home staff to interact.

But there are still problems because the clinics happen whether or not they are wanted by the staff, and staff may not necessarily respect the service or carry out the advice offered. This model also potentially lessens the engagement of GPs with the home, and yet the GP is still needed as the first port of call for front-line emergencies. Often the clinics are not sufficiently frequent for a real relationship to develop between the clinicians and the staff, especially as many care homes have a high staff turnover. This model emphasizes the treatment of problems, and does not affect the conditions within the home to prevent the situation occurring or to manage the situation better.

Nominated point of contact

This is where a specific member of the team is allocated to specific care homes. They take the referrals from that home and act as the point of contact, particularly in areas where there are not too many homes.

This model shares many of the advantages and disadvantages of outreach clinics. The reduced frequency of the visits can mean the visits are not taken for granted as much as in the outreach clinic model. It probably offers a slightly better chance that some attention will be given to providing support and training to the care home staff, but this still is rarely a significant part of what is provided. Inevitably, the main problem is of resources. The specialist team member will have other commitments, and this will be a small part of their job, so they may be unable to provide a sufficient frequency of visits and thus may not develop as much expertise as might be hoped.

Joint reviews with the GP and the specialist

A third model involves joint reviews undertaken by the GP and the specialist together. This model is more often seen in a continuing care setting, but can be used in a care home. Not only does this provide a service benefiting from the GP's medical and local knowledge but it also ensures that the GP remains engaged in the process.

However, generally this is too ambitious and difficult in scope, starting with the difficulty in finding space in the diaries of GPs and specialists. Resources are likely to limit this approach.

Process consultancy

Process consultancy is where a team goes into care homes to facilitate change. The emphasis is on facilitation—the team helps the care home management and any GPs serving the home to develop their own ideas to improve the service and to manage the necessary changes. The emphasis on involving and empowering staff and the presence of GPs makes any changes far more likely to succeed. It is cost-effective from the viewpoint of secondary services. It is not however a model for providing care to individual residents, but a process used to support the homes in making the necessary changes.

Care home support teams

Another model is based on a specialist team model of support to care homes, which often are called care home support teams, or care home liaison teams. These teams vary as to their professional mix and their specific aims and this is best illustrated by several examples as described in the Boxes 17.1 and 17.2.

To summarize, while there is wide variation in make up and in function of these teams the core features of these specialist teams are:

- Mix of staff from different disciplines
- Working together with care homes managers to encourage participation, for example the Managers' Consultative Group in South East London, and the Sheffield Care Homes Best Practice Group
- Aim to reduce hospital admission and improve the abilities of the care homes to meet the health needs of the residents
- Often produce guidelines on best practice as they relate to the care homes and disseminate relevant information. In some cases, the team is used by PCT to help disseminate best practice, for example with flu information
- Often work on transfer documents and communication of information
- Usually a focus on end-of-life issues
- Usually end up involved in providing advice/reports for safeguarding issues
- Provide support for care home staff using link nurses or champions meeting to help allow staff to share best practice with each other

Effectiveness of dedicated teams supporting care homes

Szczepura et al. (2008) studied the impact of a dedicated nursing and physiotherapy team supporting 131 residents in four residential care homes in Bath and North Somerset. Overall costs and savings ranged from a worse case scenario of £2.70 extra costs to the more likely saving of £36.90 per resident per week. The savings were mainly due to reduced use of NHS services by avoiding hospital admissions and avoiding delayed transfers to care homes with nursing. They postulated that there may be an initial increase in costs from detecting new problems but these would probably be

Box 17.1 Examples of teams supporting care homes

Sheffield care homes support team
This team consisted of general and psychiatric nurses along with a pharmacist and a speech and language therapist. One of its functions was to provide a rapid response to help residents remain in their care home during an acute deterioration.

Brighton and Hove care homes support team
This team comprises nurses, a CPN, an end-of-life care facilitator, and a physiotherapist. They are actively involved in continuing care assessments.

Partnership for older people project
A partnership project between Gloucestershire County Council, Gloucestershire PCT, and other independent organizations, set up a team consisting of general and mental health nurses, OTs, physiotherapists, speech and language therapists, and a medicines management team. It provides education, training, and hands on support to the homes, including end-of-life work and dementia care mapping.

Durham care homes team
The service consists of two nurses and two social workers working with care homes to respond to safeguarding incidents in care homes and to work proactively with providers to reduce the number of safeguarding incidents.

South West Yorkshire continuing care team
This team (1999–2007) later became the Kirklees care home liaison service. It covered about 50 homes with 1200 residents. Led by a consultant old age psychiatrist with input from a specialist GP, CPNs, part time OT, support workers, and a dietician, the team offered an open referral system and assessed and managed all cases with mental health problems in local care homes, so the community mental health team did not go into care homes. They worked with individuals for an average of 8–10 weeks and worked with 80–100 clients at any one time. They also facilitated discharges from the ward and the community into the homes, and provided advice, training, and support. An audit in 2000 revealed a substantial reduction in hospital admissions from care homes, falling from 61 in 1997 to 13 in 2000.

Newcastle challenging behaviour service
The team, based at Newcastle General Hospital, is led by a clinical psychologist and consists of nurses and psychologists. It works with 80 care homes with and without nursing. All referrals of residents displaying challenging behaviour go through this team and not the local community mental health teams. The Newcastle model provides a framework for understanding the cause of the challenging behaviour in terms of the person's needs which, in turn, drive the person's behaviour. Another team using this model is the Behavioural Sciences Team based in Belfast, a nurse-led team with input from other professional disciplines.

Box 17.2 South East London CHST

The CHST in South East London was a multidisciplinary initiative established in 2003 to strengthen NHS specialized medical and nursing to 36 care homes in Lambeth, Lewisham, and Southwark. The team consisted of older persons' specialist nurses with part time support from pharmacists, consultant geriatricians, and a consultant old age psychiatrist. The older persons' specialist nurses were allocated particular care homes and as a result established close working links built on trust with the care home staff over the years.

The role of the team involved the statutory review of every care home resident's registered nursing needs and this allowed a unique opportunity to review their physical and mental health needs and medications. Various assessment tools were used to monitor, for example nutrition, continence, falls, cognitive impairment, and depression. Antipsychotic drugs and sedatives are regularly reviewed, thus increasing the awareness of staff of their potential adverse consequences, further supported by meetings between the link nurses and care home staff to discuss best practice. The team was also involved in assessments for NHS Continuing Care funding, which often can raise issues about long-term disease management.

The other part of its work involved increasing the knowledge, skills and self–confidence, and competence of the staff by providing information (often based on Department of Health guidance), advice, training, and personal support. The role modelling done by the nurses appeared to be particularly appreciated. The team actively supported the implementation of the Gold Standard Framework and liaised with the acute sector, particularly when people were being discharged from hospital to a care home and were involved in preventing readmissions.

This team was similar in design to the Continuing Care Team in South West Yorkshire, and offered similar advantages, due the expertise offered by a specialist team dedicated full time to this area. Unlike most of the other models described, there was proactive screening of all the residents via the statutory nursing assessment, and this ensured that the problem of unrecognized needs was substantially lessened. Although this does provide a comprehensive assessment, assessing every resident does create a large workload. Another drawback of this team compared with some other examples is that the CHST did not entirely replace the role of local services, so the care homes were able to by-pass the team and refer directly to local services, occasionally causing a muddle. The team also did not cover emergencies.

offset by longer terms gains in health and well-being. The effect on a possible improvement in quality of life as a result of early detection should not be underestimated for the individual themselves. The audit also suggested that the team had a positive impact on preventing longer admissions and facilitating early discharges but the time span of 2 years was felt to be too short to demonstrate a meaningful trend in hospital stays.

Doherty et al. (2008) examined the impact of a specialist CHST based on semi-structured interviews and focus groups of staff and managers. This research was unable to demonstrate the effectiveness of the team statistically but, however, the narrative evidence indicated that the team had successfully empowered the care home staff and supported them in the systematic management of long-term conditions. It was also felt that the team promoted more rapid access to services for care home residents and improved the quality of life for residents by promoting changes in the culture of the participating homes. The importance of sharing knowledge and experience was particularly noted.

An audit by the Hartlepool care homes liaison service (National Mental Health Development Unit, 2010) found that admissions to mental health inpatient beds from care homes were reduced. In the year prior to the service (employing one liaison nurse), there were 13 admissions, which decreased to 5 admissions in the next 3 years, an average of 1.6 per year.

Disadvantages of these models

The main disadvantage is that such teams are vulnerable to financial pressure and often they are one of the first services to be cut. They maybe seen as an 'added extra', as has occurred with some of the teams I have described. Another challenge is that sometimes the teams can be asked to do work that should be within the capabilities of the staff or the GP. Another weakness is that they are often not linked closely to the commissioning of care home services and so their influence may be limited. When concerns are raised about the quality of care, a clinical perspective is required, which may put the teams, somewhat reluctantly, into the role of inspector.

Nor does it appear that specialist care home teams have official sanction. Banerjee (2009), in his report for the Department of Health, did not favour the specialist team model but expressed the view that support to care homes to reduce antipsychotic drug use could best be provided from outreach by the mental health team.

Specialist nursing home physicians

In the Netherlands, the medical long-term care of residents in care homes is provided by specially trained doctors practising in a distinct speciality. There are 330 nursing homes in the Netherlands with a total of 57,000 beds and the nursing home is comparable to a skilled nursing facility in the United States. The nursing homes usually have around 200 beds with separate units for rehabilitation, long-term physical care, and residents with dementia. Most nursing homes also have day clinic facilities and they all have a fitness training facility.

Specialist staffing in a nursing home consists of one full time nursing home physician per 100 patients along with physiotherapists, occupational therapists (OTs), speech therapists, dieticians, music therapists, and psychologists, all employed by the home. There is a low referral rate of residents to hospital because of the presence of the nursing home physicians since diseases that elsewhere might need hospitalization can be managed within the home.

The nursing home physicians have a 3-year specialist training, affording specific knowledge and skills regarding the detection, management, and treatment of chronic diseases and mental health conditions. Their work involves diagnostic assessment and medical care for the individual patient, including laying down the priorities for the care plan as well as palliative care discussions and planning. They also have input into the management of the nursing home as an institution and formulating an overall medical policy for the nursing home (see Hoek et al., 2003 for further information).

Staff training and the way forward

Several reports over the last decade, including the National Dementia Strategy, have highlighted the need for care home staff to have an appropriate level of skills, especially for working with people with dementia. Some research has looked at effective ways of delivering training to care homes but the understanding remains limited as to what kind of training and support is effective when the contact from health is intermittent.

Work on dementia training from the University of Bradford has shown that workplace mentoring is of variable success. While it can be a very positive experience, this depends on the culture of the organization and its commitment to change. The most effective form of training appears to be by using actual cases rather than made up vignettes and involving the person with dementia in the training if at all possible. It is also essential to provide the training in a student-centred way to meet their learning needs rather than having a fixed curriculum. The training needs to take into account the individual's needs (especially as the carer's first language may not be English), roles, and study time available, and it must be flexible. A review of studies of dementia training for care workers has shown generally positive results but not in every case. Training has ranged from 30 minutes with video examples to 20 hours of lectures and 18 hours of group discussions over 1 week along with 3 months on the job guidance. There is not always a correlation between length of training and effect on behaviour or knowledge of staff.

Meehan et al. (2002) used an action research approach to identify the training and development needs of staff in 25 care homes. They found that the main challenges to the training related to staff issues in general, such as difficulties in releasing staff to attend.

Providers of secondary services often complain that care staff are not sure how to deal with physical health problems and this may then impact on the resident's mental health. Often care staff do not even have access to reference texts. To help address these problems, several teams (e.g. Sheffield, Somerset, and the South East London CHST) have developed guidance on recognition and treatment of common minor illnesses and conditions. This guidance also contains information about some of the various drugs used in the care home, including antipsychotics or sedatives, so that staff can be aware of what side-effects to look for. However, written guidance can only achieve so much; it is essential that there is clinical and managerial leadership and to allow enough time for change.

In conclusion, residents in care homes have complex physical and mental health needs but often do not have full access to the specialist services that would be available if they lived in their own homes. This is currently being addressed by statutory bodies such as the Care Quality Commission in its audit of services available to care home residents, but it also needs commissioners of health and social care to invest in services that can demonstrate how they can improve care for residents. Commissioners also need to be clear about the responsibilities of the rest of the NHS in providing health-care and support to residents in care homes. This can only come about through closer collaborative working between health and care home staff for the benefit of residents.

References

Badger, F., Clifford, C., Hewison, A., & Thomas, K. (2009). An evaluation of the implementation of a programme to improve end-of-life care in nursing homes. *Palliative Medicine, 23*, 502–511.

Banerjee, S. (2009). *The Use of Antipsychotic Medication for People with Dementia: Time for Action*. London: Department of Health.

Barber, N.D., Alldred, D.P., Raynor, D.K., et al. (2009). Care homes' use of medicines study: prevalence, causes and potential harm of medication errors in care homes for older people. *Quality and Safety in Health Care, 18*, 341–346.

Bowman, C., Whistler, J., & Ellerby, M. (2004). A national census of care home residents. *Age and Ageing, 33*, 561–566.

Bright, L. (2008). The cheek of it: problems accessing GP services persist. *Nursing Older People, 20*, 12. Available at: http://www.relres.org/pdf/press-releases-articles/NOP_Nov_08.pdf (accessed 15 March 2010).

Burns, E. (2010, Spring). *Prescribing in Care Homes: The Role of the Geriatrician*. Retrieved from http://www.bgs.org.uk/powerpoint/spr10/burns_prescribing_care_homes.pdf (accessed 16 February 2011).

Care Quality Commission (2008). *Guidance for Inspectors: Short Observational Framework for Inspection*. Available at: http://www.cqc.org.uk/_db/_documents/20081212 SOFI Guidance for Inspectors v 1.01 104–08.doc (accessed 13 June 2010).

Care Quality Commission (2010). *Review of 'Meeting the Healthcare Needs of People in Care Homes' 2009/10*. Available at: http://www.cqc.org.uk/aboutcqc/whatwedo/improvinghealthandsocialcare/specialreviewsandstudies/reviewofhealthcareforpeopleincarehomes2009/10.cfm (accessed 16 February 2011).

Cowan, D.T., Roberts, J.D., Fitzpatrick, J.M., & While, A.E. (2003a). Need for effective assessment of pain among people in care homes. *Reviews in Clinical Gerontology, 13*, 335–341.

Cowan, D.T., Roberts, J.D., Fitzpatrick, J.M., While, A.E., & Baldwin, J. (2003b). Nutritional status of older people in long term care settings; current status and future directions. *International Journal of Nursing Studies, 41*, 225–237.

Doherty, D., Davies, S., & Woodcock, L. (2008). Examining the impact of a specialist care homes support team. *Nursing Standards, 23*, 35–41.

English Community Care Association (2008). *'Can we Afford the Doctor?' GP Retainers and Care Homes*. London: ECCA.

Fahey, T., Montgomery, A., Barnes, J., & Protheroe, J. (2003). Quality of care for elderly residents in nursing homes and elderly people living at home: controlled observational study. *BMJ, 326*(7389), 580. doi:10.1136/bmj.326.7389.580.

Fossey, J., Ballard, C., Juszczak, E., et al. (2006). Effect of enhanced psychosocial care on people with severe dementia: clustered randomised trial of antipsychotic use in nursing home residents. *BMJ, 332*(7544), 756–761. doi:10.1136/bmj.38782.575868.7C.

Furniss, L., Burns, A., Craig, S.K., Scobie, S., Cooke, J., & Faragher, B. (2000). Effects of a pharmacist's medication review in nursing homes: randomised controlled trial. *British Journal of Psychiatry, 176*, 563–567.

Gladman, J., Donald, I., Archard, G., & Morris, J. (2009). *Interface between Primary and Secondary Medical Care*. Available at: http://www.bgs.org.uk/Publications/Compendium/compend_4-14.htm (accessed 16 February 2011).

Glendinning, C., Jacobs, S., Alborz, A., & Hann, M. (2002). A survey of access to medical services in nursing and residential homes in England. *British Journal of General Practice*, *52*, 545–548.

Goodman, C., Woolley, R., & Knight, D. (2003). District nurses' experiences of providing care in residential care home settings. *Journal of Clinical Nursing, 12*, 67–76.

Groom, L., Avery, A.J., Boot, D., et al. (2000). The impact of nursing home patients on general practitioners' workload. *British Journal of General Practice, 50*, 473–476.

Hoek, J.F., Ribbe, M.W., Hertogh, C.M., & van der Vleuten, C.P. (2003). The role of the specialist physician in nursing homes: the Netherlands' experience. *International Journal of Geriatric Psychiatry, 18*, 244–249.

House of Commons Health Committee (2004). *Elder Abuse*. London: Stationery Office.

Lyne, K.J., Moxon, S., Sinclair, I., Young, P., Kirk, C., & Ellison, S. (2006). Analysis of a care planning intervention for reducing depression in older people in residential care. *Aging & Mental Health, 10*, 394–403.

Meehan, L., Meyer, J., & Winter, J. (2002). Partnership with care homes: a new approach to collaborative working. *Journal of Research in Nursing, 7*, 348–359.

National Audit Office (2009). *Improving Dementia Services in England: An Interim Report*. London: Stationery Office.

National Mental Health Development Unit (2010). *Hartlepool Care Home Liaison*. Retrieved 13 June 2010, from http://www.nmhdu.org.uk/our-work/mhep/later-life/communities-of-interest/care-homes-liaison-/hartlepool-care-home-liaison (accessed 15 March 2010).

National Prescribing Centre (2000). *Prescribing for the Older Person*. MeReC Bulletin. Retrieved 25 June 2001, from http://www.npc.co.uk/ebt/merec/other_non_clinical/resources/merec_bulletin_vol11_no10.pdf.

Perry, M., Carpenter, I., Challis, D., & Hope, K. (2003). Understanding the roles of registered nurses and care assistants in care homes. *Journal of Advanced Nursing, 42*, 497–505.

Proctor, R., Burns, A., Powell, H.S., et al. (1999). Behavioural management in nursing and residential homes: a randomised controlled trial. *Lancet, 354*, 26–29.

Proctor, R., Stratton Powell, H., Burns, A., et al. (1998). An observational study to evaluate the impact of a specialist outreach team on the quality of care in nursing and residential homes. *Aging and Mental Health, 2*, 232–238.

Steves, C., Schiff, R., & Martin, F. (2009). Geriatricians and care homes: perspective from geriatric medicine departments and Primary Care Trusts. *Clinical Medicine, 9*, 528–533.

Szczepura, A., Nelson, S., & Wild, D. (2008). In-reach specialist nursing teams for residential care homes: uptake of services, impact on care provision and cost-effectiveness. *BMC Health Services Research, 8*, 269.

Wild, D., Szczepura, A., & Nelson, S. (2010). *Residential Care Home Work Force Development: The Rhetoric and Reality of Meeting Older Residents' Future Care Needs*. York: Joseph Rowntree Foundation Report. Available at: http://www.jrf.org.uk/publications/care-workforce-development (accessed 16 February 2011).

Chapter 18

Working with minorities in care homes

Jill Manthorpe and Jo Moriarty

Abstract

The most pervasive recreational activity . . . was bingo, something most men said they avoided. When asked if there were activities he was interested in, one resident flatly replied, 'No. They play bingo'.

(Park et al., 2009: 777)

[My dad] also forgot how to speak. He used to speak English very well, but it disappeared completely [with his dementia]. It just went. Then his Urdu started to go. In the home they couldn't understand what he was saying. They would say, 'Can you translate for us?'

(The Malik family, 2010: 90)

Michael . . . was a gay man suffering from an extreme form of dementia and a number of other life-threatening illnesses. He and I were not 'partners' but had a very close and affectionate friendship which had lasted over 40 years . . . I have no doubt that I had a unique role in Michael's life and in his care . . . He was able to co-operate and respond to me in ways in which he could not communicate with the care staff and others. I was the unique link enabling him to access the bits of remembered past experience.

(Bayliss, 2007)

Introduction

Only around 5% of older people live in care homes (Dening and Milne, 2009), so the decision to move into a care home means that every care home resident becomes part of a minority. It is, therefore, self-evident that people from minority groups in care homes will be a minority within a minority. For many years, little was known about their experiences and how these might impact upon their mental health but there is now an emerging literature, mostly based upon the accounts of family carers and practitioners, but rarely older residents themselves, about ways of promoting good practice. There is also a limited amount of evidence based on empirical research. However, we still know very little about whether residents from minorities are more or less likely to experience mental health problems compared with other residents. This chapter draws together some of the main messages about the mental health of men, older people from Black and minority ethnic (BME) groups, and lesbian, gay, bisexual, and transgendered (LGBT) people living in care homes and suggests ways in which practice with these groups can be improved. In focusing on these three groups, we recognize that there are other ways in which older people can experience minority status in care settings, such as coming from a different socioeconomic group (see Tester et al., 2005) but this is an area in which there is even less research. We also recognize that some people will experience multiple minority status, such as being an older LGBT and BME person. Nevertheless, we hope that this way of discussing some of the key issues will help to identify shared issues and those that may be specific to a particular group.

Men in care homes

Women are generally the majority of care home residents and comprise the bulk of practitioners in health and social care. Their longer life span, greater prevalence of long-term disability, and likelihood of outliving a male partner and thus being left on their own puts them at enhanced risk of care home entry. Local contexts are also likely to be important in residents' demographic profiles. For example, in areas where early male mortality is high, notably in poorer and former industrialized localities, men may be a very small minority of care home residents.

We know that widowed, divorced, and never married men often have more restricted social networks, engage in more risky health behaviours, and are more materially disadvantaged than their married counterparts (Age Concern Surrey, 2006). They may move to care home settings and, for many, this may be very welcome with real improvements in their quality of life, mood, diet and nutrition, self-care, and a reduction of loneliness. Studies of the experiences of being widowed in later life have found that some men find it hard to sustain their former contacts and friends and that their support networks may also decrease in size as they age (Davidson, 2000; Chambers, 2005). As the opening quotation to this chapter suggests, many men prefer different forms of social involvement than women, of a type that seems useful and supports their identity (Davidson et al., 2003) but this may need to be proactively maintained, with access to transport, for example. Furthermore, some men have never been 'joiners' and are unlikely to become so when older. Indeed, men often consult health professionals at a very late stage (Davidson and Arber, 2003). Masculinity thus continues to structure male experiences and activities even in care home settings.

In this section, we consider the ways in which care home settings can support the well-being of men who are living in care homes; this may be by recognizing and responding to risk factors for mental health problems and developing services in wider communities that may be particularly welcome to men and their family supporters. Matters such as access and acceptability may be just as relevant to minorities such as men as they are to other cultural or ethnic minorities. Furthermore, taking gender into account when thinking of providing good quality and person-centred services to other minority groups is now emerging as a key way to ensure services can meet equalities standards, fulfil inspection requirements, and comply with legal obligations. Being a minority in any group may be a cause of anxiety, for example the only man may feel very isolated or self-conscious, the more so if he is gay, or from a minority ethnic or religious group. Manthorpe and Moniz-Cook (2009) suggest that more thought needs to be given to how men are welcomed into early dementia services and the images that such services convey in terms of their publicity and illustrative activities. This point could be carried through to all services. The voluntary sector in England has recently observed that its activities are often perceived as 'feminized' and that there are few front-line male staff or volunteers (Ruxton, 2006). Again, this point is more widely applicable.

Promoting men's mental well-being

Within care homes, men may be at risk of loneliness; indeed this may have been the overt or underlying factor behind their move. It may be a mistake though to see that living in a care home necessarily reduces feelings of loneliness and other risks for developing depression, such as pain or declining health (National Collaborating Centre for Mental Health, 2009b). Life in a care home may not be rich in relationships and physical symptoms, such as pain, may be overlooked or not communicated.

All staff need to ensure that support or care plans are alert to mental as well as physical well-being indicators (changes in appetite, development of apathy, and so on) and that key workers are familiar with signs of depression in terms of recognition but also response and monitoring (National Collaborating Centre for Mental Health, 2009a). Sleep problems may be observed by night staff or feelings of being 'fed up' might be identified by other residents who may draw it to someone's attention if the home has an ethos of 'looking out for each other'. For all residents the contents of a care plan need to include biographical details such as information on personal background, preferences, and life history. In the case of men, particular information about employment, hobbies, sporting interests, and wartime or armed services experiences may be worth seeking out. And, to avoid stereotypes, the lack of interest in sport, a disinclination to go to the pub, or a strong interest in embroidery all need to be mentioned and should influence care practice and choices.

In some homes social activities are female dominated—with emphases on domestic skills, female crafts, and interests. Being conscious of this, some care settings have developed men's rooms, or areas, recreating, for example, the setting of a pub or a workshop. Others have developed men's groups, often facilitated by men—sometimes residents but also male members of staff, students, or volunteers.

Men in care homes may include visitors who have been former carers and these have been identified as a group who may be vulnerable if they feel guilty or bereft. In the examples of a husband visiting his wife, there may be symptoms of depression that may explain why the person feels so anxious about leaving his partner and appears to be so argumentative or disruptive to care staff.

For male residents in care settings there are risks of behaviour being seen as so challenging that care practices become overcontrolling and the resident becomes stigmatized. In a feminized environment, expressions of sexualized behaviour or disinhibition may be seen as distressing or 'abnormal' and the man may be at risk of becoming known as the 'dirty old man'. This may, in turn, cause distress to family members who visit and become aware of how their relative is perceived.

Care practices that address gender dynamics and the needs of men as minorities need to ensure men have the space to express aspects of their masculine identities. Archibald (1994) reports that 'special' places for men in service settings may help them feel less constrained and may enable them to talk about shared interests or backgrounds. The creation of opportunities to do what men might value and recreate aspects of their social roles, whether this relates to sport, games, socializing, or other parts of their biography, is also valued. This may be assisted by the presence of male workers. Attention to informants' accounts at the time of moving to a care home may be particularly important if an older man is losing his memory and/or if informants may not have continued involvement. Records of the details of work, involvement in armed services, sporting or hobby interests, activities and pastimes, are difficult to recreate if a person is no longer able to communicate well.

Not all men, of course, wish to socialize with other men and a cautionary note is made by Age Concern Surrey that sometimes practitioners may overemphasize men's desire to mix in male company:

> Professionals were inclined to stress the need for men to be able to meet other men, but many (by no means all) of the men interviewed were keen to meet with women as they missed female companionship.

(Age Concern Surrey, 2006: 13)

Finally, there is considerable evidence that older men are at greater risk of suicide and that care home services and others need to be aware of threats to older men's mental health. All staff need to know that expressions of a wish to take one's own life, the hoarding of items that might suggest a person is making plans (or starting to make preparations) to take an overdose, should be reported to managers and to mental health services. Within homes, if a suicide takes place staff have responsibility to see that the effects of this do not add to the problems of other residents. Responses to suicide need to encompass older people, caregivers, and staff (Manthorpe and Iliffe, 2005) and should be able to draw on pre-existing policies, such as policies covering communication, support, and involvement in the funeral and during the inquest process, and provision of supervision or debriefing. The rarity of suicide in settings such as nursing homes (Menghini and Evans, 2000) may mean that such plans need to include providing staff and other residents with support at a time when they are feeling particularly shocked.

Older people from Black and minority ethnic groups

Ethnicity is a self-defined and fluid concept, which can embrace a number of features such as skin colour, national or regional identity, cultural, religion, country of birth, language, dress, and political affiliation. The term 'Black and Minority Ethnic' refers predominately to people who migrated to Britain after the Second World War and whose ancestral roots can be traced to countries in the former British colonies in Africa, the Indian subcontinent, China and the Far East, and the Caribbean (Katbamna and Matthews, 2007: 5). It also applies to 'Other White' groups who identify themselves as having either an Irish or other White background, to people from the various traveller communities, and to people without strong historical ties to the United Kingdom, such as Iraq and Afghanistan where world events have shaped new patterns of migration.

In the past, and at the time of writing, most ethnic groups in the United Kingdom have younger populations than the majority White British population. This will gradually change and by 2051 the ethnic groups with the highest proportions of people aged 50 years and over will be 'Other White', Chinese, 'Other Asian', White British, Indian, 'Other', and 'White Irish' (Lievesley, 2010). Prevalence rates of depression and dementia among BME older people are broadly similar to those for the UK White population (Shah et al., 2009) but, given the association between ageing and dementia (Knapp et al., 2007) and ageing and depression (Osborn et al., 2003; McDougall et al., 2007), the number of BME people with dementia and/or depression is likely to rise particularly quickly as first generation migrants enter their 70s and 80s. As other chapters in this book have shown, high proportions of people admitted to care homes (Bowman et al., 2004; Macdonald and Cooper, 2007; Sutcliffe et al., 2007) have dementia and/or depression and so care homes are likely to see a corresponding increase in the number of BME residents with both these conditions.

Having said this, it is hard to know whether BME older residents are more or less likely to experience mental health problems. Historically, data on the ethnic origin of care home residents have not been good (Netten et al., 2010), partly because of variable ethnic monitoring and recording and partly because of differences in the way that ethnicity is defined. In addition, existing studies on the prevalence of mental health problems among care home residents have either not been reported by ethnicity or have not obtained sufficient numbers of BME people to enable separate analysis.

However, Bebbington and colleagues (2001: 58) dispute that BME older people are underrepresented in care homes and suggest that, among publicly funded residents, their admission rates are almost *twice* as high when differences in the age structure of the populations are taken into account. They go on to suggest that, in general, BME people admitted to care homes:

- are younger;
- are more likely to be men;
- are more likely to have been living with their family prior to admission;
- have a higher incidence of cognitive impairment/dementia and incontinence; and
- are more dependent, scored on the Barthel scale (a commonly used way of measuring how well a person can undertake activities of daily living such as washing and dressing).

Bebbington and colleagues also found that the interval between admission and death was shorter for BME people, suggesting that BME older people are likely to be admitted to care homes at a later stage in their illness trajectory than their White counterparts. Laing's (2005) survey of care home admissions in London found a similar pattern of overrepresentation among BME older people.

Promoting the well-being of BME older people

Despite this evidence of increased risk of admission, BME older people and their family carers tend to look unfavourably on the idea of moving into a care home (Mold et al., 2005; Banks et al., 2006; Badger et al., 2009). The biggest barriers to using care homes—and other health and social care services more generally—among BME older people are lack of information and fears that they will not provide culturally acceptable care (Butt and O'Neil, 2004; Sharif et al., 2008; Manthorpe et al., 2009).

A combination of experience in dealing with greater ethnic diversity among residents, training, regulation, and legislation has improved care home providers' awareness of the need to provide more culturally sensitive care, especially around the provision of food, assistance with personal care, such as bathing and dressing, and religious worship. Alongside these improvements lies the risk that unquestioning attention to the 'food and faith' agenda (Manthorpe et al., 2010) could, in itself, contribute to stereotyping and a tendency to ignore other aspects contributing to well-being. For instance, while adherence to a formal religion is higher among BME groups than the White British population, the highest proportion of people stating that they do not have a religion are Chinese (Office for National Statistics, 2004). In the same way, when asked where they wanted to go on an outing, a group of older Asian women attending a mental health day centre chose to visit a pizza restaurant (Manthorpe et al., 2010).

Although much of the good practice in identifying depression and promoting well-being described above in the section on men, applies equally to BME residents, some different factors need to be considered. BME people, family carers, and practitioners all identify the sense of isolation that can occur for BME residents in homes in which the overwhelming majority of residents are White (Manthorpe et al., 2010). Given that levels of fluency in English vary among this generation of BME older people, these feelings can be accentuated when no other residents or staff members speak their language, as in the opening quotation to this chapter. Although homes specializing in services for different ethnic and faith groups do exist, they are mainly situated in major conurbations. BME older people may either not have the choice of moving to one of these homes or may decide that the advantages of moving to a home in their own neighbourhood is preferable to moving many miles away to a home specializing in care for people from their own ethnic group. Although bilingual staff and access to DVDs and satellite television stations can help prevent isolation, it is very important that care home staff help support the maintenance of links with the resident's wider community. For example, the manager of one home who took part in a study of social care practice with BME older people (Manthorpe et al., 2010) explained:

> We have a peripatetic activities coordinator that visits our homes—she's very much trained up and in touch with community groups—she would look at what we can bring in . . . We had [a] traveller in . . . He always worked with horses . . . He got out of the home a couple of times—he was looking for a horse [so] we approached the organisation that did . . . [riding for the disabled] and arranged for him to go over once a week as part of his care plan, that was his big thing.

Another factor for practitioners to bear in mind is the different levels of awareness and understanding of mental health issues that exist among BME people and their family carers (Bowes and Wilkinson, 2003; Adamson and Donovan, 2005; Seabrooke and Milne, 2009). It is worth remembering that many people with dementia never receive a formal diagnosis (Department of Health, 2009), and so even at the stage at which people are admitted to a care home there can still be considerable variation in residents' and family members' understanding of dementia and so sensitive probing may be required.

Practitioners also need to be alert to the different ways in which BME people may describe feelings of depression. For example, Asian and Black Caribbean older people may talk about 'worrying' or 'thinking too much' rather than describing feeling 'hopeless' or 'low' (Lawrence et al., 2006).

The experience of racism (Karlsen and Nazroo, 2002) or fear of racial harassment (Karlsen and Nazroo, 2004) can, in itself, contribute to poor mental health. Care home procedures and staff training sessions need to include how to respond to racist behaviour by other residents, staff, and visitors.

Lesbian, gay, bisexual, and transgendered residents

Most care homes include LGBT people, but they are often 'invisible'. While no published research has looked at LGBT residents in care homes, emerging evidence from syntheses of the research literature suggests that LGBT people are at significantly higher risk of suicidal behaviour, mental disorder, substance misuse, and substance dependence than heterosexual people (King et al., 2008; Addis et al., 2009). There is, of course, a possibility that heterosexism may have influenced the way in which some of this research itself was framed. However, they are still real risks and risks that may result in, or at least contribute to, the likelihood of admission to a care home. On this basis alone, the researchers suggest that the mental health needs of LGBT people should become standard in training for all health and social care professionals.

King and colleagues (2006: 4) further recommend routine inclusion of sexual orientation in data collection to assist in identifying these high-risk groups and therefore being more alert and responsive to the risks. They suggest that agencies and professionals who have particular expertise with gay and lesbian service users should be publicized across local networks, adding 'There is an urgent need for mental health services to develop LGB sensitive services and an obvious initial step would be the incorporation of LGB issues into diversity training for staff'. For homes specializing in mental health support, risks may have been identified in care plans; however older people who have multiple health problems or frailty may move to care homes without such detailed records. The combined evidence that a high number of lesbian and gay people (Warner et al., 2003) live alone after retirement and that there is a link between living alone and entering long-term care (e.g. Kendig et al., 2010), further suggests that older gay men and lesbians may be at enhanced risk of care home admission.

Disclosure and preferences for care

There is often no attempt to distinguish provision of care for this group from those of heterosexual people and LGBT residents may not wish to expose themselves to possible negative reactions by asserting themselves and appearing to be different. Only a small number of studies have been able to include the experiences of care home residents who are from LGBT groups. Price (2008, 2010) is one of the few who has sought accounts from carers of gay and lesbian older people with dementia, including those with experience of the person they were supporting moving into and living in care homes. She found that carers, both lesbian women and gay men, mediated disclosures of their sexualities to health and social care service practitioners. For many carers, initial professional responses to these disclosures and hints of disclosure affected their decisions about 'coming out' further. She concluded that service providers' reactions were at best accepting of gay and lesbian people, but generally there was 'pervasive disregard' of their needs. In relation to care homes, while people living in the community might have supportive networks which are largely of their choosing, on moving to a care home reactions may not be positive and people may understandably be guarded for fear of hostile and homophobic attitudes and treatment. For gay and lesbian people with dementia, declining cognitive impairment may mean that fears of losing abilities to keep aspects of their lives private may surface, compounding distress.

Other studies reveal that many lesbian and gay men express a wish to live in a care home run by lesbian and gay providers of care if they were to need such support (Heaphy and Yip, 2006). Of the 226 lesbians and gay men who responded to their survey, 120 considered this would be desirable or highly desirable. In this study, focus group participants voiced their fears about discrimination, stigma, and harassment in non-specialist care homes and other social care settings. Heaphy and Yip (2006) raise the importance of training for care home staff (among others), of adherence to anti-discriminatory practice, and suggest that a system of 'kite-marking' might be helpful in enhancing confidence among prospective residents that a home promotes equalities. Assurances of confidentiality may be particularly important around record keeping and access to personal information.

Impact of legislation and regulation

There have been major legislative changes in the United Kingdom in recent years: the introduction of the Employment Equality (Sexual Orientation) Regulations (2003), Civil Partnership Act (2005), Equality Act (2006), and the Equality Act (Sexual Orientation) Regulations (2007) prohibiting discrimination in public life and providing a statutory framework for the equalities for LGBT people (Cocker and Hafford-Letchfield, 2010). These changes, and the inclusion of sexuality and transgender in the six equality strands of the Equality and Human Rights Commission, suggest that care providers will be increasingly under the spotlight to provide assurances that their staff respect and promote non-discriminatory practice. However, these will take time to have effect; Mitchell and colleagues (2008) suggest that the care and support concerns of lesbian, gay, and bisexual (LGB) people as they grow older relate to loss of independent living in a context where they might be forced to rely on care home provision that could be heterocentric, potentially isolating, or even homophobic.

The specifics of what inspectors and regulators will be looking for are spelled out by the former Commission for Social Care Inspection (CSCI) (2008: 6) which describes how care providers should ensure that LGB people receive an equal service by:

- creating an ethos in the service where LGB people are valued;
- reviewing policies and procedures and assessment/admission processes to ensure that they do not discriminate;
- providing training and support to staff;
- positive action to make LGB people feel welcome and able to come out, for example by including them in publicity;
- ensuring that LGB people have a choice of which staff support them;
- enabling LGB people to have contact with their communities and friends;
- valuing LGB people's relationships;
- taking appropriate action when discrimination does happen; and
- listening to the views of LGB people and monitoring progress.

As one example of this, Davies and colleagues (2006: 58) suggest that service providers should not assume heterosexism when older people wish to appoint surrogate decision-makers. They recommend, on the basis of their literature review, that service providers should build trust with the partner of a sick, dying, or deceased LGBT person so that grief (bereavement) counselling might be extended to them. In addition, they suggest that practitioners should be aware of how 'homophobic, heterosexist, and ageist attitudes may converge to sanction any forms of affection or love-making between LGBT residents and residents and visitors'. In their view, care facilities, may through ignorance or prejudice, undermine residents' support and so contribute to stress and anxiety. Further, they recommend that homophobia, biphobia, and transphobia should be recognized as forms of abuse and addressed in policies and procedures to safeguard older LGBT people from harassment and intimidation. There are therefore emerging studies and training materials relevant to care home practitioners and managers (Fish, 2007) who may wish to improve or sustain good practice in this area.

Discussion

This chapter has tried to identify some of the shared and specific issues around working with minorities in care home settings. The need for staff to be alert to changes in well-being and to find ways of enabling residents, whatever their ethnicity, gender, or sexual orientation, to maintain purpose and fulfilment in their lives are among those issues that are shared. Equally, the need for access to training in understanding the issues faced by different minorities and how to provide culturally sensitive care are cross-cutting themes. By contrast, while the negative effects of discrimination on mental health is something that BME (Karlsen and Nazroo, 2002) and LGBT residents (King et al., 2008) both share, for White heterosexual men, moving into a care home may be the first time they experience being in a minority. Although we know a limited amount about how living in a care home may replicate 'old' issues, we know very little about how it may create new challenges that impact upon the health of residents from minority groups.

Some of the debates about promoting well-being raise wider issues about the role of specialist provision for various groups of residents. As already mentioned, in the United Kingdom, specialist homes already exist for some ethnic and faith groups. In the United States, this practice has spread to include the development of LGBT provision (Gross, 2007). Although developments such as these are likely to expand to the United Kingdom, it is clear that most care homes will continue to be generic—albeit with the inclusion of separate areas, as mentioned earlier in this chapter. From an optimistic standpoint, this may mean that some of the issues faced by particular minorities may be ameliorated. For instance, younger gay and bisexual men are more open about their sexuality with family, friends, and colleagues than their older counterparts (Warner et al., 2003) and so the fear of disclosure mentioned here may gradually prove to be less of an issue in the future. Turning back to the present, the views of older people themselves about better ways of working with minorities are strikingly absent; it is important that we make more efforts to listen to their ideas about creating environments in which all minorities can receive equally good care and have their well-being nurtured and promoted.

References

Adamson, J. & Donovan, J. (2005). 'Normal disruption': South Asian and African/Caribbean relatives caring for an older family member in the UK. *Social Science & Medicine, 60*, 37–48.

Addis, S., Davies, M., Greene, G., MacBride-Stewart, S., & Shepherd, M. (2009). The health, social care and housing needs of lesbian, gay, bisexual and transgender older people: a review of the literature. *Health & Social Care in the Community, 17*, 647–658.

Age Concern Surrey (2006). *Investigation into the Social and Emotional Wellbeing of Lone Older Men*. Guildford: Age Concern Surrey.

Archibald, C. (1994). The trouble with men. *Journal of Dementia Care, 2*, 20–22.

Badger, F., Pumphrey, R., Clarke, L., et al. (2009). The role of ethnicity in end-of-life care in care homes for older people in the UK: a literature review. *Diversity in Health and Care, 6*, 23–29.

Banks, L., Haynes, P., Balloch, S., & Hill, M. (2006). *Changes in Communal Provision for Adult Social Care: 1991–2001*. York: Joseph Rowntree Foundation. Available at: http://www.jrf.org.uk/sites/files/jrf/9781859354865.pdf (accessed 2 August 2010).

Bayliss, B. (2007). Having dementia and being gay: fighting the system. *Mature Times*. Available at: http://www.maturetimes.co.uk/node/3265 (accessed 2 August 2010).

Bebbington, A., Darton, R., & Netten, A. (2001). *Care Homes for Older People Volume 2: Admissions, Needs and Outcomes*. Canterbury: Personal Social Services Research Unit. Available at: http://www.pssru.ac.uk/pdf/chop2.pdf (accessed 2 August 2010).

Bowes, A. & Wilkinson, H. (2003). 'We didn't know it would get that bad': South Asian experiences of dementia and the service response. *Health & Social Care in the Community, 11*, 387–396.

Bowman, C., Whistler, J., & Ellerby, M. (2004). A national census of care home residents. *Age and Ageing, 33*, 561–566.

Butt, J. & O'Neil, A. (2004). *'Let's Move On': Black and Minority Ethnic Older People's Views on Research Findings*. York: Joseph Rowntree Foundation. Available at: http://www.jrf.org.uk/bookshop/eBooks/185935176X.pdf (accessed 2 August 2010).

Chambers, P. (2005). *Older Widows and the Lifecourse: Multiple Narratives of Hidden Lives.* Abingdon: Ashgate.

Cocker, C. & Hafford-Letchfield, T. (2010). Out and proud? Social work's relationship with lesbian and gay equality. *British Journal of Social Work, 40,* 1996–2008.

Commission for Social Care Inspection (2008). *Putting People First: Equality and Diversity Matters 1. Providing Appropriate Services for Lesbian, Gay and Bisexual and Transgender People.* London: Commission for Social Care Inspection. Available at: http://www.cqc.org.uk/_db/_documents/putting_people_first_equality_and_diversity_matters_1.pdf (accessed 2 August 2010).

Davidson, K. (2000). What we want: older widows and widowers speak for themselves. *Practice: Social Work in Action, 12,* 45–54.

Davidson, K. & Arber, S. (2003). Older men's health: a life course issue. *Men's Health Journal, 2,* 63–66.

Davidson, K., Daly, T., & Arber, S. (2003). Older men, social integration and organisational activities. *Social Policy and Society, 2,* 81–89.

Davies, M., Addis, S., MacBride-Stewart, S., & Shepherd, M. (2006). *The Health, Social Care and Housing Needs of Lesbian, Gay, Bisexual and Transgender Older People: Literature Review.* Cardiff: Centre for Heath Sciences Research, University of Cardiff.

Dening, T. & Milne, A. (2009). Depression and mental health in care homes for older people. *Quality in Ageing and Older Adults, 10,* 40–46.

Department of Health (2009). *Living Well with Dementia: A National Dementia Strategy.* London: Department of Health. Available at: http://www.dh.gov.uk/prod_consum_dh/groups/dh_digitalassets/@dh/@en/documents/digitalasset/dh_094051.pdf (accessed 29 July 2010).

Fish, J. (2007). *Reducing Health Inequalities for Lesbian, Gay, Bisexual and Trans People— Briefings for Health and Social Care Staff.* London: Department of Health. Available at: http://www.dh.gov.uk/en/Publicationsandstatistics/Publications/PublicationsPolicyAndGuidance/DH_078347 (accessed 2 August 2010).

Gross, J. (2007). Aging and gay, and facing prejudice in twilight. *New York Times.* Available at: http://www.nytimes.com/2007/10/09/us/09aged.html (accessed 2 August 2010).

Heaphy, B. & Yip, A.K.T. (2006). Policy implications of ageing sexualities. *Social Policy and Society, 5,* 442–451.

Karlsen, S. & Nazroo, J.Y. (2002). Relation between racial discrimination, social class, and health among ethnic minority groups. *American Journal of Public Health, 92,* 624–631.

Karlsen, S. & Nazroo, J.Y. (2004). Fear of racism and health. *Journal of Epidemiology and Community Health, 58,* 1017–1018.

Katbamna, S. & Matthews, R. (2007). *Ageing & Ethnicity in England: A Demographic Profile of BME Older People in England.* London: Age Concern England. Available at: http://www2.le.ac.uk/departments/health-sciences/archive/extranet/research-groups/nuffield/project_profiles/Ageing%20%20Ethnicity%20Briefing.pdf (accessed 2 August 2010).

Kendig, H., Browning, C., Pedlow, R., Wells, Y., & Thomas, S. (2010). Health, social and lifestyle factors in entry to residential aged care: an Australian longitudinal analysis. *Age and Ageing, 39,* 342–349.

King, M., Semlyen, J., Tai, S.S., et al. (2006). *Mental Disorders, Suicide, and Deliberate Self Harm in Lesbian, Gay and Bisexual People: A Systematic Review of the Literature.* London: University College London, Department of Mental Health Sciences, Royal Free and University College Medical School.

King, M., Semlyen, J., Tai, S., et al. (2008). A systematic review of mental disorder, suicide, and deliberate self harm in lesbian, gay and bisexual people. *BMC Psychiatry, 8,* 70. Available at: http://dx.doi.org/10.1186/1471-244X-8-70 (accessed 2 August 2010).

Knapp, M., Prince, M., Albanese, E., et al. (2007). *Dementia UK. A Report to the Alzheimer's Society on the Prevalence and Economic Cost of Dementia in the UK Produced by King's College London and the London School of Economics.* London: Alzheimer's Society. Available at: http://www.alzheimers.org.uk/News_and_Campaigns/Campaigning/PDF/Dementia_UK_Full_Report.pdf (accessed 2 August 2010).

Laing, W. (2005). *Trends in the London Care Market 1994–2024.* London: King's Fund. Available at: www.kingsfund.org.uk/document.rm?id=5522 (accessed 2 August 2010).

Lawrence, V., Murray, J., Banerjee, S., et al. (2006). Concepts and causation of depression: a cross-cultural study of the beliefs of older adults. *Gerontologist, 46,* 23–32.

Lievesley, N. (2010). *The Future Ageing of the Ethnic Minority Population of England and Wales.* London: Runnymede Trust/Centre for Policy on Ageing. Available at: http://www.runnymedetrust.org/publications/147/32.html (accessed 2 August 2010).

Macdonald, A. & Cooper, B. (2007). Long-term care and dementia services: an impending crisis. *Age and Ageing, 36,* 16–22.

Manthorpe, J. & Iliffe, S. (2005). *Depression in Later Life.* London: Jessica Kingsley Publishers.

Manthorpe, J. & Moniz-Cook, E. (2009). Developing group support for men with mild cognitive difficulties and early stage dementia. In: J. Manthorpe & E. Moniz-Cook (Eds.), *Psychosocial Interventions in Dementia: Evidence-based Practice* (pp. 174–185). London: Jessica Kingsley Publishers.

Manthorpe, J., Iliffe, S., Moriarty, J., et al. (2009). 'We are not blaming anyone but if we don't know about amenities, we cannot seek them out': Black and minority older people's views on the quality of local health and social services. *Ageing & Society, 29,* 93–113.

Manthorpe, J., Moriarty, J., Stevens, M., Sharif, N., & Hussein, S. (2010). *Practice Enquiry: Supporting Black and Minority Ethnic Older People's Mental Wellbeing: Accounts of Social Care Practice.* London: Social Care Institute for Excellence.

McDougall, F.A., Kvaal, K., Matthews, F.E., et al. (2007). Prevalence of depression in older people in England and Wales: the MRC CFA Study. *Psychological Medicine, 37,* 1787–1795.

Menghini, V.V. & Evans, J.M. (2000). Suicide among nursing home residents: a population-based study. *Journal of the American Medical Directors Association, 1,* 47–50.

Mitchell, M., Howarth, C., Kotecha, M. & Creegan, C. (2008). *Research Report 34: Sexual Orientation Research Review 2008.* London: Equality and Human Rights Commission. Available at: http://www.equalityhumanrights.com/uploaded_files/sexual_orientation_research_review.pdf (accessed 2 August 2010).

Mold, F., Fitzpatrick, J.M., & Roberts, J.D. (2005). Minority ethnic elders in care homes: a review of the literature. *Age and Ageing, 34,* 107–113.

National Collaborating Centre for Mental Health (2009a). *National Clinical Practice Guideline 90: Depression: The Treatment and Management of Depression in Adults (Update).* London: National Institute for Health and Clinical Excellence. Available at: http://www.nice.org.uk/nicemedia/live/12327/45913/45913.pdf (accessed 2 August 2010).

National Collaborating Centre for Mental Health (2009b). *National Clinical Practice Guideline Number 91: Depression in Adults with a Chronic Physical Health Problem: Treatment and Management.* London: National Institute for Health and Clinical Excellence. Available at: http://www.nice.org.uk/nicemedia/live/12327/45913/45913.pdf (accessed 2 August 2010).

Netten, A., Beadle-Brown, J., Birgit Trukeschitz, B., et al. (2010). *PSSRU Discussion Paper 2696/2: Measuring Outcomes for Public Service Users' Project.* Canterbury: Personal Social Services Research Unit. Available at: http://www.pssru.ac.uk/pdf/dp2696.pdf (accessed 2 August 2010).

Office for National Statistics (2004). *Focus on Religion.* London: HMSO. Available at: http://www.statistics.gov.uk/downloads/theme_compendia/for2004/FocusonReligion.pdf (accessed 2 August 2010).

Osborn, D.P.J., Fletcher, A.E., Smeeth, L., et al. (2003). Factors associated with depression in a representative sample of 14 217 people aged 75 and over in the United Kingdom: results from the MRC trial of assessment and management of older people in the community. *International Journal of Geriatric Psychiatry, 18*, 623–630.

Park, N.S., Knapp, M.A., Shin, H.J., & Kinslow, K.M. (2009). Mixed methods study of social engagement in assisted living communities: challenges and implications for serving older men. *Journal of Gerontological Social Work, 52*, 767–783.

Price, E. (2008). Pride or prejudice? Gay men, lesbians and dementia. *British Journal of Social Work, 38*, 1337–1352.

Price, E. (2010). Coming out to care: gay and lesbian carers' experiences of dementia services. *Health & Social Care in the Community, 18*, 160–168.

Ruxton, S. (2006). *Working with Older Men: A Review of Age Concern Services.* London: Age Concern England. Available at: http://www.menshealthforum.org.uk/files/images/AgeConcernoldermenservices.pdf (accessed 2 August 2010).

Seabrooke, V. & Milne, A. (2009). Early intervention in dementia care in an Asian community. *Quality in Ageing and Older Adults, 10*, 29–36.

Shah, A., Adelman, S., & Ong, Y.L. (2009). *Psychiatric Services for Black and Minority Ethnic Older People. College Report 156.* London: Royal College of Psychiatrists. Available at: http://www.rcpsych.ac.uk/files/pdfversion/CR156.pdf (accessed 13 May 2010).

Sharif, N., Brown, W., & Rutter, D. (2008). *The Extent and Impact of Depression on BME Older People and the Acceptability, Accessibility and Effectiveness of Social Care Provision.* London: Social Care Institute for Excellence. Available at: http://www.scie.org.uk/publications/map/map03.pdf (accessed 2 August 2010).

Sutcliffe, C., Burns, A., Challis, D., et al. (2007). Depressed mood, cognitive impairment, and survival in older people admitted to care homes in England. *American Journal of Geriatric Psychiatry, 15*, 708–715.

Tester, S., Hubbard, G., Downs, M., MacDonald, C., & Murphy, J. (2005). *Full Research Report ESRC Grant L480254023: Exploring Perceptions of Quality of Life of Frail Older People During and After their Transition to Institutional Care.* Swindon: Economic and Social Research Council. Available at: http://www.esrcsocietytoday.ac.uk/ESRCInfoCentre/ (accessed 2 August 2010).

The Malik family (2010). Our mum had to be the man of the house. In: L. Whitman (Ed.), *Telling Tales about Dementia: Experiences of Caring* (pp. 88–92). London: Jessica Kingsley Publishers.

Warner, J.P., Wright, L., Blanchard, M., & King, M. (2003). The psychological health and quality of life of older lesbians and gay men: a snowball sampling pilot survey. *International Journal of Geriatric Psychiatry, 18*, 754–755.

Chapter 19

Physical health issues

Clive Bowman

Abstract

The purpose of this chapter is to encourage a proactive approach to the physical health needs of the care home resident with mental health problems through a consideration of some common clinical issues. The key point is that many problems are not complicated but just need a clear-minded approach and methodical resolution with clear communication. Admission to long-term care in a care home signals a transition in a person's life and an opportunity to review their health needs and simplify the medications that they are receiving. The approach is a palliative one that aims to promote mental and physical well-being where possible, and to see the resident through to the end of their life in peace and dignity.

Introduction

The care home was originally a housing solution for predominantly older people and carried all the stigma of the poor laws and workhouses. Homes have evolved through a period where they provided communal living with some personal care, often over many years. The current situation, however, is that they are facilities providing care, support, and sanctuary for people with major disabilities arising from chronic diseases of which the dementias and mental illnesses are the most common, often complicated by comorbidities and frailty.

Not only has the dependency and vulnerability of older people using care homes increased but so too has the 'intensity of care' (the level of dependency compounded by the activity of admissions, death, and discharges). Lengths of stay have fallen both through a combination of improved community care and rationing of access. These factors have meant that admissions to care homes now occur later in the life course and therefore there are shorter lengths of stay in long-term care. In addition, temporary admissions for respite and various strategies for avoiding acute hospital admission or promoting early discharge have exacerbated these trends. Though the commissioning of care homes and the healthcare support they receive is nominally based on long-term care with expected stays measured in years rather than months, the reality is of a much more demanding, transient, vulnerable, and frail population. Furthermore, care homes are often mistakenly thought only to provide long-term care with death being the usual outcome, but for many years the rate of transfer and discharge from care homes has exceeded mortality, reflecting a more dynamic role than is commonly appreciated.

The admission of older people with mental health problems to care homes frequently follows escalating care needs and increased involvement of health and care services in the community. In around half of such cases, a relatively minor intercurrent illness, which probably reflects more the stage of the patient's life and illness than the severity of the presenting illness itself, precedes the admission to care homes. Although the admission to care may have been anticipated, it is in the event usually poorly planned and hallmarked by disappointment, defeat, frustration, and bewilderment by exhausted carers and family.

Care home admission is also often accompanied by the transfer of care to a new general practitioner who may be provided some information regarding the precipitating 'acute' event but relatively little about the nature of chronic disease and disability that are at the root of the patient's need for care. Although care home residents are likely to have long-term medical conditions, simply referring to them as such carries insufficient information for attending doctors to be able to take decisions.

Typically, considerable health and care support is provided to sustain an individual in the community but following admission to a care home there is, at least medically, often a relative withdrawal, the patient having been admitted to a 'place of safety'. Admission to a care home should not prejudice an individual's rights to have access to medical opinion though there may well be limits to what can be expected from medical interventions. Nonetheless, there are real opportunities to improve well-being and avoid complications.

Logically, admission to care should be seen as a watershed that should prompt a reappraisal of long-term medical conditions and the objectives of treatment(s) and their consequence(s). There is, at present, little consistent structure to health support for care home residents and, as adequate clinical information is often lacking, receiving doctors may be reluctant to make appropriate revisions to patients' treatment. After the initial admission period, the impetus for review often becomes lost, and medicines (and their consequences) are simply continued uncritically.

The treatment objectives of long-term conditions may significantly change following admission, for example, from maintaining mobility at the expense of cognitive function or using sedation at night to provide carers with some rest time. Similarly, episodes of acute illness should lead to a critical questioning of the potential benefit of hospitalization against the risks and opportunities for in situ care within the care home. Although the medicine of the care home resident is probably the greatest Cinderella in healthcare today, it is worth reflecting that in the United Kingdom for every NHS (National Health Service) hospital bed of all types there are between three and four care home beds. This chapter will not seek to emulate a comprehensive textbook of clinical medicine but highlight some selected issues, opportunities, and common problems in care home medicine that hopefully will encourage a positive, proactive approach to clinical practice.

Assessment and review of health status

The healthcare needs of care home residents remain poorly understood, partly because of the failure to adopt a consistent approach to measurement through standardised assessment. It is nearly a decade since the English government published the National Service Framework for Older People which championed the need for, yet failed to establish, a single assessment process. What does exist is an industry of assessments that centre on eligibility and funding entitlement (either for Fully Funded NHS Care or for Registered Nursing Care Contribution) and means testing (eligibility for local authority funding). None of this assessment 'industry' actually provides into a specific care plan for the individual. Arguably, a rational system would determine needs, plan care, and then determine funding. The system of care and its funding remains unresolved, and currently inequalities in healthcare support for older citizens with physical and mental illness persist.

In many countries it is mandatory to have a pre-admission assessment. This provides an opportunity for the attending doctor to consider all the conditions that the person may have been diagnosed with, so that they can decide which treatments should be continued, when to review the patient's condition, and what the appropriate level of response should be in the case of acute illness. Although multiple pathologies are common, there is usually a dominant or principal diagnosis which may significantly influence the approach to other illnesses. For example, the presence of severe dementia may dominate the picture and affect all the decisions that are made on behalf of that individual. Comorbidities may significantly change the course of the principal diagnosis but they are usually secondary. On occasion, the pursuit of highly specialist treatments and interventions may detract from the management of the principal condition, which is particularly important during acute illness or following a major tissue injury such as a fracture. Without clear information about the principal diagnosis and comorbidities, it is not surprising that many vulnerable older people are seemingly indiscriminately referred or sent to accident and emergency departments when either chronic disease slides out of control or acute events occur.

In summary, medical assessment that facilitates good care requires a record of:

◆ principal clinical problems;
◆ comorbidities;
◆ functional and mental capacities disabilities;
◆ likely prognosis and expectations of admission;
◆ medicines and other treatments and their rationale; and
◆ personal preferences and directives.

Once someone is living in a care home, reassessment should be routinely considered at least 3 monthly or more often in the event of a significant change in health status. At present, there is no statutory planned reassessment for resource allocation and so good practice dictates that any significant change in care needs be alerted to commissioners to ensure that funding care keeps pace with actual needs. Increasing dependency and frailty require increased care and if only a low level of personal care has been purchased it is unlikely to prove sufficient for escalating care needs.

Communication

On transfer from the community or acute hospital to a care home, it should be mandatory to provide a summary of the individual's clinical status with sufficient medical information to enable a receiving doctor to take over routine care and plan any response to future acute events. Given the absence of standardized assessments and tools, the following case study provides the bare minimum for newly attending doctors to take clinical responsibility with confidence.

Case study 1

Mr X, an 85-year-old widower, has been transferred to St. Erstwhile's specialist dementia care home following an acute hospital admission for multiple falls and urinary incontinence. These appear to have been related to an *Escherichia coli* urinary tract infection that has been successfully treated.

Mr X has received increasing support in the community for 3 years because of his Alzheimer's disease which had been diagnosed by the Memory Clinic. In spite of escalating care by social services and his daughter, it has become apparent that he was approaching the point of needing 24/7 care because of his disorientation and failure to care for himself when unsupervised.

The acute admission has provided an opportunity to pursue a care placement. During his hospital admission, he became very agitated and a danger to himself and others and was sedated with antipsychotics. It is expected that following a period to settle into the care home this medication could be reduced and withdrawn. Mr X also has long-standing hypertension; the need for his continued treatment for this was not reviewed in the acute admission.

Prior to his hospital admission he was ambulant, continent, and largely self-caring. He fed himself but was disorientated and could easily become frustrated. He now needs to be prompted to take adequate fluids. At discharge, Mr X was regaining his mobility but still required a steadying hand. He was regaining continence with a regular toileting regime and typically having one episode of incontinence a day.

His daughter, Mrs Y, lives nearby and has a lasting power of attorney. While he was an inpatient, the multidisciplinary team and family agreed that Mr X should not be subject to resuscitation and that the stance to his care should be palliative.

Before an older person moves to a care home, it is important to communicate in a realistic way with the individual and with his or her family and carers, to avoid unrealistic expectations arising. For example, hospital staff sometimes suggest that admission to a care home may 'make things better'. It is of course inappropriate for a patient with dementia to remain in an acute hospital any longer than necessary, but being in a care home is certainly not focused on active treatment and cure. It may be that such advice is offered to soften the impact upon families of making difficult decisions for their relatives. The trouble is that this can often give rise to unreasonable expectations.

However, it is more sensible to be realistic and explain that now the person has reached the limits of care in the community and that the issues causing hospital admission have now been resolved, admission to a care home is now a sensible step that reflects the severity of disease and the person's care needs. A positive perspective would be to suggest that admission to care offers new opportunities for family and friends through being relieved of the 24/7 burden of care and support but perhaps yielding time for socialization which simply did not exist before. When the older person has lived alone, there are new opportunities for company and a release from the pressures of domestic organization.

As well as medical information, there also needs to be an up-to-date care plan and/ or nursing assessment, with clear written advice and guidance to care home staff. This needs to be transferred to the care home records as soon as possible so that an appropriate care plan can be established and communicated to all the staff involved in that person's care. As well as this, such records should also include concerns, complaints, or indeed regulatory or criminal investigation. If an investigation is ever required, the time spent writing contemporaneous notes will prove to have been well worthwhile in understanding what went wrong.

The confidentiality of medical records should be most carefully managed. Care home records are the property of the care home. Care home staff, particularly more professional and senior staff, do work to similar standards to those in the health service but, until electronic records with graded security of information become a reality, it is incumbent of all health and social care staff to be mindful of what can be exquisitely sensitive information.

Examining the care home resident

The usual physical examination often proves difficult in the care home for a whole variety of reasons, but basic medicine should be adapted to the circumstances. It might sound all too obvious but, before embarking on an examination, does the resident require his or her hearing aid or glasses? Declaring an individual aggressive or confused when in truth they are fearful of assault seems a dreadful error!

Vital signs are helpful as always, particularly if there are 'normal resting' values against which to compare. Respiratory rate may be particularly useful in a resting patient. Observation of the respiratory rate and the pattern of breathing of a sleeping or resting patient from the end of the bed is useful, as well as noting the colour both centrally and peripherally. Respiratory rates of 10–20 per minute are normal, and certainly a rate of 25 or above should raise concern but, as with so many physical signs in older people, a normal rate does not rule out abnormalities.

Core temperature may be helpful particularly if hypothermia is being considered, but don't be misled by cold peripheries. The person's core temperature, oral or tympanic, should be measured. If a thermometer is not available, simply place a hand on the abdomen: assuming the examiner's sense to be normal, a very cold feeling abdomen should raise concern for hypothermia. The absence of fever does not reliably exclude illness.

If the resident is bedfast, a methodical examination of limbs for fractures should be performed, by means of gentle palpation of each limb before putting them through a range of movement. It is especially easy to miss the shortened externally rotated femur of a fractured hip. At all times, the examiner should be aware of the patient's facial expression or any other signs of discomfort.

The state of hydration should be not be considered simply on the basis of skin turgor. A very dry tongue is likely to be of significance and oral thrush should always be considered.

If a resident is ambulant, observing walking or even taking the resident for a walk can be hugely instructive. For example, when a confused resident maintains a conversation without breathlessness while walking, a great deal has been learnt about his or her fitness and cardiopulmonary reserve.

If someone is bedfast, it can be easy to overlook a pressure tissue injury through inadequate examination. It doesn't need a full thickness pressure sore to cause symptoms. A dusky reddened non-blanching area of skin over a pressure area should be considered significant. Large breast tumours and overt abdominal masses or lymphadenopathy are all missed from time to time but clearly should not be and constipation can be so easily confirmed with a rectal examination. And finally, it really should not require specialist referral to diagnose scabies! Always consider this in an excoriated patient.

Chronic physical disease

In the community, treatment, particularly medication, is often pushed very hard to maintain sufficient functional capacity or behavioural control to cope with living at home. Following admission to a care home, reappraisal may lead to a change of priorities, for example with the aim of improving mental well-being rather than prevention of physical disability. Clearly, when a patient has been on treatment for a condition for a long period of time both the patient and often his or her relatives and carers will have been very involved in the 'therapeutic journey' and may be very wary of sudden changes by unfamiliar doctors. It is therefore paramount to discuss the rationale for making revisions in a resident's medication.

Two examples:

◆ **Parkinson's disease and Parkinsonism**—New residents with long-standing Parkinson's disease may have acquired a hugely complex regime of medication. This results from attempts to maintain sufficient mobility to enable a spouse or family to cope with everyday care needs such as transferring and maintaining mobility to facilitate toileting. The consequence of this may be troublesome medication-related hallucinations and even overt psychosis.

Admission to a care home may result from motor or mental impairment, or commonly a combination of the two. This presents an opportunity to review the priorities of treatment. It is relatively rare for someone who is both cognitively intact and still physically responsive to medication to be admitted though, if they are, medicine administration times may be very specific. For those who have had treatment pushed to the limit and beyond in an attempt to maintain their independence, it may be reasonable to reduce their treatment in order to lessen hallucinations and improve social engagement, even if that is at the cost of reducing their mobility.

In practice, it is often found that reduction of treatment does not cause a significant reduction in physical capacity. This signifies that the disease has progressed to being largely insensitive to treatment. Some cases actually benefit in complete drug withdrawal, the 'Parkinson's disease' actually being another form of Parkinsonism that is not responsive to treatment. Probably, the least problematic treatment regimes are based on modest doses of L-dopa with a decarboxylase inhibitor and they are possibly least toxic in controlled release formulations.

◆ **Treatment of hypertension**—Heightened awareness and more assertive diagnosis and treatment of hypertension mean that increasing numbers of older people continue to take medication. However, the need for treatment is often not adequately reviewed and patients may not be offered the opportunity of a test withdrawal of treatment. Obviously, the point of entering a care home is a good opportunity to consider this.

Blood pressure can be measured daily in a care home if required but it is worth suggesting some rules. For ambulant residents, blood pressure measured standing is most likely to disclose postural hypotension (and the risk of falling) and it seems sensible to measure it postprandially. For the immobile, blood pressure can be measured while sitting and, for those who are bedfast, semi-recumbent. A significant proportion of patients are able to discontinue hypotensive treatment which may reduce the likelihood of falls but also they may improve mentally, not only because of improved cerebral perfusion but also because commonly used drugs such as beta-blockers may have adverse effects on a person's cognitive functioning.

Acute illness and delirium

A common acute referral from a care home may be that a patient is simply not right, in itself hardly a diagnosis. In fact, the early symptoms of delirium may be protean, such as 'off their food' or 'aggressive'. The key to making an effective response is to obtain clear information about the patient's normal functional status and the nature and time course of change.

Delirium, the sudden onset of a fluctuating deterioration of mental function such as a loss of attention, alertness, inability to think clearly, disorientation, and usually reversible disturbance of mental function, may be a common presentation for any underlying condition or indeed the product of several comorbidities. It is important to make the diagnosis of delirium, rather than dismissing its symptoms and signs, but the crucial act is the urgent consideration and establishment of the precipitating cause and its treatment. Sometimes the underlying cause is not obvious, in which case it must be considered whether to perform further investigation or treat on a balance of probability.

A pragmatic checklist of common clinical issues may be helpful. In other words, could this be due to:

◆ infection, typically urinary, but also chest and pressure sore(s);

◆ infarction or haemorrhage, particularly cerebral or cardiac;

◆ unintended consequences of medication;

◆ dehydration;

◆ constipation/retention;

◆ metabolic disturbance typically related to diabetes or renal failure; and

◆ fractures.

Clearly, this is not comprehensive but having gone through this list and undertaken a general examination of the patient many cases will have been resolved. The more difficult decision-making then surrounds the appropriate level of further investigation and really this has to be considered in the context of the individual's overall condition.

Delirium is associated with mortality as well as behavioural disturbance and the awareness of this and communication is important. The Royal College of Physicians of London has published excellent guidance on the prevention, diagnosis, and management of delirium in older people which is recommended (Royal College of Physicians, 2006).

Nutrition and hydration

A common concern is individual weight change in care homes, usually related to weight loss. Generally speaking, weight loss is a consequence of one or more of the following:

- inadequate diet;
- inadequate assistance with feeding; and
- cachexia related to chronic disease.

It is rare for new metabolic or gastrointestinal diseases to appear in care home residents. Care homes should weigh residents regularly unless this is inappropriate, for example in an individual receiving end-of-life care.

Care homes have increasingly adopted the Malnutrition Universal Screening Tool (MUST toolkit available at BAPEN (2004)). This tool identifies risk of malnutrition but it is important to realize that it does not indicate whether malnutrition is the root of a patient's illness or even that it is contributory, let alone whether supplemental feeding will be beneficial. This point is stressed because expecting diets or dietary supplements to correct illness and frailty in the majority of cases is often misconceived. It is important that clinical assessment determines the underlying basis of patients' malnutrition and, more importantly, what if anything should be done. Simple questions about whether meals are consumed and what help is provided at mealtimes are likely to be more relevant than complex investigations or exhaustive dietary assessment. It is quite revealing to quietly observe mealtimes in care homes, as it readily shows whether staff are using good proactive approaches or whether they are less committed to ensuring that residents are well fed.

All care homes should be capable of presenting appetizing food of sufficient quantity to maintain or restore nutritional status, at least when this is physiologically and psychologically possible. Furthermore, all homes should be capable of providing appetizing modified meals. For example, it should be possible to offer a meal with individual components pureed. Regrettably, the common response to identifying malnutrition risk is a knee jerk provision of supplemental feeding, which almost certainly is an unnecessary complication and a distraction from the person's basic care needs.

Hyperactivity may render a standard diet inadequate. It is not uncommon for an individual with early dementia to be 'on the go' around the clock. In such circumstances, a standard diet is unlikely to sustain the patients, and they will need additional nutrition. This clearly does not have to be through expensive prescribed dietary supplements but simply by offering frequent snacks and by careful attention to mealtimes, ensuring that the person does eat good size portions of rich food. Once again, the language used here is determinedly not technical. These residents simply need diets adequate to match their activity.

Help with feeding may be necessary in various ways. Most obviously, there are individuals whose frailty means they have to be fed. There has to be adequate carer time to do this: put simply, if 10 out of 30 people need assistance with feeding and there are 5 staff on duty, mealtimes will need to be staggered or some residents will not get fed properly. For people whose attention is easily distracted, undisturbed mealtimes can lead to better food intake.

With so much emphasis on diet and the risk of malnutrition, it is worthwhile reflecting that often over 20% of care home residents are being prescribed statin drugs, whose therapeutic intent is to disturb nutrition by impairing lipid metabolism. There is no evidence that these drugs are generally beneficial in frail elderly patients with malnutrition but their potential for adversely affecting individuals seems high. It is likely to be in an individual patient's best interest to discontinue statins unless he or she has a clearly documented hyperlipidaemia and/or vascular disease.

It is interesting to note that many admissions to care homes are followed by weight gain. This is because a proportion of people admitted to care homes from the community or hospitals are malnourished. For individuals with limited mental capacity there should be no doubting the pleasure that eating wholesome food can bring. However, ageing bodies do not perform well with significant weight gain and so weight monitoring should also be used for identifying inappropriate gain as well as loss.

When oral intake is insufficient there is the option of enteral feeding. The occasions when invasive feeding can genuinely improve the quality of life and well-being of an individual are much less common than the opportunities to deploy such approaches. Therefore, the goals of embarking upon enteral feeding need to be very carefully considered. The Royal College of Physicians report 'Oral feeding difficulties and dilemmas—a guide to practical care', particularly towards the end of life is strongly recommended as an up-to-date set of guidance (Royal College of Physicians and British Society of Gastroenterology, 2010).

Maintaining hydration can be difficult and, particularly in warm weather, insensible loss can mean that regular drink rounds and encouragement with drinking are very important. Unless swallowing has become unsafe or the patient has become severely unwell, dehydration should not be permitted to occur. Medically, the ubiquitous use of diuretics often in a misguided attempt to manage postural oedema should be avoided. The prescription of these drugs needs to be reviewed critically. For example, diuretic doses that were justified for treating heart failure in active well-nourished individuals need to be reviewed when weight loss and general frailty and reduced mobility occur.

Medicines and medicines management

Much concern is expressed regarding medication in care homes. There are three principal areas of concern:

1 The indications for medicines and their prescription by doctors
2 The dispensing of medicines by pharmacists
3 The storage and administration of medicines by care homes

Though it is clear that doctors prescribe, pharmacists dispense, and care homes have to comply with the administration of dispensed medication, the focus continues to be mainly on the management of medication in homes. Although at some point this will change, at present the pressure on the regulation of medicines storage and administration has meant that inappropriate medicines are administered much reliably than they are in the community or even NHS hospitals (though it is unlikely that adherence to any form of regime is routinely monitored let alone regulated).

A 30-bedded care home unit may use most of the professional time of one nurse in medicines management, ordering repeat scripts, checking dispensed medicines, and reconciling paperwork. Care home residents typically may have seven or more prescribed items with often four dosing times in a day. Often several different general practitioners will prescribe on different cycle times and may ask of a retail pharmacist for a dispensing volume (over 20 routine monthly scripts for a 30-bed facility) quite at odds with the retail model of typical pharmacies.

Clearly, seeking high institutional standards of medicines management is right and proper. But, in fact, although care homes make errors from time to time in medication management, these are usually relatively minor and they are not the weakest link in the system. Residents are probably at more risk from inappropriately prescribed and inadequately reviewed medications than any deficiency in the storage and administration of medication.

Particular concern has been raised with regard to the use of sedation and the use of antipsychotic drugs. Although there may be a professional consensus that these drugs can, in the short term, bring control to a situation that poses a risk to the individual and those around them, their use in this way is 'off licence'. Good practice must surely be that the use of these drugs should be accompanied by documentation of the intended result and proposed duration of treatment.

In specialist dementia homes, the range of usage of antipsychotic drugs varies unacceptably in relation to case mix. Typically, half the prescriptions for these drugs will have been commenced prior to admission. It is difficult to set targets for levels of prescribing, but rates of prescribing to 25% or more of residents should be subject to careful scrutiny and review. It is not simply of course the rate of prescribing but the dosage and while a low dose may attenuate symptoms and be beneficial in the medium to longer term, often the doses used are excessive and unjustified. At every review, sedation, particularly antipsychotic prescribing, should be critically considered and whenever feasible reduced with a view to discontinuing over time.

The so-called 'PRN' (as required) prescriptions of drugs, such as analgesics and night sedation, without clear guidance for actual administration are undesirable. Analgesia for chronic pain is best provided continuously rather than waiting for pain to 'break through' and then seeking control. There is no doubt that the professional consequences of the tragic Shipman-related deaths have led doctors to be wary about prescribing opioid drugs. As with all medicines, there should be a clearly documented rationale for using opioids. They should be started in low doses and frequently reviewed, carefully increasing the dosage until adequate pain control is achieved. However, medicines such as simple laxatives and analgesics such as paracetamol should generally be available as required.

Infection and infection control

The most common medical problem in care homes is infection. Immobility, poor protection of the airway, and long-standing chest disease all predispose to low-grade chest infection and occasional severe exacerbations, while poor hygiene, poor fluid intake, and incontinence predispose to urinary tract infection. Very often the first sign of infection will be relatively minor, such as loss of appetite, or, less often, delirium. What is important is a prompt diagnosis and commencement of treatment before the infection becomes so severe that it requires hospitalization.

For urinary tract infections, while it is desirable to have a urine sample the practicalities in procuring one are often insurmountable and should not delay the start of treatment. If a patient is catheterized, then seeing clear urine in the catheter bag, for practical purposes, rules out a urinary tract infection. Recurrent chest infections should lead to prompt consideration as to whether the person is inhaling his or her food and drink or about the possible presence of specific chest pathology. Recurrent infections more generally are often a sign of increased frailty and failing immune competence, and therefore should prompt a review of the patient's status.

Antibiotic use in care homes is poorly controlled compared with hospitals but increasingly local microbiologists are providing guidelines which should be sought and followed. Particular risks arise when multiple course of antibiotics are used raising the risk of a multiple-resistant infection. As with all institutions, there is a high risk of outbreaks of infection. Although care homes have the advantage of many single rooms that enable a degree of confinement, it is important that whether the outbreak is flu, gastroenteritis, MRSA (methicillin-resistant *Staphylococcus aureus*), or other infectious disease, the public health services (in England, the Health Protection Agency) should be alerted and asked for guidance.

Skin care and tissue damage

With frailty comes the heightened risk of pressure injury and overt sores. Generally, in care home medicine 50% of pressure sores are acquired before admission to the home and 50% in the home. Clearly, most but not all pressure sores are preventable and they run the risk of becoming more extensive if not properly managed. There are some useful scales such as the Waterlow score (Waterlow, 2005), which raises awareness of risk, and the European Pressure Ulcer Advisory Panel classification system of pressure ulcer grades, which describes the nature of injury (European Pressure Ulcer Advisory Panel and National Pressure Ulcer Advisory Panel, 2009).

However, neither of these helpful tools gives insight to the probability of healing of established sores. If an older patient with advanced disease and increasing frailty develops an extensive deep full thickness sacral sore in spite of adequate diet and good general care, the likelihood of healing is low and the event may be a sign of the onset of a terminal decline. Before commissioning or condoning highly disruptive and disturbing care (for many vulnerable elderly), such as a specialist low air loss mattress, it is important to clinically stand back and consider carefully the patient's prospects. NICE has produced useful guidance for treatment of suitable cases (National Institute for Health and Clinical Excellence, 2005).

End-of-life care

One of the most difficult clinical decisions is determining whether an individual has made the transition from living with his or her condition(s) to dying. Making these judgements is an imprecise science. But increasing frailty, weakness, weight loss, disengagement, and low-level chest infection collectively should raise awareness of this transition. These changes are often so insidious that the onset of dying is often most clearly made in retrospect and even then, after careful consideration, most clinicians managing older people will have the experience of the 'miraculous recovery' of a patient who appeared by all reasonable indicators to be in a terminal state. These circumstances tend to make clinicians cautious about prognostication. However, when there is a general consensus or a clinical concern that dying has commenced, it is important to communicate this so that carers and family are aware. It is of course quite acceptable to recognize that an individual patient may have rallied and important to revise the status of the patient. It is equally important to ensure that this has been communicated too.

Dying and death are of course to be anticipated in care homes and for many individuals there will be no need for particular medical interventions, just dignified care and support. Arguably, most deaths in chronic disease can be reasonably anticipated even if the actual timing is unclear and an intense 'medicalization' of dying is inappropriate. However, other cases will need prescribed medications for symptom control and the use of protocols such as the Liverpool Care Pathway can greatly increase quality of care, timeliness, and share clinical accountability between visiting doctors and care home staff.

The Liverpool Care Pathway has been well tested in practice but the existence of an evidence-based pathway does not abrogate clinical responsibilities. Like all protocols, it requires that all participating clinicians, medical and nursing, are properly trained and understand their responsibilities (Marie Curie Palliative Care Institute Liverpool, 2010).

Conclusion

This chapter has argued through examples that well-organized approaches to the ongoing and emerging physical healthcare needs of the care home resident with mental health needs are possible, desirable, and likely to be simple, often remarkably beneficial to the individuals well-being and will most probably have a positive impact on resource utilization. This is probably the most unexplored area of modern medicine relative to its scale and emerging importance!

References

BAPEN (2004). *The Malnutrition Universal Screening Tool.* Redditch: BAPEN. Available at: http://www.bapen.org.uk/must_tool.html (accessed August 2010).

European Pressure Ulcer Advisory Panel and National Pressure Ulcer Advisory Panel. (2009). *Treatment of Pressure Ulcers: Quick Reference Guide.* Washington, DC: National Pressure Ulcer Advisory Panel. Available at: http://www.epuap.org/guidelines/Final_Quick_Treatment.pdf (accessed August 2010).

Marie Curie Palliative Care Institute Liverpool (2010). *Liverpool Care Pathway for the Dying Patient*. Liverpool: Marie Curie Palliative Care Institute. Available at: http://www.liv.ac.uk/mcpcil/liverpool-care-pathway/ (accessed August 2010).

National Institute for Health and Clinical Excellence (2005). *The Prevention and Treatment of Pressure Ulcers*. London: NICE. Available at: http://www.nice.org.uk/nicemedia/live/10972/29883/29883.pdf (accessed August 2010).

Royal College of Physicians (2006). *The Prevention, Diagnosis and Management of Delirium in Older People: National Guidelines*. London: Royal College of Physicians. Available at: http://www.rcplondon.ac.uk/pubs/books/pdmd/DeliriumConciseGuide.pdf (accessed August 2010).

Royal College of Physicians and British Society of Gastroenterology (2010). *Oral Feeding Difficulties and Dilemmas: A Guide to Practical Care, Particularly towards the End of Life*. London: Royal College of Physicians. Available at: http://bookshop.rcplondon.ac.uk/contents/68e931b6-e3bf-41bd-99a4-3900569d4973.pdf (accessed August 2010).

Waterlow, J. (2005). *Waterlow Pressure Ulcer Prevention/Treatment Policy*. Available at: http://www.judy-waterlow.co.uk/downloads/Waterlow%20Score%20Card-front.pdf (accessed August 2010).

Chapter 20

Palliative care and end-of-life care

Elizabeth L. Sampson and
Karen Harrison Dening

Abstract

Care homes are major providers of end-of-life care as a high
proportion of their residents are frail and have multiple medical
comorbidities, often with advanced dementia. Residents are often
transferred to the acute hospital during their final illness and die
there; they frequently receive poor quality palliative care. A major
barrier to providing end-of-life care to frail older people is
identifying those reaching the end stages of their life. The symptoms
experienced by this group are common and can be relatively simple
to manage, for example pain, constipation, and swallowing
difficulties. Therefore, good generalist palliative care can be provided
in care homes if staff are adequately trained. Several initiatives have
been developed to improve end of life, such as the Gold Standards
Framework (GSF) and Liverpool Care Pathway. These help staff to
recognize that a resident is reaching the end of life and to plan for
and provide better care.

Dying in care homes

Approximately one-fifth of deaths in the United Kingdom occur in care homes.
Despite this, the provision and quality of end-of-life care in care homes is patchy and
inconsistent. Although some homes provide excellent palliative care, others do not
and care is poorly coordinated and provided. Despite the fact that most people say
they would like to die in their own home, usual place of residence, or care home,
the proportion of deaths occurring in the acute hospital (currently 60%) is set to
increase (Gomes and Higginson, 2008). Care home residents are often transferred to
the acute hospital where they die in unfamiliar surroundings and receive poor quality
care (Sampson et al., 2006). There is little research on the experiences of frail care
home residents at the end of life and how best to improve care. More work has focused
on those with advanced dementia, and given how common this is in residential
settings, much of the following chapter will focus on this.

'Terminal illness' in care home residents

Nursing homes are major providers of end-of-life care. In contrast to hospices, less than 10% of residents will die from a diagnosed cancer (Sidell et al., 1997). Instead, many residents will die from multiple medical pathologies such as stroke, respiratory illnesses, and neurodegenerative disorders such as Parkinson's disease. Many will have comorbid dementia and much evidence indicates that this is a 'life limiting' illness and an independent cause of mortality in its own right. Many care home residents have advanced dementia which has a median survival time of 1.3 years; a life expectancy similar to that of well-recognized terminal diseases such as metastatic breast cancer (Mitchell et al., 2009). The median length of stay in UK nursing homes is 18 months and therefore the majority of residents will die within 2 years of admission (Watson et al., 2006). Medical and nursing home staff consistently overestimate how long people are likely to live. An American study found that on nursing home admission only 1.1% of residents were perceived to have a life expectancy of less than 6 months but, in the event, 71% died within that period (Mitchell et al., 2004).

Common symptoms at the end of life

The symptoms that older people suffer from at the end of life differ from those in younger populations. Constipation, problems with bowel and bladder control, and visual and hearing impairment affect nearly half of those over 75 years old who are dying and the frequency of these problems increases further with age (Davies and Higginson, 2004).

Patients with advanced dementia suffer a range of symptoms, similar to those found in the terminal stages of cancer, for example, pain and dyspnoea (McCarthy et al., 1997). Pressure sores, agitation, and eating problems are very common (see Table 20.1).

Table 20.1 Prevalence of symptoms in nursing home residents with advanced dementia

	Mitchell et al. (2009)	Di et al. (2008)	Aminoff and Adunsky (2005)
Study details	Proportion of patients with symptoms 18 months prior to death (prospective study) n = 323	Proportion of patients in the last 30 days of life (retrospective study) n = 141	Proportion of patients in the last week of life (prospective study) n = 71
Dyspnoea	46%	39%	~
Pain	40%	26%	18%
Pressure ulcers	39%	47%	70%
Agitation/restlessness	54%	20%	72%
Aspiration	41%	~	~
Eating problems	86%	~	95%

Pain

Older people tend to underreport pain and it is often undertreated (Davies and Higginson, 2004). Most nursing home residents complain of pain, this is not well-managed and sometimes not treated at all (Landi et al., 1998). In one American study, a quarter of nursing home residents who had cancer and reported daily pain did not receive pain medication (Bernabei et al., 1998). Residents with advanced dementia will have difficulties in communicating that they are in pain and this often manifests as behavioural change such as agitation, distress, social withdrawal, or resistive behaviour (Scherder et al., 2009).

Eating and swallowing

Nursing home residents often develop problems with eating. People with Parkinson's disease, strokes, or advanced dementia often develop swallowing difficulties. The decision to use enteral (artificial feeding tube) feeding is particularly difficult if a resident has had a stroke or suffers from dementia and he or she lacks the capacity to make an informed decision. Two methods of enteral tube feeding are used: a nasogastric tube (a tube that is passed through the nose and into the stomach) or a percutaneous endoscopic gastrostomy (PEG), where the tube is inserted through the abdominal wall. A recent Cochrane Review (Sampson et al., 2009a) found inconclusive evidence that enteral tube feeding provides any benefit in dementia patients in terms of survival, mortality, quality of life, nutrition, and improvement or reduced incidence of pressure ulcers. PEG is an invasive surgical procedure with significant risks including aspiration pneumonia and wound infection. The decision to use enteral tube feeding is emotive and the culture of a care home can have a profound influence on this. Lopez et al. (2010) found that tube feeding was far more likely to be used in care homes where there was an 'institutional' environment, poorly staffed mealtimes, and staff believed feeding tubes avoided aspiration or perceived that regulators expected such interventions. Nursing homes with lower use of enteral feeding had a more homely environment and staffed mealtimes with nursing assistants who were willing to spend time feeding residents by hand.

Behavioural and psychological symptoms of dementia

Behavioural and psychological symptoms of dementia (BPSD) are common in dementia, affecting 90% of people at some time during the course of their illness. They are extremely distressing for the person with dementia and his or her family and carers. They are a strong predictor of admission to a care home and thus very common in this setting. In the advanced stages of dementia, over half of patients remain agitated and distressed (Mitchell et al., 2009). The management of these symptoms is complex and requires a structured approach, using a range of therapeutic approaches. Aggression may be an indicator of unmet need such as undertreated pain. Residents therefore require a full assessment and this can be challenging in advanced dementia when verbal communication is limited.

Infections

Acute illnesses, such as pneumonia or urinary tract infection, are common and they are often indicators of imminent death in frail older people. Over 18 months, 53% of nursing home residents with advanced dementia will have a febrile episode, and 41% will have pneumonia (Mitchell et al., 2009). Often this results in transfer to the acute hospital, although studies have shown that many nursing home residents and their families would prefer that pneumonia is treated in the nursing home (Carusone et al., 2006). People with advanced dementia are often immobile and bed bound, and may have impaired immunological function. They are at risk of aspiration and pneumonia will be the immediate cause of death in up to 71% of cases (Burns et al., 1990).

The use of antibiotics to treat fevers and recurrent infections is controversial. Withholding antibiotics increases the level of discomfort (van der Steen et al., 2009), but it has also been argued that antibiotics might delay death, leaving the patient exposed to the risk of further pain and suffering and prolonging the dying phase. In this situation, discussion with families and the care team may lead to a 'palliative approach' and adequate symptomatic control through the use of analgesia.

Identifying care home residents approaching the end of life

One of the major barriers to providing good quality end-of-life care for frail older people is prognostic uncertainty. When considering frailty and complex comorbidities, it can be difficult to identify when someone may enter the final stages of his or her life. Cancer, congestive heart failure, renal failure, and dementia or Alzheimer's disease are most strongly predictive, particularly when accompanied by symptoms of shortness of breath, weight loss (particularly more than 10% over 6 months) poor appetite, a serum albumin of less than 25 g/dl, and dehydration. Functional performance for activities of daily living has been found to be a strong independent marker of end-stage illness, particularly a Karnofsky performance score (KPS) of less than 50% (100% indicates maximal functional ability and 10% indicates lowest ability). In practice, a score of less than 50% represents dependence in most activities of daily living (Gold Standards Framework, 2008; Porock et al., 2005). Acute illness such as pneumonia is a key indicator that a palliative care approach should be considered.

Challenges to providing good end-of-life care

Research in the United Kingdom shows that nursing homes can become isolated from recent innovations, especially those regarding pain control and palliative care (Sidell et al., 1997). A number of factors have been identified that may act as barriers to providing good quality end-of-life care (Henry and Young, 2006). Good communication between care homes and primary care or general practice is of key importance. Some care homes may be served by multiple general practitioners or surgeries, all of whom may offer differing levels of palliative care support. Acute illness often occurs at night and on-call doctors may not have the information necessary to make the decision that a resident is for palliative care and not active intervention. This can lead to the distressing situation where a resident is admitted to the acute hospital and dies there. A related issue is that of anticipatory prescribing. For example, care homes may not hold drugs, particularly opiates, which are commonly held by palliative care teams and hospices. Because care homes that have been designated as 'nursing homes' employ registered nurses, their residents may not be able to access palliative care nurses, and thus provision may be inconsistent or patchy, as is access to hospices and specialist palliative care.

Some care home staff have reported concerns that they will be 'blamed' for deaths and fear regulatory authorities or having to attend coroners' inquiries; this is another driver of unnecessary acute hospital admission (Sampson et al., 2009b). Care homes may have high rates of staff turnover so that training and supporting staff to provide emotionally demanding care at the end of life is especially challenging. However, most of the symptoms experienced by frail older people at the end of life, such as pain or difficulties with swallowing, do not require specialist palliative intervention but good generalist care (Department of Health, 2008).

How can end-of-life care be improved?

Several initiatives, in the United Kingdom and worldwide, have aimed to improve end-of-life care for care home residents. However, the evidence base on how care may be improved is somewhat limited, particularly when compared to research for people dying from cancer. Palliative care uses a team approach and is not just provided by specialists; it can take place in any care setting. Good person-centred care requires a rounded approach and a number of 'multicomponent' complex interventions and pathways have been developed. For example, in Australia and New Zealand, increasing specialist medical support to nursing homes and 'Hospital at Home Schemes' for residents with acute medical illness have been shown to reduce deaths in the acute hospital, have significant cost savings, and most importantly are associated with high levels of patient and carer satisfaction. Some specific interventions and care models are discussed below (see Boxes 20.1 and 20.2).

Box 20.1 Useful resources

Preferred priorities for care (PPC): http://www.endoflifecare.nhs.uk/eolc/ppc.htm
Gold Standards Framework (GSF): http://www.goldstandardsframework.nhs.uk/
Liverpool Care Pathway: http://www.endoflifecare.nhs.uk/eolc/lcp.htm
National Council for Palliative Care: http://www.ncpc.org.uk; http://www.ncpc.org.uk/policy/dementia.html
Dementia UK: http://www.dementiauk.org

Admiral Nursing *DIRECT*
0845 257 9406
Telephone information and support line for family carers, people with dementia, and professionals.
direct@dementiauk.org

Box 20.2 Useful publications

National Council for Palliative care (NCPC)

- ◆ Exploring palliative care for people with dementia (2005)
- ◆ Progress with dementia—moving forward: addressing palliative care for people with dementia (2007)
- ◆ Creative partnerships: improving quality of life at the end of life for people with dementia (2008)
- ◆ Out of the shadows: end-of-life care for people with dementia (2009)
- ◆ The power of partnerships (2010)
- ◆ Focus on care homes—improving palliative care provision for older people in care homes (2004) (all available from http://www.ncpc.org.uk/)

Other publications:

- ◆ NHS End of Life Care Programme. Advance Care Planning: a guide for health and social care staff. London, 2007 (available from http://www.endoflifecare. nhs.uk/eolc/eolcpub)
- ◆ Royal College of Physicians, National Council for Palliative Care, British Society of Rehabilitation Medicine, British Geriatrics Society, Alzheimer's Society, Royal College of Nursing, Royal College of Psychiatrists, Help the Aged, Royal College of General Practitioners. *Advance Care Planning.* Concise Guidance to Good Practice series, No. 12. London: RCP, 2009 (available from http://bookshop. rcplondon.ac.uk/details.aspx?e=267)

Advance care planning

Advance care planning (ACP) is understood in a variety of different ways. The term is often used without definition or explanation and different emphases are placed upon the different elements of the care planning. The discussion and process of formulating an advance care plan may be more valued than the final document that is produced.

ACP usually involves a process of discussing and recording priorities and wishes for future care and treatment between the person and health and/or social care providers. It attempts to anticipate the future deterioration of a person's condition so that when a person is no longer able to communicate, for whatever reason, wishes and preferences that have been recorded earlier can be met (Froggatt et al., 2008).

Froggatt et al. (2008) surveyed 500 managers of care homes in an attempt to understand the ACP practices in care homes. Although the majority of managers viewed ACP as a beneficial process, the number of completed ACPs remained generally low with the end-of-life tools promoted by the government not widely used. Froggatt et al. identified several barriers to ACP in care homes: lack of staff confidence; the difficulty in ascertaining the wishes and priorities of older people at the transition point of entering a care home; and the lack of external healthcare support to care homes carrying out an ACP.

In contrast to those with cancer and other advanced chronic disease, residents with severe dementia have profound cognitive impairment and lack the capacity required to make decisions about their care and treatment. People with dementia are significantly less likely to have an ACP compared to those with cancer although uptake of the process in cancer remains variable (Mitchell et al., 2004). Ideally, ACP should be attempted in the earlier stages of dementia when a person is still competent to make decisions. In current UK clinical practice, it remains rare for a person with advanced dementia to have an advance care plan.

In the United Kingdom, the Mental Capacity Act 2005 provides a legal framework for this process. The Act gives competent adults in England and Wales the legal right to refuse treatment (i.e. artificial feeding and resuscitation) through the writing of an 'advance decision'. People can also make an 'advance statement' which reflects their general beliefs and personal values about the sort of care they would like to receive in the future.

Lasting Powers of Attorney (LPA) were also introduced through the UK Mental Capacity Act 2005 and enable the appointment of an attorney to make proxy decisions when the person with dementia no longer has the capacity to do so. A 'Personal Welfare' LPA allows the attorney to give or refuse consent to medical treatment, if such preferences have been expressed in the document. Similar frameworks are available in other countries to facilitate advance care decisions, for example the 'Let Me Decide' programme from Australia has led to a significant decrease in the transfer of nursing home residents to acute hospital with no changes in overall mortality (Caplan et al., 2006).

The Gold Standards Framework

The UK GSF is a multidimensional programme that supports and trains staff to identify patients requiring palliative or supportive care towards the end of life and improve their care. This is the largest UK programme undertaken to improve end-of-life care in care homes. Currently, over 1,000 homes have undertaken training in the programme and a further 100 homes per year are joining the scheme and being accredited.

The GSF for care homes aims to overcome many of the barriers to better end-of-life care, through a systems change approach, at an individual level with staff members, within the organization of the care home, in the community, and in relation to national guidance and policy. The key aims are:

1 Improving the quality of care for people nearing the end of life
2 Improving the collaboration between care homes and general practitioners (GPs), primary care teams, and other specialists
3 Reducing hospitalization in the last stages of life.

It uses a structured approach to recognize when the last year of life may have begun, to assess patients' needs, symptoms, and preferences and to plan care around these, in particular supporting people to live and die where they choose. A structured training programme through four workshops is provided to care home staff. This includes teaching on identifying those who may be entering the last phase of life, ACP, assessing and meeting needs, care in the final days of life (through integrated care plans and the Liverpool Care Pathway), spirituality and improving continuity, and out of hours care. The programme takes account of issues of staff turnover and is designed to embed and sustain these changes in the practice and culture of the home and maintain continuous quality improvement (Gold Standards Framework, 2008).

The GSF has been independently evaluated and has been found to ensure a more consistent quality of care and improve the culture of the home. Staff report feeling more confident in communicating with relatives about death and dying and become better at recognizing dying. It improves communication and collaboration with primary care. Hospital deaths have been shown to reduce by 50% and crisis hospital admissions decease by 30–40%.

Preferred priorities for care (formerly preferred place of care)

Developed by the Lancashire & South Cumbria Cancer Services Network, the preferred place and priorities of care plan is a patient-held record designed to facilitate patient choice in relation to end-of-life issues. The Preferred Priorities for Care (PPC) aims to promote both patient and carer choices through good communication and clear documentation. It records an individual's preferences with respect to different aspects of the care including his or her preferred place of care and death (Pemberton et al., 2003). Originally developed and used to support people with cancer to die in a place of their choice, it is now adapted for use in other life limiting conditions and can help residents in care homes to indicate their preferences. The PPC provides the opportunity to discuss difficult issues that may not otherwise be addressed. The explicit recording of patients' and carers' wishes can form the basis of care planning in multidisciplinary teams and other services, minimizing inappropriate admissions and interventions. As with most ACP tools, the PPC also records what services are available, what services are being accessed, and any reasons for changes in the care pathway.

The Liverpool Care Pathway

The Liverpool Care Pathway was originally developed to improve care in hospital for cancer patients during the last 48 hours of life (Ellershaw, 2007). The pathway has three phases: initial assessment of the patient, ongoing assessment, and care after death. The pathway attends to medical needs, such as stopping inappropriate interventions and medications, and the provision of comfort measures, for example mouth care. It also enhances person-centred care by assessing the patient's insight into their situation, their psychological and spiritual needs, and those of their family. The pathway is flexible and it is appropriate that sometimes residents are moved from the pathway back to more 'active' management should their clinical condition improve. Using an integrated care pathway for the last hours of life can significantly increase openness and team work around death and dying (Watson et al., 2006). A specific version for care homes is now being developed and tested.

Supporting carers and relatives

Over the course of the dementia, carers may be required to cope with various practical and physical aspects of the illness: dealing with difficult and puzzling behaviours, providing physical care, dealing with financial and legal aspects, etc. Some will adapt to the caring role easily whereas others will require more support. A common approach in working with carers in any care context where the person with dementia resides is to improve their knowledge, understanding, and problem-solving skills. When information and guidance is provided within the context of continuing professional support, as in the case of Admiral Nursing (specialist dementia care nurses), this is more successful in supporting family carers and reducing anxiety levels (Wills and Woods, 1998). A distinct advantage of the Admiral Nurse service is the long-term nature of the work with families of people with dementia and the support offered throughout the trajectory of the illness; this support is of particular value during transitions from community to care home (Harrison Dening, 2010).

Family members and carers are often required to make difficult decisions for the older person they care for. These can range from day-to-day matters such as the paying of bills to more complex and emotionally charged decisions such as placing a relative in a care home or deciding whether a feeding tube is inserted or whether the person with dementia should be resuscitated. These decisions are noted for the particular challenges they present; Baldwin et al. (2005) refer to this as an 'ethical burden' carers face in an attempt to decide what is the right thing to do. Baldwin et al. state that while many carers may feel well supported by professionals and care home staff, in practical ways they feel unprepared for the decisions required around end-of-life care. Educating the carers of people with dementia, particularly with the use of video vignettes, about the clinical features and implications of advanced disease increases the likelihood that they will choose 'comfort care' for their relative rather than aggressive medical interventions. When healthcare proxies are aware of the poor prognosis and the high risk of clinical complications, their relatives with dementia are less likely to receive burdensome interventions at the end of life (Volandes et al., 2009).

There has been little research on carers of people with advanced dementia and their experiences of caring at the end of life. Carers and families are described as experiencing 'anticipatory' or 'pre-death' grief: the cognitive deterioration of dementia leads to the loss of personhood often long before actual bodily death (Meuser and Marwit, 2001). This grief is distinct from depression and may be related to the quality of care that the person with dementia received.

Supporting care home staff

When considering the workforce within care homes, it is important to note the huge variation not only between different types of home but also in the range of qualified and unqualified staff, whether these are from a health or social care background. Some care homes also have volunteer workers. The majority of hands on care is likely to be delivered by unqualified care workers and so this is likely be the case when a person is nearing the end of life. Caring for people who are dying is often emotionally charged (Froggatt, 1998), so it is important for care home management to recognize the needs of staff members who may be affected emotionally by elements of providing care for people who are dying. As we have noted earlier, Froggatt et al. (2008) found that staff members lacked confidence in addressing ACP, which may also reflect a lack of confidence in delivering end-of-life care. Training and educational programmes on end-of-life care for nursing home staff also appear to be effective in improving knowledge and increasing satisfaction with end-of-life care in bereaved family members (Arcand et al., 2009).

Conclusions

Care home residents have high mortality rates and complex medical, social, and psychological needs. Care provision at the end of life is often patchy. There are challenges to providing good quality end-of-life care but recent innovative national programmes such as the GSF are aimed at supporting not only the residents but also their families and the staff who care for them.

References

Aminoff, B.Z. & Adunsky, A. (2005). Dying dementia patients: too much suffering, too little palliation. *American Journal of Hospice and Palliative Care, 22*(5), 344–348.

Arcand, M., Monette, J., Monette, M., et al. (2009). Educating nursing home staff about the progression of dementia and the comfort care option: impact on family satisfaction with end-of-life care. *Journal of the American Medical Directors Association, 10,* 50–55.

Baldwin, C., Hope, T., Hughes, J., Jacoby, R., & Ziebland, S. (2005). *Making Difficult Decisions.* London: Alzheimer's Society.

Bernabei, R., Gambassi, G., Lapane, K., et al. (1998). Management of pain in elderly patients with cancer. SAGE Study Group. Systematic assessment of geriatric drug use via epidemiology. *JAMA, 279*(23), 1877–1882.

Burns, A., Jacoby, R., Luthert, P., & Levy, R. (1990). Cause of death in Alzheimer's disease. *Age and Ageing, 19*(5), 341–344.

Caplan, G.A., Meller, A., Squires, B., Chan, S., & Willett, W. (2006). Advance care planning and hospital in the nursing home. *Age and Ageing, 35*(6), 581–585.

Carusone, S.C., Loeb, M., & Lohfeld, L. (2006). Pneumonia care and the nursing home: a qualitative descriptive study of resident and family member perspectives. *BMC Geriatrics, 6,* 2.

Davies, E. & Higginson, I.J. (2004). *Better Palliative Care for Older People.* Europe: World Health Organisation.

Department of Health (2008). *End of Life Care Strategy: Promoting High Quality Care for all Adults at the End of Life.* London: Department of Health.

Di, G.P., Toscani, F., Villani, D., Brunelli, C., Gentile, S., & Spadin, P. (2008). Dying with advanced dementia in long-term care geriatric institutions: a retrospective study. *Journal of Palliative Medicine, 11*(7), 1023–1028.

Ellershaw, J. (2007). Care of the dying: what a difference an LCP makes! *Palliative Medicine, 21*(5), 365–368.

Froggatt, K. (1998). The Place of Metaphor and language in exploring nurses' emotional work. *Journal of Advanced Nursing, 21,* 319–332.

Froggatt, K., Vaughan, S., Bernard, C., & Wild, D. (2008). *Advance Planning in Care Homes for Older People: A Survey of Current Practice.* Lancaster: International Observatory on End of Life Care.

Gold Standards Framework (2008). The Gold Standards Framework. England: NHS End of Life Care Programme.

Gomes, B. & Higginson, I.J. (2008). Where people die (1974–2030): past trends, future projections and implications for care. *Palliative Medicine, 22*, 33–41.

Harrison Dening, K. (2010). Admiral nursing: offering a specialist nursing approach. *Dementia Europe, 1*, 10–11.

Henry, C. & Young, E. (2006). *Introductory Guide to End of Life Care in Care Homes.* Leicester: Department of Health.

Landi, F., Gambassi, G., Lapane, K.L., et al. (1998). Comorbidity and drug use in cognitively impaired elderly living in long-term care. *Dementia and Geriatric Cognitive Disorders, 9*(6), 347–356.

Lopez, R.P., Amella, E.J., Strumpf, N.E., Teno, J.M., & Mitchell, S.L. (2010). The influence of nursing home culture on the use of feeding tubes. *Archives of Internal Medicine, 170*, 83–88.

McCarthy, M., Addington-Hall, J., & Altmann, D. (1997). The experience of dying with dementia: a retrospective study. *International Journal of Geriatric Psychiatry, 12*(3), 404–409.

Meuser, T.M. & Marwit, S.J. (2001). A comprehensive, stage-sensitive model of grief in dementia caregiving. *Gerontologist, 41*(5), 658–670.

Mitchell, S.L., Kiely, D.K., & Hamel, M.B. (2004). Dying with advanced dementia in the nursing home. *Archives of Internal Medicine, 164*(3), 321–326.

Mitchell, S.L., Teno, J.M., Kiely, D.K., et al. (2009). The clinical course of advanced dementia. *New England Journal of Medicine, 361*(16), 1529–1538.

Pemberton, C., Storey, L., & Howard, A. (2003). The Preferred Place of Care document: an opportunity for communication. *International Journal of Palliative Nursing, 10*, 439–441.

Porock, D., Oliver, D.P., Zweig, S., et al. (2005). Predicting death in the nursing home: development and validation of the 6-month Minimum Data Set mortality risk index. *Journals of Gerontology Series A: Biological Sciences and Medical Sciences, 60*(4), 491–498.

Sampson, E.L., Gould, V., Lee, D., & Blanchard, M.R. (2006). Differences in care received by patients with and without dementia who died during acute hospital admission: a retrospective case note study. *Age and Ageing, 35*(2), 187–189.

Sampson, E.L., Candy, B., & Jones, L. (2009a). Enteral tube feeding for older people with advanced dementia. *Cochrane Database of Systematic Reviews, 2*, CD007209.

Sampson, E.L., Harrison Dening, K., Greenish, W., Mandal, U., Holman, A., & Jones, L. (2009b). *End of Life Care for People with Dementia.* London: Marie Curie Cancer Care UK.

Scherder, E., Herr, K., Pickering, G., Gibson, S., Benedetti, F., & Lautenbacher, S. (2009). Pain in dementia. *Pain, 145*(3), 276–278.

Sidell, M., Katz, J., & Komaromy, C. (1997). *Dying in Nursing and Residential Nursing Homes for Older People: Examining the Case for Palliative Care. Report for the Department of Health.* Milton Keynes: Open University.

van der Steen, J.T., Pasman, H.R., Ribbe, M.W., van der, W.G., & Onwuteaka-Philipsen, B.D. (2009). Discomfort in dementia patients dying from pneumonia and its relief by antibiotics. *Scandinavian Journal of Infectious Diseases, 41*(2), 143–151.

Volandes, A.E., Paasche-Orlow, M.K., Barry, M.J., et al. (2009). Video decision support tool for advance care planning in dementia: randomised controlled trial. *BMJ*, *338*, b2159.

Watson, J., Hockley, J., & Dewar, B. (2006). Barriers to implementing an integrated care pathway for the last days of life in nursing homes. *International Journal of Palliative Nursing*, *12*(5), 234–240.

Wills, W. & Woods, B. (1998). *Report for the NHS Executive North Thames R&D Directorate: An Evaluation of the Admiral Nursing Service: An Innovative Service for the Carers of People with Dementia*. London: HMSO.

Part 4

Promoting health and well-being

Chapter 21

Promoting health and well-being: good practice inside the care homes

Dawn Brooker

Abstract

The quality of caring relationships between staff and residents living in care homes is a key factor in promoting health and well-being. How this is achieved is a function of leadership at many levels within the care home. The VIPS framework of person-centred care is provided as a means of helping care homes to reflect on their strengths and weaknesses in relation to having a strong set of systems in place to ensure health and well-being are maximized for residents. Examples are provided from a study of 100 care homes that looked at the well-being of residents with dementia (CSCI, 2008).

Introduction

By suggesting that care homes can promote the health and well-being of residents is not to suggest that we can reverse the causes of their frailty or confusion or to underestimate their experience. We do know, however, that supportive skilled care can enable many residents to experience well-being and enjoy their life on a day-to-day basis. When we talk about promoting health and well-being in this context it is about eradicating the excess disability that residents experience because their care does not support their needs. Good quality care can make a great deal of difference to whether the person experiences good mental health.

Person-centred care rests on a value-base that recognizes the personhood of all persons (Kitwood, 1997; Brooker, 2004). People are treated as individuals, recognizing that each of us has a unique history and personality. The perspective of the individual is seen as the starting point for care and that empathy with this perspective has its own therapeutic potential. Care is provided that recognizes that all human life is grounded in relationships and that people, particularly those living with dementia, need an enriched social environment which both compensates for their impairment and fosters opportunities for personal growth.

These ideas are not new but they appear difficult to sustain in care home practice (Hoe et al., 2006; Alzheimer's Society, 2007). Tom Kitwood, whose writing helped to shape these ideas into a coherent theory, rather chillingly, made this prediction when writing a year before his death:

> It is conceivable that most of the advances that have been made in recent years might be obliterated, and that the state of affairs in 2010 might be as bad as it was in 1970, except that it would be varnished by eloquent mission statements, and masked by fine buildings and glossy brochures (Kitwood, 1997: 133).

People in care homes face an uphill struggle to maintain a sense of health and well-being. In addition to declining cognitive powers, and arguably an increased need for familiarity and human contact, people have to cope with a novel and often unpredictable care environment. They may also be cared for by people who often know very little about them. They are at significant risk of developing behavioural and psychiatric disorders and also of developing acute confusional states if physical health problems are not addressed promptly (Brodaty et al., 2001; Evers et al., 2002; Pitkala et al., 2004).

Are we trying to achieve the impossible here? Can we go beyond the rhetoric of person-centred care to really influence the lives of people living in care homes? There is a growing evidence base to suggest that activity and occupation is important in promoting health and well-being in care homes (Marshall and Hutchinson, 2001; Brooker et al., 2007) and that psychosocial interventions (Cohen-Mansfield, 2005), person-centred interventions (Chenoweth et al., 2009), and training staff (Featherstone et al., 2004) can all have beneficial effects on residents' quality of life, health, and well-being.

In my job I get to visit a great many care homes. When I reflect on the changes I have seen, particularly over the past 10 years, I do see more care homes that are genuinely engaged in promoting health and well-being. There are homes where I see people interacting with each other with a feeling of friendship and care, where life (although not perfect) is fun and meaningful, where care staff help residents to forget their troubles and enjoy life in the moment and where families are welcomed and the home truly feels like a home. There are homes where people feel loved and accepted for who they are. These are the environments that promote health and well-being in its deepest sense.

An illustration of this can be found in the photographs in Figure 21.1.

The name of the older lady in the photographs is May Williams.[1] May has dementia and she was admitted to Lady Forrester Nursing Home from a hospital ward. In hospital, she had been nursed in bed for the last 7 weeks and had been assessed by them as 'all needs, no mobility, not eating'. In many respects, the care home could just have received her and kept her comfortable until she died. Fortunately, May had gone to live in a home that took its responsibilities around promoting health and well-being seriously. The home believed in providing an enriched environment where people can live a life worth living.

---

[1] Permission has been granted to use the photographs and details of the older woman's name and the name of the nursing home.

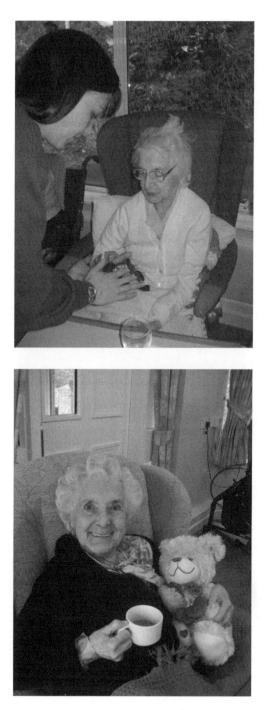

Fig. 21.1 The impact of good practice on May Williams who was deemed as 'all needs, no mobility, not eating' when she was admitted to this care home.

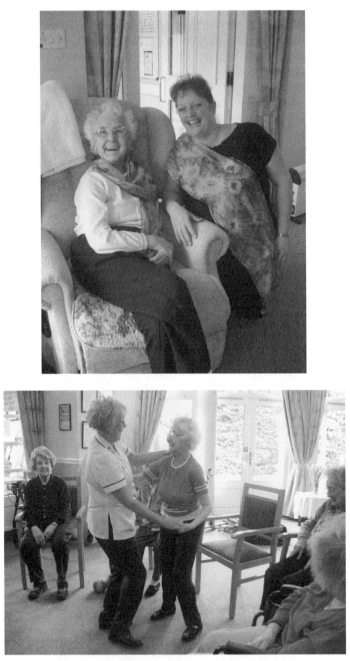

Fig. 21.1 *(continued)*

In the first photo May is sitting up and dressed but looks thin and somewhat wary. The other photos are taken about 1 month later where she is engaged in various activities such as knitting, making silk scarves, and dancing. From the photos we can see a lady whose health and well-being blossomed in an enriched environment. She looks relaxed, confident, and gaining pleasure and achievement from activities that are meaningful to her. May continued to improve and at her 12-week review her social worker could not believe she was the same person admitted 3 months previously.

The 100 care homes study

A few years ago, I led on the design of a thematic inspection of the quality of care for people with dementia for the then regulator of care home standards in England, the Commission for Social Care Inspection (CSCI, 2008). I had worked with CSCI to develop an observational tool called SOFI (Short Observation Framework for Inspection) in which care home regulators were trained to observe levels of well-being and ill-being in residents with moderate to advanced dementia and to assess the level and type of interactions over a sample 2-hour period in the middle of the day. This tool appeared to help those inspecting care homes to differentiate between those care homes that provided an enriched care environment and those that did not (Brooker et al., 2007).

During the thematic inspection (CSCI, 2008: called the '100 care homes study' in this chapter), SOFI observations were triangulated with other sources of evidence about the homes including recent inspection reports, speaking with people living in the homes and their visitors, talking with care staff and managers, reviewing policies and procedures including training records, and reviewing care plans. A broad range of care homes were involved, both specialist and non-specialist. We excluded those that were seriously underperforming. Using SOFI we observed the experience of 424 residents with dementia, capturing 840 hours of experiences of people living in care homes.

My aim in this chapter is to use some of the observations from this study to illustrate a number of the key dimensions that need to be in place for care homes to effectively promote health and well-being.

The VIPS framework for person-centred care

From a review of the literature, and from observing current ideas on best practice around the world, I developed the VIPS framework to help care providers reflect on whether their care homes were delivering best practice in person-centred care (Brooker, 2007). The VIPS definition of person-centred care encompasses four major elements:

V A value base that asserts the absolute value of all human lives regardless of age or cognitive ability.

I An individualized approach, recognizing uniqueness.

P Understanding the world from the perspective of the service user.

S Promotion of a positive social psychology in which service users can experience relative well–being.

From the evidence review, I defined six concrete indicators for each of these elements that care providers could use to benchmark how well they thought they were doing. Person-centred care requires signing up to working in this way across the whole care home organization if it is to be sustained over any length of time. Particular elements require leadership at different levels.

The first element—Valuing—requires leadership from those responsible for leading the care home at a senior level. This might be board level for bigger providers but will certainly require sign-up from the care home manager. The second element—Individual Care—requires leadership particularly from those responsible for setting care standards and procedures within the care home. The final two elements—Perspectives and Social Environment—require leadership for those responsible for the day-to-day management and provision of care, particularly shift leaders.

For each of the indicators set out below care providers are asked to reflect on how well they think they are doing. There is a choice of four ratings.

Excellent: reaching the highest standards, maintained over a period of time, and consistently applied across the whole service.

Good: achieved a high standard against the indicator but some concerns about consistency or sustainability in some areas.

OK: adequate performance most of the time or elements of good practice that could be introduced more widely.

Need to work on this: area not addressed, need to identify the blocks to it happening on a consistent basis.

Valuing statement and indicators

This care home values the life of all its residents regardless of age or ability. It also values the lives of those people who provide care and support for residents: we promote citizenship rights and entitlements and root out discriminatory practice.

- **V1 Vision** The care home has a clear shared vision about providing person-centred care services to all residents regardless of age and cognitive disability.

- **V2 Human resource management** Systems are in place to ensure staff delivering direct care feel valued by their employers.

- **V3 Management ethos** Management practice empower staff delivering direct care for them to act in the best interests of their residents at all times.

- **V4 Training and practice development** Practices are in place to support the development of a workforce skilled in person-centred care.

- **V5 The service environments** Provides supportive and inclusive physical and social environments that compensate for the whole range of impairments experienced by residents.

- **V6 Quality assurance** Continuous Quality Improvement mechanisms are in place which are driven by knowing and acting upon needs and concerns of residents and their families.

In analysing the results from the 100 care homes study, we could identify 19 homes that were providing very good levels of supportive communication and interaction for most of their dependent residents with dementia. This compared with 22 homes that were not communicating or interacting with their most dependent residents. The other 59 homes provided some positive communication.

There was no straightforward relationship between the type of home and good supportive communication. Those in the best and poorest categories included a mix of private providers, charitable trusts, and council-run. There was a tendency for the better performing homes to be smaller in size than those performing less well, but not exclusively.

Two key features were however clear. All the well performing homes had consistently invested time and resources in dementia awareness and person-centred care training, including personalized care planning. In addition, 9 of the poorly performing homes (41%) had vacant manager posts. None of the well performing homes had vacant manager posts.

As to why the homes with the poorest interaction and communication had such a high proportion of vacant manager posts was beyond the scope of the study. There is little doubt that the culture of the care home is, in large part, a reflection of the leadership within the home. As is stated in a recent CSCI report:

> Effective mangers who are good communicators themselves will find the right staff, they will know what the right training is and they will advocate for their residents with the owners (care home provider). (CSCI, 2008)

The most effective way of promoting health and well-being of residents in care homes is to recruit and retain a good care home manager. It is they who will be responsible for setting the Valuing Indicators. Providing care in a humanistic and person-centred way is a challenge. This is particularly difficult in an industry where front-line care staff often feel undervalued (Skills for Care, 2007). There is increasing evidence that care home staff routinely experience demoralization, burnout and stress, low work satisfaction or job clarity, low psychological well-being, and high workforce turnover (Moniz-Cook et al., 1997; Cole et al., 2000). Staff burnout has been shown to be associated with less willingness to help residents, low optimism, and negative emotional responses to their behaviour (Todd and Watts, 2005). In turn, high levels of staff turnover, staff shortages, and poorly trained staff exacerbated feelings of depression in care home residents (Choi et al., 2008). The key role here for the care home leadership is to ensure that staff feel valued so that they in turn can value the lives of those they care for.

Nolan et al. (2008) developed the Senses Framework which has been adopted by the *My* Home Life programme (Owen and National Care Home Research and Development Forum, 2006) with the aim of improving the quality of life for those living in, working in, and visiting care homes. The Senses Framework proposes that in order for optimal quality of life to be achieved for those living in care homes then all parties need to attain a sense of security, continuity, belonging, purpose, achievement, and significance. Achieving these senses for staff will assist in both the recruitment and retention.

When external 'rewards' such as staff pay levels are (often) set at a low level, it is the care home managers who need to value their staff. Table 21.1 shows a multiplicity of ways which a group of care home managers said that they found to show appreciation

Table 21.1 Care home managers 'ways we value staff'*

Traditional personnel processes	Everyday staff care and support	Treats	Rewards
Staff supervision	Manager speaks to staff when in care home every time	Birthday cakes and cards	Monetary rewards for full attendance at work—
Staff meetings		Christmas parties	individuals and teams
appraisals	Thank everyone for contribution to shift every day	Meals out	
Career progression		Christmas dinner, dance, and taxis home	Gift vouchers for innovations and success
Equality of opportunities	Always say please and thank you		
Critical incident analysis	Two-way communication	Special breakfast on bank holidays	Extra day annual leave for no sickness
Open door surgery once a week	Daily appreciation of each other of what went well	Ice cream and cake treats	
Team building events	On floor practical support from manager to staff	Staff nights out	Long service awards
News letters		Magic moment photographs	Staff awards— staff and resident voted for most cheerful staff, best cakes, making the residents' day
Staff surveys	Debriefing when things don't go well	Free use of gym	
Ideas board in the staff room	Control tower philosophy—if you report 'a near miss' you are not punished, you are rewarded	Secret Santa	
Pay rises		Free pens and stationery	
Financial bonuses		Annual staff celebration with gift and card	
Sick pay	Training staff to notice the end result—what you see in your residents is a result of your work		Nominations for outside awards
Pension scheme			
Health insurance			
Counselling	Praise in public, reprimand in private		
Occupational health	Role appreciation—have to experience every role in the home		
	Flexibility for special occasions		

*Dementia care leadership course, Wolverhampton City Council, 2010.

to their staff. The level of thoughtfulness showed by some care home managers was considerable; among others, it was less so. It is interesting to reflect on what would happen to the well-being of residents if all of the things in Table 21.1 were applied on a regular basis.

Achieving a valued staff team who in turn support the health and well-being of residents is difficult where staff:resident ratios are very low. When a typical care home is providing care and support for upwards of 40 residents, providing individualized care poses a real management challenge. There is an ongoing debate about whether there should be a minimum staff to resident ratio specified in care standards. Obviously, issues like skill mix and the physical layout of a care home influence this. In the 100 care homes study, inspectors noted particularly low levels of staff on duty in 15 out of the 100 care homes. This was seen to have a direct impact on residents:

> On the afternoon there was only one member of care staff on duty for up to 14 residents due to a member of staff not being able to undertake their shift. Residents were seen becoming disorientated with their surroundings, asking the inspector "Can you find someone to help me back to the lounge" and another resident was seen using a toilet, exposing themselves with no staff available to maintain that person's dignity. (CSCI, 2008)

By contrast, in another home, inspectors noted:

> There were 17 residents with four staff members present and the staff were talking to the residents in a way that was both respectful and inclusive. They were getting down to the same level as the people they were caring for and making eye contact and if one of the residents weren't joining in the conversation they were drawn into it. (CSCI, 2008)

The 100 care homes study also demonstrated a statistically significant relationship between staff training and development and people living in the home experiencing good levels of well-being.

Few care staff have specialist nursing qualifications or training in dementia care. The numbers of homes providing good quality training was very low. Only in 5 homes did inspectors rate staff training as 'excellent' and 'good' in a further 16. Training in care homes is an important area in its own right, an issue that is addressed fully in Chapter 24.

Individualized care statement and indicators

This care home recognizes that all people have a unique history and personality, physical and mental heath, and social and economic resources and that these will affect their response to living in a care home.

- **I 1 Care planning** Strengths and vulnerabilities are identified across a wide range of needs and individualized care plans in place that reflect a wide range of strengths and needs.
- **I 2 Regular reviews** Care plans are reviewed on a regular basis.
- **I 3 Personal possessions** Residents have their own personal clothing and possessions for everyday use.
- **I 4 Individual preferences** Individual likes and dislikes and preferences and daily routines are known about by direct care staff and acted upon.
- **I 5 Life history** All staff are aware of individual life histories, key stories of proud times, and these are used regularly to help people feel at ease.
- **I 6 Activity and occupation** There is a variety of activities available that meet the interests and abilities of all residents.

People's gender, socioeconomic status, ethnicity, and culture also shape their experiences of care (Marshall and Hutchinson, 2001). Tailoring care to people's needs must also involve understanding people's own cultures and developing the knowledge and skills of care staff accordingly (May et al., 2009).

In the 100 care homes study (CSCI, 2008), 25% indicated that people living in the home and their carers had played an integral part in the care planning process. The best care plans are clearly and sensitively written with detailed information regarding people's personal preferences, for example:

> I wear a light night dress, I like a cup of tea before bed and when in bed please close the door. I would prefer to be washed and dressed by a female carer. (CSCI, 2008)

However, in other homes staff were detached from the care planning process:

> The staff said, "We have nothing to do with the writing up of the care plans, or any changes made at review, the manager sees to all of this". (CSCI, 2008)

When staff are not fully involved in care planning, the quality of care was reduced. Drawing up life histories can help to involve everyone in the care planning process, including families and care staff.

> A "Life History" of the person had been drawn up by their family, and staff found these very helpful in getting to know the person and what is important to them. This information was also used to help staff plan appropriate activities. (CSCI, 2008)

Life story work is particularly important in helping people retain a sense of identity after moving into a care home. There is an ever-increasing number of resources available that can assist in the building of life stories (see http://lifestorynetwork.org.uk/lifestory/).

The residents in the study by Choi et al. (2008) reported boredom as one of their biggest challenges in keeping depression at bay. Harmer and Orrell's (2008) study focused on people living with dementia in care homes and their feelings about activity. All agreed that there was a lack of meaningful activity. The themes that emerged around what constitutes an enjoyable activity included talking about old times, music, and spending time with family and friends.

The 100 care homes study showed a significant relationship between people being in happy and relaxed mood states and being involved and engaged in the world around them. Residents who do more and communicate with others experience a greater proportion of time in a positive frame of mind. This finding underlines the importance of opportunities for meaningful activity in care homes. In just 15 of the care homes, 50–100% of residents experienced some proportion of their time in a withdrawn mood state. High amounts of time spent sleeping also clustered in the same homes. This suggests that lack of appropriate stimulation may, in part at least, account for residents being withdrawn.

Those of us providing care need to ensure that we can maintain links with the familiar touchstones in peoples' lives. We can use lifestyle and preferences as a means of building personalized activity programmes.

Although these ideas around individualized care and life story work have a proven positive impact on enhancing well-being, they are often difficult to implement without allocating specific responsibility for them to individual members of staff. Although a number of care homes employ 'Activity Coordinators' to provide a programme of activities for residents, these roles often seem to fall short of providing truly individualized care. Within the research and development programme for the Enriched

Opportunities Programme (Brooker and Woolley, 2007), a new staff role of 'Locksmith' was developed to work with individuals to help unlock their potential through individualized care and activity. The National Dementia Strategy identified a number of other similar roles such as Dementia Champions (Heath and Sturdy, 2009) to undertake this sort of work. These new staff roles require further research and development but they could provide a valuable career progression for front-line staff who wish to take on a more specialist role.

Perspective statement and indicators

This care home always tries to look at the world from the perspective of its residents: we recognize that each person's experience has his or her own psychological validity, that people act from this perspective, and that empathy with this perspective has its own therapeutic potential.

- **P1 Communication with residents** On a day-to-day basis, residents are always asked about their preferences, consent, and opinions.
- **P2 Empathy and acceptable risk** Staff show the ability to put themselves in the position of the person they are caring for and always to think about decisions from their point of view.
- **P3 Physical environment** Staff ensure that the physical environment is always managed to ensure residents feel comfortable and at ease.
- **P4 Physical health needs** Physical health needs of residents including pain assessment, sight, and hearing problems are given particular attention to ensure problems do not go unnoticed.
- **P5 Behaviour as communication** Distressed behaviour is analysed to discover the underlying reasons for it.
- **P6 Advocacy** In situations where the actions of an individual resident are at odds with the safety and well-being of others, we have a system of independent advocacy in place.

Seeing the care home from the perspective of the residents is not something that many people working in care ever consider. All of us involved in promoting good mental health need to recognize that moving into a care home is a huge transition—a normal response to this would be to feel emotionally upset and bereft. People living in care homes often have long life experience to draw upon and they already have coping strategies that have got them through hard times. We need to understand what these are and to help people build on them in the care home.

The data from the 100 care homes study confirmed that the quality of staff communication with residents had a major impact on their observed well-being. There was a strong correlation between negative staff interactions and low levels of well-being. In addition, high levels of 'neutral' interactions (where staff are just concentrating on a task to be performed) were also strongly related to low mood in residents with dementia.

On the other hand, we found a strong statistically significant relationship between positive staff interactions and positive state of well-being for people living in the homes.

When staff interact in a positive way with residents, those residents spend a greater proportion of time in a positive mood. For example:

> One carer was observed throughout the entire inspection to interact positively with residents, providing warmth, acknowledgement and respect of individual's needs. Several residents were observed to respond to this carer by either smiling, providing good eye contact or by making positive verbal comments. When questioned by the inspector, the carer was clearly knowledgeable of individual residents' care needs, personal preferences, likes and dislikes. One resident was overheard to say as the carer left the lounge area "she's lovely" and "I like her". (CSCI, 2008)

On the other hand, in the poorer performing homes the following instances were observed:

> People who needed help with their meals had a series of different members of staff stop and help them with one or two mouthfuls before moving on to either continue to give out meals or help someone else. There were no chairs for staff to sit on and this resulted in members of staff bending over people to help them eat.
>
> One person had a series of different members of staff stop by to give her a forkful of food from time to time without sitting down with her, in 45 minutes she had eaten very little. (CSCI, 2008)

By contrast,

> The staff member told the resident what was on each fork before she offered it to her. She also asked for regular feedback about whether she was enjoying it, whether she wanted more and if she would like a drink.
>
> Comments such as "is that nice?" and "are you enjoying that?" were overheard. The resident looked calm and relaxed and appeared to enjoy their meal and the 1-1 attention being provided. (CSCI, 2008)

There are various ways of improving staff empathy with residents. Helping staff think through how they themselves would respond to receiving care is a powerful tool. Spending time with staff to help them reflect on what they would want in their care plan, what would be important for others to know about their life history, what daily routines would be important for them to maintain, and what objects and possessions help them to feel at home. One care provider who uses the VIPS framework has gone even further than this and developed a reflective learning tool called Resident Experience Training (Baker, 2008). This involves staff volunteering to undertake the experience of feeling what it might be like to be a resident with high dependency needs for a period of 6 hours. This included being assisted to eat a meal in a manner where the pace is set too fast for the person to eat and drink comfortably. Baker (2008) reports that although this is a highly intensive experience it pays dividends in that it has proved to be an experience that really helps staff empathize at a very deep level with residents. In order to help staff reflect on this experience, there is an in-depth individual debriefing with a skilled dementia care trainer as part of the Resident Experience Training.

Another issue that is receiving much needed attention at long last is care at night (Kerr et al., 2008). Promoting health and well-being is a 24-hour a day activity. Night staff often feel forgotten and unimportant. Disturbed sleep greatly decreases health and well-being at any age.

Physical fitness and comfort of care home residents need to be taken seriously. As residents tend to have a number of (often complex) health problems, they are prone to worsening physical ill-health; symptoms can go undetected for a long time if staff are not vigilant about investigating causes of any changes in behaviour such as a sudden increase in confusion. Pain is often ignored in residents, particularly those with dementia (Cipher and Clifford, 2004); the manifestations of the person's discomfort may be misperceived as episodes of 'challenging behaviour' (Nygaard and Jarland, 2005). As people with dementia may have difficulty remembering episodes of pain and/or have difficulty finding the words to describe their symptoms, the onus has to be on the care staff to be proactive and alert to signs and symptoms.

Unaddressed age-related sensory impairments such as not having the correct spectacles or functioning hearing aids often lie at the root of communication problems. If residents have poor visual perception and dysphasia due to their dementia, this only gets worse if they do not have all the help they can get from physical prostheses. Again, individuals may not be able to say that they have lost their glasses or be able to complain that their hearing aid no longer functions. Care staff have to be vigilant on their behalf.

Supportive social environment statement and indicators

This care home recognizes that all human life is grounded in relationships and that people living here need a social environment which both compensates for their disabilities and fosters opportunities for personal growth.

- **S1 Inclusion** Residents are helped by staff to be included in conversations and helped to relate to others. There is a complete absence of people being 'talked across'.

- **S2 Respect** All residents are treated with respect. There is a complete absence of residents being demeaned by 'tellings off' or labelled for their shortcomings.

- **S3 Warmth** There is an atmosphere of warmth and acceptance towards residents.

- **S4 Validation** Residents' fears are taken seriously. Residents are not left alone in emotional distress unless this is their express wish.

- **S5 Enabling** Staff help all residents to be active in their own care and activity. There is a complete absence of residents being treated like objects without reference to their humanity.

- **S6 Part of the community** Residents use local community facilities and people from the local community visit the home regularly. Families are actively involved in the life of residents.

In the 100 care homes study, we found that communicating with residents in ways that demonstrated sensitivity to their emotional needs had a distinctly positive impact on them. Non-verbal communication was especially important when residents appeared anxious or distressed:

> Some staff in particular were very warm and accepting to all people who used the service. These staff members frequently held or touched people who were distressed and this seemed to provide comfort to them. (CSCI, 2008)

On the other hand, inspectors observed a number of instances when staff were insensitive to people's emotional needs and feelings:

> One resident, who was eating off her knife had it removed altogether and was told that, "she was playing with it". Another resident said she wanted her Mum and the staff member replied, "she doesn't want you".

There were a number of cases when people were treated like children:

> There were many examples of staff treating residents with dementia like children, e.g. they referred to aprons used to keep people clean during lunch openly as "bibs".

Staff found it difficult to feel a personal connection to some people:

> One member of staff was observed during the observation to ignore a resident who was trying to gain their attention and searchingly kept looking into their face. The member of staff was observed to interact with other staff members rather than with individual residents and as a result of this the resident gave up and became withdrawn and entered into their own inner world. (CSCI, 2008)

Positive interactions that are friendly and warm have a strong relationship with residents feeling happy and relaxed. Anxiety, anger, and shame are often present as the emotional undercurrents for residents who have to depend on others for personal care. Even residents who are fully aware that they require help will feel these emotions at times when receiving care. For those residents who have limited insight into the fact that they need help, these negative emotions can be very near the surface. Uncaring communication on the part of the care staff can make these negative feelings intensify. Caring communication on the other hand will provide residents with a sense of safety and acceptance. There is a responsibility upon care providers to have processes in place to ensure that this is always the case. Strong interactive care does not occur by chance. It occurs because a care culture exists where it is expected and modelled by senior staff on a day-in-day-out basis.

Tom Kitwood first described the Malignant Social Psychology (MSP) of dementia care nearly 20 years ago (Kitwood and Bredin, 1992). This was a description of the way in which the personhood of people in care homes and hospitals is undermined by the negative interactions that go unchecked. Kitwood underlined that care staff rarely do these things with malicious intent. Rather, episodes of MSP are left unchallenged and overtime become an interwoven part of care culture (Kitwood, 1997).

One of the most prominent examples of MSP is where a resident's needs are being discussed in front of him or her (or over his or her head) without any attempt made to include the resident in that discussion. The discussion may be about his or her continence or nutrition, for example. If it is assumed that residents have no awareness this sort of 'care' will occur repeatedly day-in and day-out. We know that even residents with advanced dementia often understand a lot more of what is being said than is first thought. The residents might not be able to exactly follow the conversation but they know that they are being discussed and that their feelings are being ignored. If this becomes routine, then Kitwood hypothesized that this will eat away at the resident's sense of self and psychological well-being. The net effect on a resident who is grappling with losing his or her identity is to decrease feelings of well-being. The malignancy that

Kitwood described was really about how a resident's sense of psychological well-being can get eroded by a negative care home culture.

The malignancy also makes reference to how quickly MSP spreads from one member of staff to another. If you're a new member of staff in a facility and ignoring residents is 'the norm' then you do it because everybody else does it. If it's not checked by shift leaders, care can turn from being caring and supportive to undermining of residents' health and well-being.

Care home residents are also at risk of losing contact with those they love and identify with unless the care home makes a specific effort to welcome and maintain links. This can have a profound impact on resident health and well being (Woods et al., 2007). Care home providers need to put processes in place that actively welcome families into the life of the care home. Family carers often struggle with their own overwhelming feelings when the person they care for moves into a home. When care homes do not understand and accept these feelings and carers are not made to feel welcome, they may be increasingly reluctant to visit. This can deny residents an important link with the past and their core identity. Maintaining contact with families means that the person's life has continuity between what went before and the here and now. Well-being is, in part, dependent on biographical continuity.

In some homes in the 100 care homes study, the maintenance of relationships with family members was actively supported. This included people living in the home enjoying visits out to their relatives or the relatives being invited to have meals within the home:

> The service periodically arranges what it calls "couples supper", providing a candle lit meal with gentle music for people and their spouses or partners, so that they have some quality time together. (CSCI, 2008)

Conclusion

When I first developed the VIPS framework it was primarily used as a reflective tool during training or practice development sessions to help care homes reflect on how well they felt they were doing on the different indicators and to help them identify areas for improvement. A number of care providers have gone further and now formally measure performance on these indicators and use them as a means of internal benchmarking of the quality of care they provide. Whether a home that does well on all 24 indicators has residents who enjoy a better sense of health and well-being than a care home that only does well on 12 of them is a question that requires empirical verification. Within the VIPS indicators there is much that is currently seen as best practice. Whether some of these indicators are more important than others we cannot yet say with certainty.

The VIPS framework offers care home providers a way of analysing the provision of person-centred care in the round. It highlights the respective roles of the organizational leaders, service managers, shift leaders, and direct care workers in working together to provide care that enhances the well-being of residents. Providing person-centred care for very dependent care home residents is a complex challenge.

Without a systematic analysis and understanding of how health and well-being is sustained, the challenge cannot effectively be met.

References

Alzheimer's Society (2007). *Home from Home. A Report Highlighting Opportunities for Improving Standards of Dementia Care in Care Homes*. London: Alzheimer's Society.

Baker, C. (2008). The power of learning through experience. *Journal of Dementia Care, 16*(4), 27–29.

Brodaty, H., Draper, B., Saab, D., et al. (2001). Psychosis, depression and behavioural disturbances in Sydney nursing home residents: prevalence and predictors. *International Journal of Geriatric Psychiatry, 16*(5), 504–512.

Brooker, D. (2004). What is person centred care for people with dementia? *Reviews in Clinical Gerontology, 13*(3), 215–222.

Brooker, D. (2007). *Person Centred Dementia Care: Making Services Better*. London: Jessica Kingsley Publications.

Brooker, D. & Woolley, R. (2007). Enriching opportunities for people living with dementia: the development of a blueprint for a sustainable activity-based model of care. *Aging and Mental Health, 11*(4), 371–383.

Brooker, D., May, H., Walton, S., Francis, D., & Murray, A. (2007). Introducing SOFI: a new tool for inspection of care homes (Short Observation Framework for Inspection). *Journal of Dementia Care, 15*(4), 22–23.

Chenoweth, L., King, M.T., Jeon, Y.-H., et al. (2009). Caring for Aged Dementia Care Resident Study (CADRES) of person-centred care, dementia-care mapping, and usual care in dementia: a cluster-randomised trial. *The Lancet Neurology, 8,* 317–325.

Choi, N.G., Ransom, S., & Wyllie, R. (2008). Depression in older nursing home residents: the influence of nursing home environmental stressors, coping, and acceptance of group and individual therapy. *Aging and Mental Health, 12*(5), 536–547.

Cipher, D.J. & Clifford, P.A. (2004). Dementia, pain, depression, behavioural disturbances, and ADLs: toward a comprehensive conceptualisation of quality of life in long-term care. *International Journal of Geriatric Psychiatry, 19,* 741–748.

Cohen-Mansfield, J. (2005). Non-pharmacological interventions for persons with dementia. *Alzheimer's Care Quarterly, 6*(2), 129–145.

Cole, R.P., Scott, S., & Skelton-Robinson, M. (2000). The effect of challenging behaviour, and staff support, on the psychological wellbeing of staff working with older adults. *Aging and Mental Health, 4*(4), 359–365.

CSCI—Commission for Social Care Inspection (2008). *See Me, Not Just the Dementia: Understanding Peoples' Experiences of Living in a Care Home*. London: CSCI.

Evers, M.M., Samuela, S.C., Lantz, M., Khan, K., Brickman, A.M., & Marin, D.B. (2002). The prevalence, diagnosis and treatment of depression in dementia patients in chronic care facilities in the last six months of life. *International Journal of Geriatric Psychiatry, 17*(5), 464–472.

Featherstone, K., James, I.A., Powell, I., Milne, D., & Maddison, C. (2004). A controlled evaluation of a training course for staff who work with people with dementia. *Dementia, 3*(2), 181–194.

Harmer, B.J. & Orrell, M. (2008). What is meaningful activity for people with dementia living in care homes? A comparison of the views of older people with dementia, staff, and family carers. *Aging and Mental Health, 12,* 548–558.

Heath, H. & Sturdy, D. (2009). *Living Well with Dementia in a Care Home: A Guide to Implementing the National Dementia Strategy*. Middlesex: RCN Publishing.

Hoe, J., Hancock, G., Livingston, G., & Orrell, M. (2006). Quality of life of people with dementia in residential care homes. *British Journal of Psychiatry, 188*, 460–464.

Kerr, D., Wilkinson, H., & Cunningham, C. (2008). *Supporting Older People in Care Homes at Night*. York: Joseph Rowntree Foundation.

Kitwood, T. (1997). *Dementia Reconsidered*. Buckingham: Open University Press.

Kitwood, T. & Bredin, K. (1992). *Person to Person: A Guide to the Care of those with Failing Mental Powers*. Essex: Gale Centre Publications.

Marshall, M.J. & Hutchinson, S.A. (2001). A critique of research on the use of activities with persons with Alzheimer's disease: a systematic literature review. *Journal of Advanced Nursing, 35*, 488–496.

May, H., Edwards, P., & Brooker, D. (2009). *Enriched Care Planning for People with Dementia: A Good Practice Guide to Delivering Person-centred Care*. London: Jessica Kingsley Publications.

Moniz-Cook, E., Millington, D., & Silver, M. (1997). Residential care for older people: job satisfaction and psychological health in care staff. *Health and Social Care in the Community, 5*(2), 124–133.

Nolan, M., Davies, S., Ryan, T., & Keady, J. (2008). Relationship-centred care and the "Senses" framework. *Journal of Dementia Care, 16*, 26–28.

Nygaard, H.A. & Jarland, M. (2005). Are nursing home patients with dementia diagnosis at increased risk for inadequate pain treatment? *International Journal of Geriatric Psychiatry, 20*, 730–737.

Owen, T. & the National Care Home Research and Development Forum (Eds.) (2006). *My Home Life: Quality of Life in Care Homes*. London: Help the Aged.

Pitkala, K.H., Laurila, J.V., Strandberg, T.E., & Tilvis, R.S. (2004). Behavioral symptoms and the administration of psychotropic drugs to aged patients with dementia in nursing homes and in acute geriatric wards. *International Psychogeriatrics, 16*, 61–74.

Skills for Care (2007). *National Survey of Care Workers. Final Report*. London: Skills for Care.

Todd, S.J. & Watts, S.C. (2005). Staff responses to challenging behaviour shown by people with dementia: an application of an attributional-emotional model of helping behaviour. *Aging and Mental Health, 9*, 71–81.

Woods, B., Keady, J., & Seddon, D. (2007). *Involving Families in Care Homes: A Relationship-centred Approach to Dementia Care*. London: Jessica Kingsley Publications.

Chapter 22

Good practice outside the care homes

Claire Goodman and Sue L. Davies

Abstract

How health services work with care homes and provide support to residents lies at the heart of 'good healthcare' for this frail population. This chapter provides an overview of how healthcare services can, and do, work with care homes and what models of integrated working achieve positive outcomes. Research demonstrates a long history of erratic and inequitable approaches to healthcare delivery by both primary and secondary healthcare agencies and practitioners. Although there are examples of innovation and good practice, these tend to be time-limited, discretionary, and locally determined; often they depend on an individual practitioner's interest. The majority of interventions are reactive, problem specific, narrowly defined, and do not consider the priorities of the older person or how the culture of the home should influence approaches to care. There is an overarching need to involve older residents in healthcare decision-making and to develop strategies that allow care homes to be equal partners in setting priorities. Only then can healthcare providers work with them effectively to improve the well-being and health of residents, however complex the needs.

Introduction

Care homes are often isolated and sequestered away from the communities in which they are situated (Field and Froggatt, 2003). Although people living in care homes have complex needs and represent the oldest and most frail of the older population in the United Kingdom, for many primary and specialist health services providing support to care homes is not seen as a priority. This is at least in part because care homes provide 24-hour care (Darton et al., 2003; Bowman et al., 2004; Froggatt et al., 2009). However, increasing emphasis on improving the quality of care and avoiding unnecessary hospital admissions for care home residents, has led to multiple initiatives to promote integrated working between care homes and health services. These range from NHS funded beds in care homes, through specialist support teams, shared care planning, and documentation to individual practitioners working directly with care home staff. Despite this, research consistently demonstrates that people living in care homes have erratic and inequitable access to NHS (National Health Service) services, particularly those that offer specialist expertise in areas such as dementia and end-of-life care (Jacobs et al., 2001; Glendinning et al., 2002; Goodman et al., 2003, 2005; Alzheimer's Society, 2007).

This chapter focuses on how care homes are supported by health services and local community resources. It considers what is known about the healthcare needs of older people living in care homes, how they define health, the range of healthcare services they receive, and what professionals, residents, relatives, care home staff, and policy makers think about how care homes should be supported. Then, drawing on a recently completed systematic review of integrated working between healthcare and care homes (Davies et al., 2010), it describes what is known about the benefits of different approaches and the facilitators and barriers to effective collaboration between care homes and health services. The focus of the chapter is then broadened to consider the training needs of staff working in care homes. Finally, the chapter concludes by asking what the future challenges might be for how services should work with care homes and what strategies are needed to sustain models of care that encourage integrated working between homes and their local healthcare economy and communities.

Health needs as an indicator for external support

Over 10 years ago, a joint report from the Royal College of Physicians, Royal College of Nursing, and the British Geriatrics Society (2001) argued that unless older people in care homes are recognized by healthcare practitioners as a discrete population it is likely their health needs will be overlooked.

This report recommended greater involvement of geriatricians and nurse specialists in the care of residents, recognizing that this population has complex healthcare needs. One census of 244 care homes from a major care home provider found that 76% of residents had reduced mobility, 64% were confused or forgetful, and 27% were confused, immobile, and incontinent (Bowman et al., 2004). A review (Evans, 2008) of national and regional UK studies on older people's health status reinforced previous work by Goodman and Woolley (2004) about the range of health needs and limited life expectancy that characterize this population. She concluded that the evidence shows there is an overlap in older people's level of dependency between those in care homes that offer residential and nursing care, that older people's health status is characterized by relative stability with steady rather than acute decline in well-being, and that the optimal management of chronic disease is a missed opportunity to promote and maintain residents' well-being. Box 22.1 summarizes the key characteristics of care home populations.

How older people define health and healthcare needs

To focus only on particular conditions or levels of dependency as a way of defining 'health' and by implication need for support from healthcare services is potentially

Box 22.1 Disease and disability in care home populations

- **Mortality**: Residents in residential homes have a longer average length of stay compared with those in nursing homes (25 months and 10.5 months, respectively) (Bebbington et al., 2001)
- **Admission to care:** A medical condition AND associated disability influence most care home admissions (Bowman et al., 2004)
- **Long-term conditions and disability:** Dementia, arthritis, stroke, and depression are the most prevalent conditions experienced by residents of care homes (Falaschetti et al., 2002; Mozley et al., 2004). Few residents have a single disability and a significant proportion have progressive loss of physical function (Forster et al., 2010) and continence-related problems (Goodman et al., 2007)
- **Medication:** Polypharmacy is the norm for this population. Differences between older people in care homes and private households indicate higher use of laxatives and antidepressants and hypnotics in care homes (Falaschetti et al., 2002)

misleading. Older people in care homes live with cumulative risks to their health, which means that the experience of being 'healthy' is often transient (Evans, 2008). Nevertheless, studies in care homes consistently highlight that feeling well is not just reliant on physical health but is closely linked to the extent to which older people readjust and compensate to threats to their health to maintain a sense of control and achieve personal goals (Nolan et al., 2004; Personal Social Services Research Unit [PSSRU], 2006). This does not contradict the need for health professionals to consider how they can support older people as they experience a reduction in functional ability, but it changes the focus of how care is provided and (importantly) whose goals are being addressed. Older people do not have to be defined by what they cannot do or their vulnerability, instead healthcare practitioners can work with care home staff to identify older people's strengths and the kind of support they need to achieve what is important to them. Health service professionals should ask if the organization and delivery of services to care homes consider:

- older people living in care homes as a discrete population who, because of the complexity of their health needs, will benefit from proactive approaches to providing healthcare and
- how the individual's experience and definition of health informs what his or her priorities are, and how the interventions can help older people retain control and achieve their goals and priorities.

Access to healthcare services

Older people in care homes are likely to require treatment and care from a range of healthcare professionals and services. Residential care homes provide personal care only, have no on-site healthcare, and are dependent on primary health professionals to meet their residents' healthcare needs. Care homes that offer nursing care will have nursing support on-site but still rely on primary care for review of medical and nursing needs and referral and access to specialist services.

In theory, care home residents are entitled to the same access to health services as older people who live in their own homes. However in practice, access to primary and specialist healthcare provision varies considerably between care homes, with some care homes receiving only basic services such as the general practitioner (GP) and district nurse and others accessing a wide variety of services. One study (Falaschetti et al., 2002) found different patterns of service use between care home and community-based older people of the same age, with a higher percentage of the latter group using outpatient services but a higher percentage of care home residents using inpatient services. This difference may not only reflect care home resident's higher level of frailty, but also the influence of care home staff and healthcare practitioners as gate-keepers of residents' healthcare use. Also, care home staff may not always be aware of the full range of services that are available for their residents.

Most care home research has been carried out with nursing homes, and where residential care homes are involved there has often been no attempt to separate the findings. The first national survey of access to medical services for care homes including nursing, residential, and dual registered care homes was a telephone survey of care home managers, based on a one in four stratified random sample of care homes across England (Jacobs et al., 2001). It focused on service provision to care homes, identifying which homes had the widest access to externally provided healthcare and how services were paid for, by the home or the NHS. It achieved a 75% response rate.

They found that care homes had contact with a wide range of service provision but it was variable. The number of GP practices providing services to care homes ranged from 1 to 20 with a median of 4; only 10% of the homes were registered with one GP practice. The majority of care homes (83%) could access a geriatrician when needed, mostly via the GP. Care homes that paid financial retainers had better access to services than those that did not. Some residents were also charged for physiotherapy services through their home fees. Payment was made in return for medical services by 8.5%, with three-quarters of them doing so as part of a formal contract with the GP concerned. Homes that paid for medical services were significantly more likely to receive services including visits on request, regular surgeries, medical, and medication review than care homes that did not pay for medical services. Nearly 10 years later, in 2008, the English Community Care Association (ECCA—www.ecca.org.uk) asked its membership about the payments (retainers) made to GPs by a care home. The survey found that there were various reasons for care homes paying a retainer, to:

♦ ensure that a GP would commit to visiting residents in the care home;

♦ secure the services of one GP for all residents, thus making appointments and home visits more easy to arrange, and/or

♦ make it easier to arrange visits from a GP on set days.

Payments, when they were made, were wide ranging and one major provider stated 12% of its care homes were paying from £897 to £24,000 per year, with the average payment being about £7,000 per year. Some care homes also paid additional charges for other services seen as 'extra', such as night visits. As with the national survey, it demonstrated that while access to a GP is a universal entitlement some residents of care homes made additional payment for this through their fees.

In the national survey of Jacobs et al (2001), all residential homes had access to a district nurse when necessary but access to specialist nurses was more variable. Less than a fifth of homes had access to specialist nurses such as tissue viability and diabetic nurse specialists. Ten per cent did not have access to a physiotherapist, 10–25% to a speech and language therapist, and 25% to an occupational therapist (OT). However, 95% of homes had access to a community psychiatric nurse (CPN), 92% to a psycho geriatrician, 84% to a psychiatrist, and 68% to a psychologist. Other essential services were almost universal: chiropody (96%), dental (97%), and optician (98%) with a high level of audiology provision at 80%. A significant minority (7.5%) of homes received no pharmacy services, but 92% had some kind of arrangement for pharmacy support, including supplying medication, education, training, and advice for staff. However, it was not possible to determine the frequency of input and the pattern of contact. One study by Crosby et al. (2000) noted that care homes that received regular and lengthy input from primary care were more likely to have few residents with a high level of dependency and specific nursing needs. High service use is therefore not necessarily an indicator of close working between the care home and primary care but may simply reflect frequent contact with a few high need residents.

More recently, the APPROACH[1] study was funded by the National Institute for Health Research Service Delivery and Organisation (NIHR-SDO) to investigate integrated working with care homes. It employed an online survey to describe current primary health service provision to residential care homes in England, and their experiences of integrated working including perceived barriers and facilitators. The online survey was sent out to a sample of managers (from one in four homes randomly chosen from the nine Care Quality Commission regions). Following a disappointing response rate, the survey was extended to include all the care homes of one large provider which achieved a 78% response rate. A comparison of the findings between these two surveys found very few differences in their responses; this strengthened the findings of the initial survey despite the low response rate. The findings reported here relate to the initial survey and it is interesting to compare these with those collected 10 years ago from the last national survey.

Managers were asked about healthcare services their care home had received in the last 6 months, whether or not they used integrated working with healthcare professionals, shared documentation, joint training, and what helped and/or hindered collaborative working. Findings are reported using percentages, but response rates varied between questions. The majority of care homes worked with more than one GP practice, ranging from 2 to 10. Less than 10% paid a retainer for this service. A quarter had

---

[1] APPROACH: A study to develop integrated working between primary health care services and care homes. Funded by the NIHR-SDO Programme (project number 08/1809/231). Disclaimer: The views and opinions expressed herein are those of the authors and do not necessarily reflect those of the Department of Health.

GPs who ran regular clinics in the home, at least fortnightly. Furthermore, just over a half of the homes had clinics run by other healthcare professionals, most commonly chiropodists, district nurses, or community psychiatric nurses (CPN).

Managers were also asked to indicate which other healthcare professionals had visited the care home within the last 6 months (from a list of 26 possible NHS services/professionals). Almost all care homes had been visited by a GP, district nurse, chiropodist/podiatrist, CPN, and pharmacist; there was less contact with specialist nurses and allied health professionals. Despite recent policy initiatives (Department of Health, 2008), palliative care services had the least contact with care homes, and the number of homes that had seen a dietician, clinical psychologist, or falls prevention service was under 50%. With the exception of the chiropodist/podiatrist and pharmacist, most homes reported that services were provided on a resident-by-resident basis rather than to the home as a whole.

Three main changes have occurred since Glendinning et al.'s survey (2002). Care homes have increased (and are continuing to increase) in size; in the APPROACH survey the number of beds ranged from 22 to 72 in care homes offering residential care compared with 15 to 35 in Glendinning et al.'s survey. There has been a reduction in the number of GPs working as sole practitioners, and there has been a change in the type of care home provider: large private companies are supplying a greater proportion of all care home places. There were some similarities in GP service provision between the two surveys; the majority of care homes were registered with more than one GP, but the range was higher for the 2001 survey, 1 to 20 compared with 1 to 10 for the APPROACH survey. In addition, the same percentage of care homes paid a retainer to GPs for their services (8%) and a similar proportion (25% and 21%) had GP clinics held in the home. In general, there were higher proportions of care homes receiving NHS services in the 2001 survey than in the 2010 although some services were comparable including district nursing, speech and language therapy, occupational therapy, CPN, chiropody, optician, and audiology. Given the difference in the size, response rates, and methodology of the two surveys, only tentative comparisons can be made. Nevertheless, these findings suggest that primary care service provision is more limited now than it was 9 years ago.

Initiatives to support and improve care by external services to care homes

Healthcare providers are very aware of the need to improve how they work with care homes. Services are often initiated, or improved, by healthcare agencies because of: an incident that highlights the need for closer working (such as an avoidable injury or death of a resident), the existence of a 'clinical champion', or a need to support older people who 'fall between' services (or are in transition), or not well enough to be at home, but not ill enough to be in hospital. Initiatives include NHS funded intermediate care beds in care homes, respite care, and joint budgets to support continuing care of people with high levels of dependency, or as they approach the end of life. It also includes schemes that are problem specific such as falls prevention, activity promotion, infection prevention, and continence and nutrition specialist support.

A review of such initiatives undertaken in five different primary care providers in 2002 revealed a 30-year history of specially created schemes, forums, new roles, and teams all dedicated to improving care for older people in care homes (Goodman et al., 2003, 2009). However, what they all had in common was a history of short-term funding and a time-limited existence. There were demonstrable achievements but no evidence of a coherent approach that addressed issues of equity, coverage, access and, most importantly, sustainability. It remains an ongoing challenge as to how to embed partnership working within existing systems of care and as part of the everyday focus and workload of healthcare professionals involved in the care of older people.

An extensive review by Szczepura et al. (2008a) summarized the evidence on improving care in residential care homes. The authors concluded that medical care could be improved by making it more proactive and preventative, and that district nurses should also work on a more strategic basis with care homes. The current bias towards individualized as opposed to whole care home provision of healthcare, works against opportunities to improve the health and well-being of care home residents as a discrete population. Despite highlighting many areas of care where there was unmet need (e.g. dementia care, identification, and treatment of depression), studies were identified that did improve the quality of care provided to care homes. For example, staff training appears to produce improvements in diabetes and nutritional care in residential homes. Interventions to reduce medication errors and adverse events through the introduction of a pharmacist's medication review in nursing homes show a positive effect and multidisciplinary case conferences and a pharmacy coordinator have also been reported to improve medication. Introducing a geriatric nurse practitioner into a nursing home can lead to a reduction in hospital admissions, improvements in pressure ulcers, incontinence, depression, and aggressive behaviour, but it has little impact on residents' functional status, physical condition, or levels of satisfaction.

A few studies describe the establishment of nursing in-reach teams to improve clinical care in care homes, and an older people's specialist nurse in a multidisciplinary team is reported to have benefits, especially in managing the interface between nursing homes and primary care. There is a reasonable evidence base to suggest that targeted support by healthcare services will improve outcomes for older people in care homes. However, as a recent Cochrane review (Forster et al., 2010) concluded, while most physical rehabilitation interventions to residents in care homes are worthwhile and safe, reducing disability and improvement in physical condition, there is insufficient evidence to make recommendations about the best intervention, improvement sustainability, and cost-effectiveness. This is a conclusion that is mirrored in work in other areas where interventions are planned and organized by healthcare staff in collaboration with care homes.

Models of integrated working between healthcare services and care homes

How healthcare services work with care homes is as important as what is actually being offered. If the motivation for local healthcare agencies to develop new services or provide extra training for care homes is so they can transfer care from hospital or reduce the need for their input in the long term, this might not be in the best interest of the care homes or residents. The Sczcepura review (2008a) included a discussion of the different approaches to care improvement, including integration/partnership working, but did not compare them in terms of their relative advantages and disadvantages for care homes and health services and the costs involved. A recently completed systematic review of integrated working between primary healthcare and care homes (Davies et al., 2010) aimed to describe what is known about the benefits of different approaches, and the facilitators and barriers to effective collaboration between care homes and health services. One of the key inclusion criteria was that the intervention did not involve the creation of a new post to deliver the intervention, and that it could be delivered within existing patterns of service provision.

Electronic database searches identified 1633 studies, only 17 of which fitted the study criteria; 10 were quantitative, mainly trials. As with Sczcepura's review, most of the studies were conducted in nursing rather than residential homes, and where both types of home were included, distinctions were rarely reported upon. Integration was classified according to three levels (Rosen and Ham, 2008):

- **Micro:** Close collaboration between practitioners and care home staff
- **Meso:** Organizational/clinical structures and processes designed to enable teams to work collaboratively, for example integrated health and social care teams
- **Macro:** Integration of structures/processes that link organizations and support shared strategic planning and development, for example NHS beds in care homes.

The majority of the studies were UK based: participants included care home staff, both nursing and non-nursing and a variety of healthcare professionals including district nurses, GPs, pharmacists, and mental health staff. The issues explored were healthcare orientated. There was minimal involvement from the older residents or care home staff. Most studies took a disease-specific or outcome-specific approach as opposed to improving the quality of care for the care home population as a whole or addressing the priorities of the home. Outcome measures reflected either priorities of healthcare professionals or service preoccupations with reducing cost and/or inappropriate demands on hospital services.

Each study was categorized according to its level of integration: 12 studies showed close collaboration between healthcare professionals and care homes (micro); and five studies showed higher levels of integration (meso/macro). For example, one UK study operated at the macro integration level where there was evidence of joint funding and planning, with NHS palliative care funded beds in the care home, two US studies on nurse practitioners used managed care.

Barriers to integrated working were identified from the qualitative data. These included:

- healthcare staff not valuing care home staff's expertise and knowledge;
- older residents lack of access to healthcare services; and
- high levels of turnover of care home staff and limited availability of training.

Facilitators to integrated working included:

◆ the inclusion of all levels of care home staff in training and support by NHS staff and

◆ the care home manager's endorsement of initiatives and training by providing dedicated time for care staff to be involved.

The heterogeneity of methodology, specific topic area, data collection, and outcomes used in the studies made it difficult to report findings collectively or draw any conclusions about the impact of integrated working on care home resident's care and quality of life. For the trials—although there were some positive outcomes as found in the Szczepura review—most interventions had mixed or no effects when compared with the control group. However, an economic evaluation of an integrated in-reach team found that it resulted in savings through reduced hospitalizations, earlier discharges, delayed transfers to nursing homes, and illness recognition (Szczepura et al., 2008a,b). Interdisciplinary care including nurse practitioners in nursing homes in the United States also reduced residents' hospital use (Joseph and Boult, 1998).

A number of the qualitative studies also showed the potential of integrated working to increase quality of care for older people through staff training and support. In particular, some interventions increased care home access to services (e.g. Avis et al., 1999; Doherty, 2008) and enhanced care home staff skills for example, in managing end-of-life care (e.g. Hockley et al., 2005). Some care home staff reported that the projects helped to overcome barriers to working with healthcare professionals, which subsequently decreased their sense of isolation in managing health problems (Avis et al., 1999; Hasson et al., 2008). Despite the wide variation in both focus and methodology across the studies, those that showed positive potential for integrated working tended to be longer in duration (at least 2 years or ongoing) (e.g. Joseph and Boult, 1998; Avis et al., 1999; Szczepura et al., 2008a,b). Healthcare professionals led the other studies, but these projects had a higher level of care home staff training and/or support or intensive input over a shorter time. For example, in the study by Proctor (1999), there were weekly visits to care home staff by a nurse specialist over 6 months, which resulted in an increase in their positive interactions with residents.

Ongoing needs for support and training of staff

As residents of care homes live longer, their health needs increase, leading to considerable overlap in the nursing care needs and dependency of residents who live in care homes that do, and do not, provide onsite nursing. The assumption is that once someone moves into a care home it is for the remainder of their life, but a move from residential care to a nursing home and/or to hospital/hospice may be necessary for them to receive the care and support they require. When older people reach the limits of their functional capacity there is increased uncertainty around symptom causation and what kind of care decisions might be in their best interests. How to manage and live with this kind uncertainty can be a major challenge for care home staff, particularly when they are often caught between the wishes of family members, the resident, the advice of healthcare professionals, and what they think is best for the older person.

Too often it is the older person who has to fit with what is available as opposed to services adapting to the changes in their condition. This is partly because there is a dissonance between the level of complexity of healthcare needs that residents live with, how resources are allocated between health and social care, and the education, training, and support that care staff receive and their ability to maintain continuity of care. In one study on end-of-life care. Decision-making about whether to keep residents in the care home when they were dying was based on care home managers' confidence in the skills of their staff, the level of support they received from generalist and palliative care services, resources and staffing levels, and how they interpreted the division between personal and nursing care (Goodman et al., 2010). Work by Wild et al. (2010) for the Joseph Rowntree Foundation on workforce development has suggested that, as the distinction between residential and nursing home clients blurs, social care staff will have to develop basic clinical skills to be able to support residents in their preferred place of care. The authors suggest that good basic health/nursing care can be delivered in a residential home in collaboration with community nurses, when there is a sound practice-driven relationship, and care home staff know when to seek nurse-led support. This raises questions about how care homes will be able to maintain their ethos of providing care in an environment and manner 'as close to living in the residents' own home' as possible. Once care home staff—by necessity—become more medicalized and oriented to healthcare and the management of health risk, there is a danger that these preoccupations will dramatically alter the culture and focus of care homes. Furthermore, any initiative that seeks to increase the skills and knowledge of the care home workforce is likely to lead to a call for greater recognition and regulation of their work and perhaps additional pay. It is also a problem if the primary aim of healthcare professionals in supporting care home staff is substitutability, that is, to reduce or withdraw their own input to the care home, rather than to develop and maintain a close reciprocal working relationship with the staff and the home.

Box 22.2 summarizes what Wild and colleagues (2010) identified in their study as supporting a workforce equipped to meet the needs of older people living in care homes.

Future needs

How healthcare services provide support and work with care homes lies at the heart of how health and social care services work together and how they resolve their often competing ideas of what constitutes 'good practice' (Glasby and Peck, 2004). This chapter has considered the evidence about how health service providers work with care homes and research about which models of integrated working achieve positive outcomes for older people. As long as provision remains erratic and uncoordinated, reliant on individual practitioners' drive to work with care homes, and lacking in centralized policy direction, then health service involvement with care homes will remain discretionary and locally determined. As demonstrated by the research reviewed here, the majority of interventions are reactive, problem specific, narrowly defined, and do not consider what the priorities of the older person are or how the culture and context of the care home should influence the approach to care. In any review of work in this area very little emerges about how the older person has been involved in decision-making, even though descriptive studies show that this population (including those with dementia) has the ability to judge effectiveness and articulate their needs and priorities (Evans, 2008; Hall et al., 2009; Goodman et al., 2010).

Box 22.2 Elements that support successful and sustainable change in the care home workforce

- ◆ Leadership by care home managers and support from external stakeholders
- ◆ Integrated health and social care approaches
- ◆ Adequate staffing levels to permit acquisition of health skills without diminishing staff time for social care
- ◆ Provision of structured community nursing and medical input
- ◆ Shared vision and commitment among care home staff
- ◆ Pay incentives for staff to undertake Level 3 NVQ and clinical skills awards
- ◆ Access to NHS community nursing staff as teaching/learning support
- ◆ Development of a 'learning organization' culture in the care home
- ◆ Financial incentives for care homes to provide specific enhanced care
- ◆ Quality of resident and relative experience placed at the heart of change

Source: Adapted from *Residential Care Home Workforce Development: The Rhetoric and Reality of Meeting Older Residents' Future Care Needs* by Deidre Wild, Ala Szczepura, and Sara Nelson, published in 2010 by the Joseph Rowntree Foundation. Reproduced by permission of the Joseph Rowntree Foundation.

Ten years of research have shown that while there is a steady stream of research designed to improve the quality of care of care home residents, we seem to know less and less about how to translate those findings into everyday practice. There is also a need to discuss to a greater extent what 'health' means for a population who are very frail and often in the last years of their life.

We still do not know how to systematize and integrate evidence about how health agencies and care homes *should* work together to enhance the quality of care. New models of working are needed that allow care homes to be valued as equal partners and recognize priorities that focus on the older person and help create a home-like environment. Froggatt et al. (2009: 18) advocate an approach that is based on participatory engagement and set out four key values/principles to work by:

- ◆ **Equity**: The assumption that all people in care homes (older people, their visiting families, and staff) have equal worth and should be valued.

- ◆ **Engagement**: Ensuring that all people are involved and have the opportunity to participate as they would like.

- ◆ **Mutual learning**: The recognition that in any situation all participants can learn from each other.

- ◆ **Honesty**: The importance about being explicit about processes and recognizing the learning that can happen in any situation, even when things do not work out as planned.

Studies that have taken a more participatory approach to research are an exemplar of how healthcare services can work with care home staff to identify, plan, deliver, and review care together (e.g. Meehan et al., 2002; Hockley et al., 2005). It is an approach that is initially resource intensive but one predicated upon an ongoing, reciprocal relationship that is more likely to result in sustainable and effective change. There is also some evidence that ongoing working relationships can be improved when an explicit theoretical model of care is used (Dewing, 2009; Froggatt et al., 2009) supported by a set of tools developed for use in care homes (Goodman et al., 2007; Badger et al., 2009). *My* Home Life (www.myhomelifeenvironment.org.uk) is an initiative that promotes good practice in care homes and one of their key themes is 'working with health and healthcare agencies'. They provide pointers for how care homes can work with health services and emphasize that care home staff have expertise that is useful for health staff (e.g. in supporting people with dementia).

When the sole reason for health service involvement with care homes is the need to seek to reduce hospitalizations (or another short-term economic driver), then goals of sustainability, mutuality, and partnership working are unlikely to be achieved. Too often the health service views care homes as a 'treatment' much like a hospital; once someone is admitted to a care home then 'the home' is his or her treatment and this justifies reduced or limited access to health services. It is difficult to see how interventions can be sustained that seek to enable care homes to become surrogate hospitals or 'para hospices' *but* with fewer resources, intermittent access to clinical support and staff who do not have access to ongoing training. Unless health service providers seriously engage with ideas of partnership and shared learning, care homes and their residents will continue to be marginalized and practices that are ageist and exclusionary will persist unchallenged.

Conclusions

Evidence would suggest that innovations that promote better working between the NHS and care homes require facilitation, leadership, and mechanisms that build and sustain (and incentivise) commitment to them (Goodman et al., 2003, 2007; Davies et al., 2010). This chapter has demonstrated that it is possible for the health service to work effectively with care home providers for the benefit of residents and care home staff. However, without a model of cooperation and collaboration that can normalize methods of working (May et al., 2006) and embed a shared philosophy of how the health of older people is articulated and addressed, it is likely that 10 years from now access to services will still be ad hoc and patterns of provision reactive and unplanned. It is important to emphasize what can be done and widely disseminate examples of best practice and methods of working that sustain genuine partnership working. Only then will it be possible to create an expectation within, and without, the health service that providing healthcare support to care homes is not only essential but is pivotal to achieving good quality of life and good health outcomes in, what for many, are the last years of their lives.

Acknowledgements

Dr Angela Dickinson, Professor Christina Victor, Dr Wendy Martin, Dr Katherine Froggatt, Professor Steve Iliffe, and Dr Heather Gage are members of the APPROACH research team and contributed to the design, development, and analysis of the survey and systematic review, some of whose findings are reported in this chapter.

References

Alzheimer's Society (2007). *Home from Home: Quality of Care for People with Dementia Living in Care Homes.* London: Alzheimer's Society.

Avis, M., Greening Jackson, J., Cox, K., & Miskella, C. (1999). Evaluation of a project providing community palliative care support to nursing homes. *Health and Social Care in the Community, 7,* 32–38.

Badger, F., Clifford, C., Hewison, A., & Thomas, K. (2009). An evaluation of the implementation of a programme to Improve End-of-Life Care in nursing homes. *Palliative Medicine, 23*(6), 502–511.

Bebbington, A., Darton, R., & Netten, A. (2001). *Care homes for older people. v.2, Admissions, needs and outcomes: the 1995/96 national longitudinal survey of publicly-funded admissions.* PSSRU. Canterbury: University of Kent.

Bowman, C.,Whistler, J., & Ellerby, M. (2004). A national census of care home residents. *Age and Ageing, 33*(6), 561–566.

Crosby, C., Evans, K.E., & Prendergast, L.A. (2000). *Factors Affecting Demand for Primary Health Care Services by Residents in Nursing Homes and Residential Care Homes.* Ceredigion: The Edwin Mellen Press.

Darton, R., Netten, A., & Forder, J. (2003). The cost implications of the changing population and characteristics of care homes. *International Journal of Geriatric Psychiatry, 18*(3), 236–243.

Davies, S., Goodman, C., Dickinson, A., et al. (2010). *The Approach Survey: Integrated Working between Care Homes and the Health Care Services.* Unpublished report, CRIPPAC, Centre for Research in Primary and Community Care, University of Hertfordshire.

Department of Health (2008). *End of Life Care Strategy—Promoting High Quality Care for all Adults at the End of Life.* London: Department of Health.

Dewing, J. (2009). Making it work: a model for research and development in care home. In: K. Froggatt, S. Davies, & J. Meyer (Eds.), *Understanding Care Homes: A Research and Development Perspective* (pp. 222–241). London: Jessica Kingsley Publishers.

Doherty, D. (2008). Examining the impact of a specialist care homes support team. *Nursing Standard, 23*(5), 35–41.

Evans, C. (2008). *The Analysis of Experiences and Representations of Older People's Health in Care Homes to Develop Primary Care Nursing Practice.* Unpublished PhD thesis. London: King's College London.

Falaschetti, E., Malbut, K., & Primatesta, P. (2002). *Health Survey for England 2000: The General Health of Older People and their Use of Health Services.* London: Stationery Office.

Field, D. & Froggatt, K. (2003). Issues for palliative care in nursing and residential homes. In: J. Katz & S. Peace (Eds.), *End of Life in Care Homes* (pp. 175–194). Oxford: Oxford University Press.

Forster, A., Lambley, R., Hardy, J., et al. (2010). *Rehabilitation for Older People in Long-term Care. Cochrane Database of Systematic Reviews 2009,* Issue 1, Art. No. CD004294. DOI: 10.1002/14651858.CD004294.pub2.

Froggatt, K., Davies, S., & Meyer, J. (2009). *Understanding Care Homes: A Research and Development Perspective.* London: Jessica Kingsley Publishers.

Glasby, J. & Peck, E. (2004). *Care Trusts: Partnership Working in Action* (p. 147). Abingdon: Radcliffe Medical Press.

Glendinning, C., Jacobs, S., Alborz, A., & Hann, M. (2002). A survey of access to medical services in nursing and residential homes in England. *British Journal of General Practice, 52*(480), 545–549.

Goodman, C., Woolley, R., & Knight, D. (2003). District nurses' experiences of providing care in residential care home settings. *Journal of Clinical Nursing, 12*, 67–76.

Goodman, C. & Woolley, R. (2004). Older people in care homes and the primary care nursing contribution: a review of relevant research. *Primary Health Care Research and Development, 5*, 179–187.

Goodman, C., Robb, N., Drennnan, V., & Woolley, R. (2005). Partnership working by default district nurses and care home staff providing care for older people. *Health and Social Care in the Community, 13*(6), 553–562.

Goodman, C., Davies, S., Norton, C., et al. (2007). *Can Clinical Benchmarking Improve Bowel Care in Care Homes for Older People? Final report submitted to the DoH Nursing Quality Research Initiative PRP* Centre for Research in Primary and Community Care. Hatfield: University of Hertfordshire.

Goodman, C., Davies, S., Norton, C., et al. (2009). Collaborating with primary care: promoting shared working between district nurses and care home staff. In: K. Froggatt, Sue Davies, Julienne Meyer, et al. (Eds.), *Understanding Care Homes: A Research and Development Perspective.* London: Jessica Kingsley Publishers.

Goodman, C., Evans, C., Wilcock, J., et al. (2010). End of life care for community dwelling older people with dementia: an integrated review. *International Journal of Geriatric Psychiatry, 25*, 329–337.

Hall, L.S., Longhurst, S., & Higginson, I.J. (2009). Living and dying with dignity: a qualitative study of the views of older people in nursing homes. *Age and Ageing, 38*(4), 411–416.

Hasson, F., Kernohan, W.G., Waldron, M., Whittaker, E., & McLaughlin, D. (2008). The palliative care link nurse role in nursing homes: barriers and facilitators. *Journal of Advanced Nursing, 64*(3), 233–242.

Hockley, J., Dewar, B., & Watson, J. (2005). *Promoting end-of-life care in nursing homes using an 'integrated care pathway for the last days of life'. Journal of Research in Nursing, 10*(2), 135–152.

Jacobs, S., Glendinning, C., Alborz, A., & Hann, M. (2001). *Health Services for Homes: A Survey of Access to NHS Services in Nursing and Residential Homes for Older People in England.* Manchester: National Centre for Primary Care Research and Development.

Joseph, A. & Boult, C. (1998). Managed primary care of nursing home residents. *Journal of the American Geriatric Society, 46*(9), 1152–1156.

Meehan, M., Meyer, J., & Winter, J. (2002). Partnership with care homes: a new approach to collaborative working. *Nursing Times Research, 7*, 348–359.

Mozley, C., Sutcliffe, C., Bagley, H., et al. (2004). *Towards Quality Care: Outcomes for Older People in Care Homes.* PSSRU. Aldershot: Ashgate.

Nolan, M.R., Davies, S., Brown, J., Keady, J., & Nolan, J. (2004). Beyond 'person-centred' care: a new vision for gerontological nursing. *Journal of Clinical Nursing, 13*, 45–53.

Personal Social Services Research Unit (PSSRU) (2006). *Control Well-being and the Meaning of Home in Care Homes and Extra Care Housing.* Research Summary 38: PSSRU. Available at: www.pssru.ac.uk/pdf/rso38pdf (accessed April 2010).

Proctor, R., Burns, A., Powell, H., et al. (1999). Behavioural management in nursing and residential homes: a randomised controlled trial. *Lancet, 354*, 26–29.

Rosen, R. & Ham, C. (2008). *Integrated Care Lessons from Evidence and Experience.* London: Nuffield Trust.

Royal College of Physicians, Royal College of Nursing, and the British Geriatrics Society (2001). *The Health and Care of Older People in Care Homes—A Comprehensive Interdisciplinary Approach.* London: Royal College of Physicians of London.

Szczepura, A., Nelson, S., & Wild, D. (2008a). In-reach specialist nursing teams for residential care homes: uptake of services, impact on care provision and cost-effectiveness. *BMC Health Services Research, 8*, 269. ISSN 1472–6963.

Szczepura, A., Clay, D., Hyde, J., Nelson, S., & Wild, D. (2008b). *Models for Providing Improved Care in Residential Care Homes: A Thematic Literature Review.* Coventry: University of Warwick. Available at: http://wrap.warwick.ac.uk/438/ (accessed 12 August 2010).

Wild, D., Szczepura, A., & Nelson, S. (2010). *Residential Care Home Workforce Development: The Rhetoric and Reality of Meeting Older Residents' Future Care Needs.* York: Joseph Rowntree Foundation.

Chapter 23

Risk and choice

Sheila Furness

Abstract

This chapter outlines a number of ethical dilemmas facing care home staff in working with residents with mental health problems, particularly dementia. On a daily basis, they have to balance residents' rights to autonomy, independence, and choice against acceptable risk taking. The importance of recognizing individuals' capacity to be involved in decisions about their care, which may involve risk, and the important role that meaningful relationships with staff and a power sharing approach can play to contribute to resident well-being is highlighted. Research indicates that staff perceptions of risk can skew their responses to risk-related decisions, contributing to the development of an overprotective and highly regulated environment. Case examples illustrate how staff can work with residents and their families in a more creative and nuanced way to respect individual capacity, ability, and choice while weighing up both the dangers *and* benefits of risky activity.

Introduction

This chapter will explore the concept of risk and key principles of autonomy, choice, independence, meaningful relationships, and power with the aim of exposing their importance to resident well-being and quality of life (QoL). In addition, key messages from research about the perception and management of risk for adult social care service users will be considered to illustrate how care staff can adopt a supportive rather than overly cautious approach to risk and risk management in their work.

Principles that underpin and serve to enhance QoL and well-being include autonomy, choice, independence, meaningful relationships, and the right to take risks. The freedom and capacity to make decisions and to follow particular courses of action is often taken for granted in wider society. However, if our decisions become questionable or 'faulty' as a result of functional mental illness, dementia, or another neurodegenerative condition, then this capacity and freedom to make decisions is often overridden by others. People living in care homes are more likely than others to have their decision-making opportunities restricted. The effects of institutionalization are well documented by Goffman (1962), who pointed out that adherence to strict routines often leads to the dehumanization and abuse of residents who have little choice but to conform to oppressive regimes. If care practice in care homes is to improve, it is imperative that staff appreciate the consequences of denying residents their rights to make choices and to take risks and thus, retain some control over their own lives.

Prior to community care legislation and related policy, some people chose to move into care homes while others were persuaded to do so by well-meaning and concerned professionals and relatives. The shift to a community-based ideology that people should be supported to live in their own homes for as long as possible coupled with constraints on public finance has meant that local authorities tend to prioritize only those who fall within the 'critical' bands of the Fair Access to Care Services (FACS) eligibility framework (Department of Health, 2002). As Ray et al state, 'Specifically, need is constructed as risk (and danger) as a means of confirming that a person is eligible to receive finite and limited services' (2009: 52). In no situation is this more evident than care home admission. That admission to a home only tends to occur when informal and/or formal community care arrangements are no longer tenable is additionally noteworthy.

There are a number of reasons for an older person's admission to a care home, including: an accident; a specific episode of poor health; a generalized decline in capacity to perform daily living tasks; a breakdown in care arrangements; lack of motivation; rehabilitation; fear of crime; abuse; homelessness; loneliness/isolation; and other people's concerns and anxieties for their well-being, safety, and protection (Office of Fair Trading, 2005; Smith et al., 2009). If the person is admitted on the grounds that he or she is at 'critical' risk then it is perhaps understandable that care staff will focus on protecting the individual from further harm and pay primary attention to specific areas of identified risk such as self-neglect or falls. This is not the case to the same extent with individuals admitted for other reasons but it is a cultural norm that nevertheless permeates and pervades care home settings.

Although care staff are obliged to assess and manage risk as a core part of their role, and should aim to minimize the risk of harm, they also need to recognize that their own fears coupled with a culture of risk aversion may result in an overestimation of *actual* risks to residents. Their attempts to reduce risk can produce an overprotective environment that serves to stifle opportunities for decision-making, agency, autonomy, and choice.

What is risk?

Risk is a social construct and therefore influenced by several cultural factors (Douglas, 1992). Ryan (1999: 4) identifies risk as a dynamic concept that is shaped and received according to experience, circumstance, and context, 'risk is not only about physical harm or financial loss but can cover less observable or tangible things such as reputation and dignity'. Kemshall (2008) makes a distinction between two types of risk: risks which people pose *to* others and risks *to* vulnerable people. 'Risk assessment can be best understood as a calculation about the possible occurrence of a negative event or behaviour in the future' (Kemshall, 2008: 141). The likelihood that something *may* happen can be difficult to predict with any certainty.

In recent years, western society has responded to 'serious adverse events' by public inquiry and the introduction of a series of—mainly quantitative—measures intended to address identified shortfalls and reduce risks. This has fostered a belief that all risk is preventable and damaging, and fuelled a culture that holds people to account for a failure to stop a risk event occurring. Media coverage of serious accidents and other (rare) mishaps skew our perceptions about the likelihood of a risk situation, for example volcanic ash cloud incidents. It also serves to reinforce our fears and contributes to the development of a risk-averse culture in services (Ryan, 1999). That risk perceptions are inaccurate and fickle is also relevant. The public's perception of the likelihood of a risk event reoccurring is heightened immediately after that incident even though in real terms the probability is often no greater than prior to the event. Considering this wider context and the rather paternalistic model of care that underpins services for older people, it cannot be surprising that a safety-first approach dominates care home culture rather than an approach that accommodates risk as a healthy part of ordinary life for all citizens.

It also needs to be borne in mind that risk assessments are global, static, and fallible. Additionally, they fail to take account of the more nuanced nature of risk as experienced by individuals (Titterton, 2005). The Better Regulation Committee (2006) calls for a rethink about society's response to risk management recognizing that risk can be beneficial as long as steps are taken to minimize the risk of harm and adequate levels of protection are in place. The previous regulatory body to the Care Quality Commission (CQC)—the Commission for Social Care Inspection (CSCI)—stressed that care home residents should be encouraged to have control over their lives and make choices including those involving risk. Therefore the management, and not the elimination, of risk must be central to achieving good care outcomes. A challenge to the current situation, where defensive practice tends to be the norm in care settings, is needed in order to curtail the routine use of unnecessarily restrictive practices. Instead of risk being seen as intrinsically and primarily harmful, it should instead be viewed as having the capacity to enhance well-being and enrich QoL (Titterton, 2005). Care homes and care home staff can work towards this goal by taking into account the following principles to aid decision-making and guide actions.

Key principles

Autonomy

Autonomy can be defined as self-rule, making one's own choices and having a right to self-determination. This 'decisional' autonomy is based on the right to make personal choices irrespective of whether one has the capacity to make those choices or not. In practice, the execution of autonomy has become confused with the ability or capacity to make decisions. This can often result in care practice which limits or even denies choice, fails to engage in a risk discourse with the resident, assumes that staff 'know best', and invades privacy (Collopy, 1995 cited in Boyle, 2004). For example,

Boyle's study found that while care routines such as staff overseeing baths and requiring residents to leave their bedroom doors unlocked at night in case they fell were intended to minimize risk, they 'did not take into account an individual's level of ability or willingness to accept a degree of risk, such that the risk was often unnecessary or excessive' (Boyle, 2004: 218).

Autonomy is not simply about an individual's right to make and communicate decisions but it is about how he or she can be assisted to make decisions and choices. It is important for staff not to limit an individual's right to autonomy because that person is perceived not to have mental capacity (for whatever reason) but to find ways of facilitating expression of choice. It is also a practice consistent with the Mental Capacity Act guidance which identifies decisions as context-specific (Department of Constitutional Affairs, 2007). Helping a resident to decide whether they are comfortable with having their bath overseen is a low level and relatively straightforward decision compared to rewriting a will or going into hospital to have an operation. Most residents, however impaired, can be helped to make a choice about a bath. A blanket assumption that because someone has moderate or advanced dementia and that he or she automatically lacks the capacity to make any care-related choices is erroneous, undermines the autonomy of the individual, and contributes to the development of a risk-averse regime.

Choice

Autonomy is closely linked to the principle of choice. As far as possible, residents should be encouraged to make choices and express their preferences and wishes. Although staff has a duty to ensure that the care and support they provide to each resident is not causing harm, it also needs to be commensurate with what he or she actually wants. Of course, allowing total freedom of choice may not be realistic or safe in all circumstances and facilitating choice can present a number of challenges. For example, if a resident apparently chooses not to eat or drink, then he or she become dehydrated and ill. The home may be accused of neglecting the resident and may be held to account for this by the family and regulatory body, the CQC. There is a balance to be struck therefore, between facilitating and respecting user choice and ensuring that 'choices' are not directly detrimental to health or well-being.

Independence

Alongside autonomy and choice, independence is a third core dimension of QoL for older people (Walker and Hennessy, 2004). In a care home setting the creation of dependency is a consequence—in part at least—of a failure to engage with residents and not facilitating communication or choice. 'Best intentions' and lack of time often undermine the potential to effect engagement in decision-making. For example, a resident may wish to walk to the toilet or dining area rather than use a wheelchair. Finding this out by talking to him or her and then taking the time to walk with the resident is encouraging him or her to remain active, engaged, and occupied with 'ordinary' daily life but is likely to be challenging in an environment that is task focused and time limited.

Meaningful relationships

Meaningful relationships are pivotal to good quality care. Residential homes offer a setting in which staff and residents can build close relationships based on a sharing of space and intimate activities. Person-centred care provides the best conditions for a relationship to develop between carer and resident based on respect, interdependence, active engagement, and choice (Nolan et al., 2001). If staff can show genuine care and concern for those in their care then residents can feel safe and secure in their attachments as well as valued and respected. Caring *for* the person can engender feelings of caring *about* the person; this forms the basis of a meaningful relationship (Payne, 2009).

Power and powerlessness

Although power is not a principle per se it has a strong influence on the ways in which mental distress is understood and treated and is of core relevance to the delivery of care to those with mental disorders. It also intersects with the principles already discussed.

Critical approaches to mental health discourse argue that power exists as a social relation between people that 'may potentially open up or close off opportunities for individuals or social groups' (Tew, 2002: 165). Older women, for example, may be disadvantaged by long-term exposure to the double disadvantages of ageism and sexism which disempowers them in relation to others. Those who lack power—inside and outside services—may develop a range of coping strategies, often in subtle or unconscious ways, in response to disadvantage and in order to gain some control over their life and situation. It has been suggested that depression and anxiety represent an extreme internalization of powerlessness and that some of the behaviours people with dementia display are responses to a lack of power and/or being marginalized from decisions that affect them (Tew, 2002). Such responses are routinely perceived (or sometimes overlooked or misinterpreted) by staff as 'difficult' or labelled as 'challenging behaviour'. Labelling reinforces the dissonance between staff and residents and underpins the process of 'othering', whereby staff differentiate between 'us' and 'them': staff are constructed as normal, superior, and as having power and residents as abnormal, inferior, and powerless (Tew, 2005: 73–74). To address this negative dynamic in care homes there is a need to develop shared or cooperative power. In this model, staff work with residents, their families, and other networks and utilize tools such as care plans and directives to support the wishes of the individual, enhance their sense of empowerment, and help them maintain or gain a sense of control over their life (Tew, 2005; Furness and Torry, 2009). A core aspect of this relates to allowing residents to define and take 'risks', an activity often curtailed by well-meaning or controlling staff, as discussed above.

Messages from research findings

Mitchell and Glendinning (2007) carried out a review of empirical research conducted from 1990 onwards about the perceptions and management of risk and their consequences for adult social care service users, primarily focused on England. They concluded that, 'The majority of studies exploring risk and mental health focused on "risk and danger", especially, the idea that mental health service users are a danger to others' (2007: 87). There was an absence of research exploring the views of service users, especially around the risks their illness presents them with and the risk it poses to their psychological well-being.

Ballinger and Payne's (2002) study was based on participant observation of doctors, nurses, and occupational therapists and interviews with 15 older patients in one hospital. They found that staff rigidly controlled the environment in order to prevent risks, especially that of falling, and that no distinction was made between those patients with mental capacity and those without. This suggests that the default approach was that of 'assumed incapacity' rather than one based on individualized risk analysis. Similarly, Manthorpe (2004) in her study of marginalized groups argued that, regardless of the degree or stage of dementia, patients tend to be treated as incapable. One of the negative consequences of an early diagnosis is that public assumptions about lack of capacity tend to subsume daily life and experiences (Iliffe and Manthorpe, 2004). These, and other studies, highlight the need to ensure that staff working with patients with dementia in all care settings—hospital, primary care, care homes—assess individual capacity and ability rather than adopting a universal blanket approach to older service users.

Staff taking control was apparent in an action research study looking into the experiences of residents and staff in three care homes for older people in Scotland. The researchers identified that 'staff carried out routine and indiscriminate "checking" (for breathing, falls, and incontinence) throughout the night, due to a general culture of anxiety' (Wilkinson et al., 2008: 1). Waking night staff usually carried out checks on residents throughout the night at regular intervals. The researchers found that this not only disturbed residents' sleep patterns but was, for some, totally unnecessary. The fact that residents' wishes and preferences were unknown and not recorded in an individualized care plan was noted as an overarching deficit; that residents can be encouraged to either call for assistance or manage independently appears not to have been explored as an obvious way forward.

Three recent studies of people with dementia and their carers revealed that behaviour or actions labelled as 'irrational', 'dangerous', or 'meaningless' often has coherence and meaning when viewed from the perspective of the older person themselves (Pugh and Keady, 2003; Huby et al., 2004; Vallelly et al., 2006). For example, Vallelly et al.'s study (2006), based in extra care housing, showed that whereas staff saw 'wandering' as risky and dangerous the older people viewed it as 'exercise' and 'a chance to meet other people'. Huby et al.'s study (2004) specifically highlights the importance of listening to residents' own views and acknowledging the subjective meanings behind their actions. The danger of not doing so is the imposition of staff's interpretation; this tends to reinforce negative beliefs about residents' competence and often results in a measure of control.

A small-scale study, conducted in a group of Nordic nursing homes, examined nurses' and nurse assistants' experiences of caring for people with dementia at risk of falling (Johansson et al., 2009). Respondents identified protecting the resident from harm while balancing integrity and autonomy 'as an ever-present and difficult balancing act for staff' (p. 65). They cited specific problems relating to forgetfulness, anxiety, and confusion that often led to resident aggression and restless wandering. Although diversionary tactics such as involving residents in activities helped to lessen anxiety, different kinds of restraints and surveillance were revealed as the most common ways of dealing with 'challenging behaviour'.

Karlsson et al.'s study (2000) considered 30 nurses' reasons for using physical restraint in two nursing homes in Sweden. A vignette was used to identify attitudes. Findings revealed that nine nurses were willing to remove the restraint when asked by the patient on the grounds of avoiding harm to the patient; respecting the patient's autonomy, and the nurse's willingness to take risks. Reasons given by the 21 nurses who would use restraint included lack of time; a duty to follow a prescription; acting in the best interests of the patient; and acting in accordance with the will of others. Interestingly, they reported being less likely to use restraint if they had more time to spend with patients and there was sufficient staff cover on the ward (Sloane et al., 1991 cited in Karlsson et al., 2000).

Overall, research suggests that in care home settings the delivery of good care to people with dementia depends on:

1) assessing the individual capacity and ability of each resident and not adopting a one–size-fits-all approach that tends to limit and restrict user autonomy, independence, and choice,

2) developing greater awareness and insight into how residents construct subjective meaning in their daily experiences so that staff do not impose their own definitions of what constitutes risky behaviour,

3) weighing up *both* the dangers and benefits of certain activities and promoting a positive and accommodating environment rather than a reductionist and confining one, and

4) developing new and creative responses to perceived risks that are the least restrictive and allow greater independence and freedom for each resident.

Risks in care homes

There are inherent risks, both positive and negative, in care home settings. Simple tasks that residents do on a daily basis such as drinking hot tea from a china cup may be perceived by staff as risky and the cup may be replaced by a plastic feeding cup to avoid spillage. This not only turns a normal activity into a 'care activity' but is very likely to be less enjoyable for the residents as they would usually have used a china cup or mug before being admitted to the home. Instead of using a plastic cup—the so-called safe option—staff need to be more willing to be creative in their responses and consider what may be most promoting of dignity and choice for the resident. Knowing whether they enjoyed a cup of tea and how they drank it (how much milk, sugar, type of cup used, etc.) before admission would help considerably in this activity. If staff are primarily mindful of protection and of reducing or preventing potential 'risks', that is, falls and other mishaps, life in the home tends to becomes driven by procedures and processes that reduce any sense of normality and erode the pursuit of an 'ordinary life', one of the key aims of current policy relating to care homes (Owen and NCHRDF, 2006).

On admission, key information should be collected about the person's lifestyle, experiences, and tastes. This will include: what assistance he or she had with daily living tasks before admission, waking routines, food preferences, religion, medical history, job/work history, family/relatives, and hobbies or interests. This will form part of the care plan and will be used by staff to ensure that care is tailored to the person's individual needs and appropriate support provided. The care plan should be used as a working tool, accessible to all staff and reviewed and updated regularly. For example, if a person indicates that he or she would rather have coffee than tea (even if the person has always had tea) then the care plan will need to be amended to reflect this change.

Specialist care homes that accommodate people with dementia normally take steps to ensure that the home is secure by locking external doors to prevent residents wandering off the premises without supervision. This is a controversial issue. The implementation of surveillance devices such as electronic tagging and CCTV have prompted much debate about achieving the right balance between promoting residents' civil liberties and monitoring their potentially dangerous behaviour. Critics have argued that these devices are an invasion of personal privacy and that, often, they are the 'lazy option' substituted for good quality care. There are a number of alternative ways of allowing residents greater freedom while still promoting safety. These include, offering unsupervised access to enclosed garden or courtyard areas, staff observing from a distance, and actively involving family and friends in the support of their relative. Joe's story below illustrates well how issues of choice and independence can be balanced with protection.

Joe's Story

Joe is a 74-year-old widower who was employed as a postman. He has always lived in the neighbourhood and is a well-known figure. At lunchtime, he liked to go for a drink at the local Catholic club. His daughter was contacted by police in the early hours of a cold winter's morning when Joe had been found wandering and disorientated in the streets. He believed that he was back at work as a postman and had been out delivering letters. Joe was diagnosed with dementia and eventually admitted to a local care home. Staff noticed that around lunchtime he used to become agitated if he did not go out to the club with either a family member or friend. His key worker invited family members to come in to discuss Joe's care plan. Joe and his family wanted him to continue going to the club but supervision was a problem. It was agreed that Joe would be accompanied to the club and a risk assessment carried out to determine whether Joe would be able to go unaccompanied. The club was a short walk from the home and Joe would not have to cross any major roads. Joe was able to walk to and from the club independently and bar staff were given telephone contact details of the home. This is an example of good care whereby care home staff were able to support Joe to socialize with his friends, maintain his independence and control over his life, allowing him some freedom after losing his home, lessen his anxiety, keep him active, and give his life meaning and purpose. Staff had to weigh up these benefits with potential risks. Joe could fall and injure himself while outside the care home, he could be involved in a road accident and be injured or killed, and he could also get lost and become upset. However, on balance—and this is the important issue—the improvement to his QoL was greater than any risks inherent in his attendance at the club.

Risk assessment

Staff and managers needed to establish the level of risk, the likelihood and immediacy of harm to Joe, and the severity of the possible outcomes. These then needed to be weighed against the benefits. Risk assessment is an inexact science; it is based on probability rather than certainty (Royal College of Nursing, 1997 cited in Doyle, 1999). Best practice suggests that risk assessments need to be carried out and decisions recorded using the least restrictive method available (CSCI, 2007: 43). In the case above, the family agreed that Joe benefitted considerably by going to the club at lunchtime. Staff also observed that he was able to make his own way to and from the club. Joe continued to go to the club two or three times a week. Sadly, a few months later Joe was knocked down by a car and died as a result. While his family and staff were naturally upset about his death, they believed that allowing him his freedom to pursue an activity he hugely enjoyed was well worth the risks. Staff also felt more confident about advocating for the rights of residents to live their lives as they choose including pursing enjoyable activities, rather than fearing reprisals for taking 'unnecessary risks'.

Managing risk and choice: guidance

There are a number of publications and assessment tools designed to assist health and social care workers to assess and manage risk in different care settings (Department of Health, 2007a; Manthorpe and Moriarty, 2010). The tools have been developed to support effective and consistent risk management but are only an aid and are not a substitute for robust and coherent decision-making (Department of Health, 2007b). When making decisions the Mental Capacity Act 2005 reminds workers that most people, even those with advanced dementia (see the section on Autonomy, page 315) are able to make some decisions with support (McDonald, 2010). Principles of best practice require workers to consider the consequences of an action and the likelihood of harm balanced against the rights of the person to independence, well-being, and choice and the potential benefits of said action or activity. As we have seen from the example of Joe, this can be done well. Workers need to work with the service user and significant others such as relatives, to come to a balanced decision that builds on the service user's strengths and promotes QoL. Positive risk management is not about eliminating all risks; a risk assessment and follow-on plan of action should weigh up the potential benefits and harms of both action and inaction and make a decision that is consistent with the user's own wishes, lifestyle, and patterns.

Concerns about the inappropriate and excessive use of restraint in care homes has resulted in a number of publications exploring the nature of restraint, reasons for its use, and alternative ways of ensuring residents' safety (CSCI, 2007; Owen and Meyer, 2009; Qureshi, 2009). Restraint can take a number of forms including: physical restraint of the individual (use of belts/cords, bed rails); physical intervention by others (holding a person or preventing them from moving); denial of practical or staff resources (removing alarm bells, not taking people to the toilet); chemical restraint (misuse of drugs); environmental restraint (locked doors); electronic surveillance (tags, CCTV); medical restraint (feeding tubes and catheters); and forced care (force feeding, making people take medication). The authors of these reports point out that there are considerable tensions facing staff in balancing keeping people safe alongside their promoting residents' rights to make choices, including those that involve risk. They conclude that restraint measures should be employed rarely and only after careful consideration of alternatives as they often infringe the human rights of the older person and can do significant harm.

Managing challenging behaviours

Stanton-Greenwood (1999) identifies those factors that may contribute to the poor management of challenging behaviours in residential settings. A key element, staff beliefs about the sources of violence, can have a profound effect on the way they respond to it. Staff can fall into the following negative traps:

- Helplessness (I've tried everything);
- Victimhood (taking the assault/incident personally);
- It's their fault (blaming the individual without considering their own behaviour);
- I want to punish them (hard to admit and often legitimized as a consequence);
- The punishment works (short-term effect and does not educate the person);
- They will not change (can become self-fulfilling);
- They do not like me (may be true); and
- That's the way it has always been (so therefore they will never change) (McDonnell, 1992 cited in Stanton-Greenwood, 1999: 193).

Trying to understand the cause of the behaviour can considerably aid its management. Difficult behaviour can be triggered by external events such as the presence of another person, being told 'no', or by internal triggers such as reminders of events or past upsets. One method that concentrates on antecedents, behaviour, and consequences (ABC) has been found to be useful in helping staff to adapt their responses. As a case example, Sam Morrison was always trying to move and rearrange the furniture in the care home (behaviour). Staff feared that he would hurt himself but when they tried to stop him he responded by shouting and hitting out. Staff were encouraged to look for the possible cause and timing of the behaviour. They found out that he used to work as a caretaker and he started to 'tidy up' at the end of each day (antecedent). Staff were asked to identify the consequences and the worst outcome. He had never harmed himself. Staff were able to change their behaviour (negative response) and instead, encouraged and thanked him for helping them. Sam was content to move the furniture with support from staff.

Reframing risk

Regulation of services and the media have contributed to a culture of blame and scape-goating when incidents occur in care homes. The threat of regulatory intervention and possible litigation can heighten perceptions of risk and determine how risks are managed by staff. As is clear from the discussion in this chapter, for residents to be able to command a greater level of control, freedom, and participation in decision-making, 'risk' needs to be understood differently and the nature of relationships between staff and residents renegotiated. Staff need to support user autonomy and choice rather than acting as gatekeepers; they also need to reflect on the cumulative effect of removing the right to be involved in everyday choices on resident well-being. Routine denial of resident participation in every activities and tasks can result, over time, in the casual erosion of independence. Sharing power with residents and challenging the dominance of the current preoccupation with risk and harm prevention can not only liberate residents but is also more likely to result in improved QoL.

A reliance on 'risk assessments' has contributed to a false sense of security; that having and following a procedure will militate against harm. Risk management policies need to recognize and take account of the balancing act that care workers are obliged to achieve between the competing demands of keeping people safe while promoting independence and choice even when this includes an element of 'risk-taking'.

It is important to acknowledge that a risk assessment process can be helpful as a framework to help explore the issues and/or decisions under consideration. This process should include: identifying any principles or duties that conflict with each other and who is likely to be affected by the decision(s); discussing all possible courses of action and the pros and cons contingent upon each (especially in the light of the General Social Care Council [GSCC] and Nursing and Midwifery [NMC] codes of practice); exploring the impact of personal values and belief systems; consulting with colleagues and appropriate others, for example relatives; and then making and documenting the decision, monitoring its impact, and reviewing it at a specified later date. This can be done as a part of reviewing and updating the resident's individual care plan.

It is instructive to remind ourselves that adults have the right to remain in a risky situation or place themselves at risk as long as they have the mental capacity to do so, can understand the danger(s) inherent in that decision, and it does not put others at risk of harm (Nuffield Council on Bioethics, 2009). In the care home sector the default position tends to be that of risk avoidance and reduction without sufficient analysis of the related benefits of a decision or action to the individual resident. For a more benefits-focused agenda to substitute for the risk-oriented one, the creation of a culture needs to be developed where human error is accepted in care homes whereby good quality care is understood as allowing residents to make challenging choices, and in which staff are encouraged to learn from their mistakes, be open to changing practices, and be creative and innovative in their daily interactions with residents.

References

Ballinger, C. & Payne, S. (2002). The construction of the risk of falling among older people. *Ageing and Society*, 22(3), 305–324.

Better Regulation Committee (2006). *Risk, Responsibility and Regulation—Whose Risk is it Anyway?* Available at: http://archive.cabinetoffice.gov.uk/brc/upload/assets/www.brc.gov.uk/risk_res_reg.pdf (accessed 24 February 2010).

Boyle, G. (2004). Facilitating choice and control for older people in long-term care. *Health and Social Care in the Community, 12*(3), 212–220.

CSCI (2007). *Rights, Risks and Restraints: An Exploration into the Use of Restraint in the Care of Older People.* London: CSCI.

Department of Constitutional Affairs (2007). Mental Capacity Act 2005 Code of Practice. London: TSO. Available at: http://www.dca.gov.uk/legal-policy/mental-capacity/mca-cp.pdf (accessed 17 June 2010).

Department of Health (2002). *Fair Access to Care Services: Guidance on Eligibility Criteria for Adult Social Care LAC Circular* (2002) 13. (London: DH).

Department of Health (2007a). *Independence, Choice and Risk: A Guide to Best Practice in Supported Decision Making.* London: Department of Health.

Department of Health (2007b). *Best Practice in Managing Risk Principles and Evidence for Best Practice in the Assessment and Management of Risk to Self and Others in Mental Health Services.* London: Department of Health.

Douglas, M. (1992). *Risk and Blame: Essays in Cultural Theory.* London: Routledge.

Doyle, M. (1999). Organizational responses to crisis and risk: issues and implications for mental health nurses. In: T. Ryan (Ed.), *Managing Crisis and Risk in Mental Health Nursing* (pp. 40–56). Cheltenham: Stanley Thornes Publishers Ltd.

Furness, S. & Torry, B. (2009). Establishing 'Friends of Care Home' groups. In: K.A. Froggatt, S. Davies, & J. Meyer (Eds.), *Understanding Care Homes: A Research and Development Perspective* (pp. 136–157). London: Jessica Kingsley Publishers.

Goffman, E. (1962). *Asylums.* Harmondsworth: Penguin.

Huby, G., Stewart, J., Tierney, A. & Rogers, W. (2004). Planning older people's discharge from acute hospital care: linking risk management and patient participation in decision-making. *Health, Risk and Society, 6*(2), 115–132.

Iliffe, S. & Manthorpe, J. (2004). The hazards of early recognition of dementia: a risk assessment. *Aging and Mental Health, 8*(2), 99–105.

Johansson, I., Bachrach-Lindstrom, M., Struksnes, S., & Hedelin, B. (2009). Balancing integrity vs. risk of falling nurses' experiences of caring for elderly people with dementia in nursing homes. *Journal of Research in Nursing, 14*, 61–73.

Karlsson, S., Bucht, G., Rasmussen, B.H., & Sandman, P.O. (2000). Restraint use in elder care: decision making among registered nurses. *Journal of Clinical Nursing, 9*(6), 842–850.

Kemshall, H. (2008). Risk assessment and management. In: M. Davies (Ed.), *The Blackwell Companion to Social Work* (pp. 139–147). Oxford: Blackwell Publishing.

Manthorpe, J. (2004). Risk taking. In: A. Innes, C. Archibald, & C. Murphy (Eds.), *Dementia and Social Inclusion: Marginalised Groups and Marginalised Areas of Dementia Research, Care and Practice* (pp. 137–149). London: Jessica Kingsley Publishers.

Manthorpe, J & Moriarty, J. (2010). *Nothing Ventured, Nothing Gained: Risk Guidance for people with dementia,* London: Department of Health.

McDonald, A. (2010). The impact of the 2005 Mental Capacity Act on social workers' decision making and approaches to the assessment of risk. *British Journal of Social Work, 40*(4), 1229–1246.

Mitchell, W. & Glendinning, C. (2007). *A Review of the Research Evidence Surrounding Risk Perceptions, Risk Management Strategies and their Consequences in Adult Social Care for Different Groups of Service Users.* Working Paper No. DHR 2180 01.07. York: Social Policy Research Unit, University of York.

Nolan, M., Davies, S., & Grant, G. (Eds.) (2001). *Working with Older People and their Families Key Issues in Policy and Practice*. Maidenhead: Open University Press.

Nuffield Council on Bioethics (2009). *Dementia: Ethical Issues*. London: Nuffield Council on Bioethics.

Office of Fair Trading (2005). *Care Homes of Older People in the UK: A Market Study*. London: Office of Fair Trading.

Owen, T. & Meyer, J. (2009). *Minimising the Use of 'Restraint' in Care Homes: Challenges, Dilemmas and Positive Approaches*. Adults's Services Report 25. London: Social Care Institute for Excellence.

Owen, T. & NCHRDF (Eds.) (2006). *My Home Life*. London: Help the Aged.

Payne, M. (2009). *Social Care Practice in Context*. Basingstoke: Palgrave Macmillan.

Pugh, M. & Keady, J. (2003). Assessing and responding to challenging behaviour in dementia: a focus for community mental health nursing practice. In: J. Keady, C. Clarke, & T. Adams (Eds.), *Community Mental Health Nursing and Dementia Care: Practice Perspectives* (pp. 199–211). Buckingham: Open University Press.

Qureshi, H. (2009). *Restraint in Care Homes for Older People: A Review of Selected Literature*. Adults's Services Report 26. London: Social Care Institute for Excellence.

Ray, M., Bernard, B., & Phillips, J. (2009). *Critical Issues in Social Work with Older People*. Basingstoke: Palgrave Macmillan.

Ryan, T. (Ed.) (1999). *Managing Crisis and Risk in Mental Health Nursing*. Cheltenham: Stanley Thornes Publishers Ltd.

Smith, C., Patel, M., Easterbrook, L., et al. (2009). *Older People's Vision for Long-term Care*. York: Joseph Rowntree Foundation.

Stanton-Greenwood, A. (1999). Managing violence in residential settings. In: H. Kemshall & J. Pritchard (Eds.), *Good Practice in Working with Violence* (pp. 190–206). London: Jessica Kingsley Publishers.

Tew, J. (2002). *Social Theory, Power and Practice*. Basingstoke: Palgrave.

Tew, J. (2005). Power relations, social order and mental distress. In: J. Tew (Ed.), *Social Perspectives in Mental Health Developing Social Models to Understand and Work with Mental Distress* (pp. 71–89). London: Jessica Kingsley Publishers.

Titterton, M. (2005). *Risk and Risk Taking in Health and Social Care Welfare*. London: Jessica Kingsley Publishers.

Vallelly, S., Evans, S., Fear, T., & Means, R. (2006). *Opening Doors to Independence—A Longitudinal Study Exploring the Contribution of Extra Care Housing to the Care and Support of Older People with Dementia*. Bristol: University of the West of England/Housing Corporation and Housing 21.

Walker, A. & Hennessy, C.H. (Eds.) (2004). *Growing Older Quality of Life in Old Age*. Maidenhead: Open University Press.

Wilkinson, H., Kerr, D., & Cunningham, C. (2008). *Supporting Older People in Care Homes at Night, Summary Findings*. York: Joseph Rowntree Foundation.

Chapter 24

Dementia training in care homes

Buz Loveday

Abstract

This chapter explores the importance of dementia training in care homes, highlighting the need to address attitudes as well as practices. The author foregrounds the importance of helping staff discard myths and negative assumptions and develop knowledge, skills, insight, and an empathic awareness of the feelings and needs of residents with dementia. For staff to learn, it is necessary not only for training to engage them but for it to be relevant to their daily practice. Helping them translate learning into practice is a key feature of effective training supported by the use of real-life examples and situations. It is widely acknowledged that dementia training for care home staff has historically been far from adequate and the author proposes that whole team training is the best method for achieving the 'informed and effective workforce' specified by the National Dementia Strategy. The chapter concludes that in order to embed real improvements in the quality of dementia care, training needs to be part of a developmental strategy that is underpinned by informed and skilled leadership.

Introduction

More than 820,000 people in the United Kingdom have some form of dementia (Luengo-Fernandez et al., 2010), a figure predicted to double within the next 30 years (Department of Health, 2009). It has been estimated that over two thirds of all care home residents have dementia with the majority having advanced dementia (Alzheimer's Society, 2007). It is widely accepted that dementia training has a pivotal role to play in enabling care home staff to meet the profound and complex needs of this growing population. The Alzheimer's Society has long maintained that care homes should make good quality dementia training 'an essential part of the team's development' (Alzheimer's Society and Royal College of Nursing, 2001) and in its 'Home from Home' report (Alzheimer's Society, 2007: vii), recommended that 'Training in dementia care must be mandatory for all care home staff'.

But the provision of dementia training in care homes has historically been far from adequate. In 1997, Tom Kitwood first wrote of the 'vast training and educational deficit' in dementia care (Kitwood, 1997) and 13 years later, the situation is little different. Two reports published in 2009 identified a fundamental lack of dementia training. The Care of Elderly People UK Market Survey (Laing and Buisson, 2009) found that dementia training in care homes is 'fragmented and often ad hoc', and one-third of supposedly specialist dementia care homes provide no dementia training at all. Reinforcing this finding, 'Prepared to Care' (All-Party Parliamentary Group on Dementia, 2009) established that 'as a whole, the social care workforce has a very limited knowledge of dementia and is therefore not ready to provide high quality dementia care' (p. xi). The recommendations of the National Dementia Strategy for England for 'an informed and effective workforce for people with dementia' (objective 13) are therefore urgent and long overdue. At last, training and development in dementia care, both inside and outside care homes, is firmly on the national policy and practice agenda.

The importance of dementia training

Dementia care is a complex and challenging area of work that requires a highly skilled, deeply empathic, and strongly motivated workforce. Many staff working in the field have innate qualities that predispose them to be excellent carers, but these require nurturing if they are to be used to benefit residents with dementia. Other care home staff may be temperamentally ill-equipped for their role and informed by negative assumptions about dementia; for them, unlearning may be a prerequisite to learning. For both of these groups, and all those whose skills and attitudes lie somewhere in between, effective dementia care will not come about without good training.

Good practice in dementia care is closely linked to the quality and quantity of specialist training received by staff. Specifically, it can impact positively on staff attitudes and performance (e.g. Bryan et al., 2002; Davison et al., 2007), though a number of factors influence its effectiveness (see later), NICE (the National Institute for Health and Clinical Excellence) and SCIE (the Social Care Institute for Excellence) reported that: 'It has long been recognised that the attitudes, skills and knowledge of staff working with people with dementia have the potential to influence the person's well-being, quality of life and function' (National Collaborating Centre for Mental Health, 2007: 266). Importantly, the Commission for Social Care Inspection (2008) found a direct correlation between the quality of staff training and development and the well-being of people living with dementia in care homes.

Enhancing the quality of life of people with dementia is profoundly important, but the benefits of a well-trained and well-supported workforce go further. Training contributes to increased confidence (Schindel-Martin et al., 2003), lowers levels of worker frustration (Feldt and Ryden, 1992), and improves staff retention (Noel et al., 2000). Families and friends of care home residents are much happier when staff have the skill to interact with residents, support them to maintain their abilities, and treat them with respect; their satisfaction with the quality of care correlates strongly with their rating of how well the home understands the needs of residents with dementia (Alzheimer's Society, 2007). Good dementia care also makes good business sense. The business guru Gerry Robinson (BBC, 2009) has shown how staff training and high quality care create sustainable businesses because happier residents mean happier relatives, a higher quality grading by the Care Quality Commission (CQC), and ultimately full beds. So everyone benefits from improved dementia care.

Key objectives for dementia training

Training staff to meet the needs of people living with dementia is a very different process from much of the other training delivered in care homes. Learning about moving and handling or food hygiene, for example, equips staff with essential facts, skills, and guidelines. These issues—unlike dementia care—are not intrinsically bound up with assumptions, prejudices, deep-seated fears, and personal needs. There are some very special considerations that need to be taken into account when considering dementia-related training.

The late Professor Tom Kitwood described dementia training as 'a process of profound personal transformation, involving the development of a very high level of interpersonal awareness and skill' (Loveday and Kitwood, 1998: 7). This is not, then, a matter of learning a particular technique or set of rules. In fact, dementia training needs to touch the hearts as well as the minds of those participating. Bringing about sustained improvements in care practice will not be possible without tackling the attitudes that lie beneath. Training needs to root out the deeply buried mistaken beliefs that have historically informed bad care practice, and replace them—at an equal depth—with new convictions. Since each person with dementia, and each situation involving a person with dementia, is unique, dementia training cannot hope to teach staff what to do in a potentially infinite number of interactions. The focus, then, is not to teach staff *what* to do, but to teach staff *how to work* out what to do for themselves. The process of person-centred dementia care should, in itself, be seen as a process of learning, in which staff reflect on their practice, learn from their experiences, and develop the ability to 'reflect in action' (Schon, 1987). This means that they are able to adapt the nature of their communication and actions to meet the individual's needs.

Grounded in reality

For this deep level of learning to take place a number of issues need to be recognized. Firstly, in order for training to be effective, it has to focus on issues that are of current concern to staff and their roles, responsibilities, and experiences. It should be made clear to participants, from the outset of any training programme, that it is about them and their work. Training should strive to be simultaneously visionary and pragmatic—keeping focused on the best possible outcomes for people with dementia while also exploring the potential of 'small steps' to effect change quickly. Defining ideals can help to inspire a vision of 'good care', but if not counterbalanced by realism, an approach that is overly idealistic can be demotivating for staff who are painfully aware of the constraints that face them every day. So training needs to focus on what can feasibly be achieved within the time and resources available to the staff team at that time. Also, every small achievement should be celebrated and viewed as bringing the team one step closer to realizing the vision.

An appropriately focused training course should also empower staff to find the most effective ways of using time. For example, care staff often report that virtually all of their time is devoted to addressing residents' essential bodily needs (e.g. hygiene, nutrition, elimination, movement). In many care homes this results in a functional culture of care, where the completion of tasks becomes the priority. In seeking to shift the staff group towards a person-centred culture, a trainer needs to temporarily accept these time constraints and work with participants to find ways in which psychological and emotional needs can be addressed simultaneously during these caregiving activities. For example, a resident's self-esteem could be bolstered by encouraging him or her to carry out parts of the task himself or herself; a person's strong love for his or her family could be the basis of ongoing conversations that care staff initiate each time they assist with personal care. Such interventions do not require extra time, but maximize the benefit of the time that staff do spend with an individual.

Keeping the training real also means avoiding a reliance on theory and drawing instead on real-life experiences. For example, using examples and sharing anecdotes that help to bring learning points to life, providing case studies and scenarios to help to generate learning through discussion and reflection, and—essentially—encouraging care home staff to talk about the residents they work with and the issues that are challenging them. Listening to the narratives of participants is an important route through which a trainer can create a climate of support and respect, showing that they value the experience of staff and care about the problems they are facing. This, in turn, will help participants feel safe enough to open themselves up to real learning.

Readiness to learn

It is important to recognize that, for many care home staff, being open to learning is actually quite challenging because it often means facing up to the fact that, unwittingly, they have failed to meet the needs of residents with dementia for many years. In the absence of training or guidance—common in the care sector—staff have had to develop their own practice, often through copying longer-serving staff. The prevalent view, inherited from a medical model of dementia, has been that there's little that can be done to help people with dementia, since their neurological impairment will continue to progress. Thus, many staff have seen their work as unrewarding and unimportant, an attitude reinforced by low remuneration.

At the beginning of a training course, their position may be described as one of 'unconscious incompetence' or 'not knowing they don't know' (Gordon Training International, c. early 1970s). If a trainer is able to gently help participants recognize that there's a lot they need to learn, then potentially, people will begin to expose deep-seated attitudes that have guided their care practice for many years and (if the training is successful) may gradually come to realize that these attitudes and practices have been unhelpful or even abusive. Some of the key messages delivered in good dementia training are painful; it is often easier for staff to raise their defences and say what they think should be said without engaging with the content on an emotional level. The creation of a safe and non-judgmental environment is a prerequisite of training that aims to reach hearts as well as minds. Care home staff should not be criticized or made to feel inferior for expressing negative opinions within a training context. Indeed, it is only through airing such views that recognition of the dissonance between their current practices and new learning becomes evident. This realization, together with supportive and constructive challenge, can empower trainees to discard old attitudes and approaches and adopt new ones.

Knowledge

In recent years, attempts have been made to establish a consensus about the key areas of knowledge and skill required for dementia care. In 2006 for example, Skills for Care published the 'Knowledge Set for Dementia', a document identifying key learning outcomes to be addressed in any learning provision on dementia (Skills for Care, 2006). In 2010, these learning outcomes have evolved into a dementia qualification, part of the Qualifications and Credit Framework. An outline of important topics for dementia training is shown in Box 24.1.

Many unhelpful care practices have, at their roots, a lack of understanding about dementia. Therefore, it is vital that all training should provide information about dementia as a baseline expectation. Helping care home staff to understand the nature of dementia and recognize some of the effects of what is, essentially, an invisible disability, helps them appreciate some of the difficulties that individuals might have. This means that they are more likely to recognize the help that they may need. Further, mistaken assumptions (e.g. that a person is being deliberately awkward or 'putting it on') can be overcome and empathy can begin to develop.

But knowledge about dementia is only one side of the equation. Unfortunately, too many short courses on dementia, or talks provided by 'experts', focus solely on the clinical aspects of the condition. Trainees are left with knowledge about the process of neurological impairment but no understanding about how to support people who have it or how to develop 'good practice'. Care home staff are not working with brains in laboratories; they are working with living, breathing, sentient individuals who, while struggling to cope with their changed situation, also 'have a life' (see Department of Health, 2010). The lack of knowledge among care home staff goes much further than a knowledge deficit about the disease process. A key contributor to negative attitudes that pervade much dementia care is a lack of understanding about *the person*. Knowledge about each individual—the person's background, his or her likes and dislikes, job, hobbies and interests, culture, religion, and sexuality, routines, achievements, emotional needs, and everything else that defines the person as a unique human being—is central to the provision of effective care. Thus, any training course on dementia needs to inspire staff to recognize the pivotal importance of gathering information about the men and women who live in the care home, and provide guidance on ways of doing so. A variety of published methodologies exist for this purpose (e.g. 'Personal fact-file' in Loveday and Kitwood, 1998). When training is provided

Box 24.1 Sample outline of a standard 3-day course in a person-centred approach to dementia care (as provided by Dementia Trainers)

Day 1:
- Introductions and objectives
- The experience of dementia
- Facts about dementia: types, symptoms and their causes, statistics, risk factors
- Factors which can cause or contribute to difficulties in dementia
- Establishing guidelines for good practice
- Individual responses to dementia
- Developing knowledge about people with dementia as individuals
- Meeting the needs of the whole person
- Well-being in dementia
- Identifying and monitoring well-being
- Key points and action planning

Day 2:
- The range of difficulties and abilities of individuals
- Compensating for difficulties caused by dementia
- Environment and dementia
- Making the most of remaining strengths
- Caring in partnership
- Basic principles of communication
- Non-verbal communication
- Communication problems
- Guidelines for good communication
- Responding to different realities of people with dementia
- Understanding messages behind challenging behaviour
- Responding to strong feelings
- Key points and action planning

Day 3:
- Working with family carers
- Reasons behind challenging behaviours
- Understanding and preventing aggressive behaviour
- Responding to challenging behaviour and meeting needs
- Understanding and responding to walking ('wandering')

> **Box 24.1 Sample outline of a standard 3-day course in a person-centred approach to dementia care (as provided by Dementia Trainers)** *(continued)*
>
> ◆ Basic rights of people with dementia
> ◆ Medication and person-centred care
> ◆ Assessing and managing risk
> ◆ The purpose of occupation for people with dementia
> ◆ Suiting occupations to individual needs
> ◆ Key points and action planning

in-house—for example, by a team leader—there are additional opportunities within the course itself to help staff understand the essential personhood of each resident.

Negative beliefs

Since negative beliefs about dementia play a major part in fostering task-focused, depersonalized care, this is another area that needs to be addressed in training. Care staff have often been exposed to messages that dementia is a 'living death' (Woods, 1989), that people with dementia are 'zombies' (Aquilina and Hughes, 2006) or 'empty shells' (Thacker, 2007), and that when someone has dementia his or her body is all that is left (Kitwood, 1997). It is not surprising that they will prioritize caring for the corporeal body, without considering the holistic needs of the sentient individual. These damaging beliefs also contribute, in a profound way, to the previously mentioned lack of understanding about individual residents' life histories. Too often, staff believe that the person has been so fundamentally changed by dementia that they are not even related to the person they were when they were neurologically intact. Further, once somebody has dementia, the tendency is to treat the dementia itself as the defining aspect of that person's identity, subsuming all other characteristics and features (Goffman, 1963).

Dementia training must challenge this stigmatizing misinformation. Care home staff need to be encouraged to recognize everything that each person with dementia can still do as well as the things he or she can't, to understand how much the person is still aware of, and—above all else—to realize that dementia does not strip an individual of his or her capacity to experience a full range of human emotion. Often, negative emotions are the result of unthinking care practice, and therefore staff must learn to strive to understand the perspective of the person with dementia, using observational and listening skills and then responding to the message communicated through the person's expression of emotion. This capacity for empathic insight can often be prompted by quite simple experiential teaching methods: for example, asking participants to consider how they would feel in the situations that people with dementia often face. Carrying out structured observations—such as those involved in Dementia Care Mapping—can also assist in the development of an understanding of the subjective reality of being a person with dementia (Brooker, 2007).

In certain, carefully managed, situations, more intense experiential training exercises can also be used to provide powerful learning. For example, Caroline Baker (2008) describes giving staff the experience of living a day in the life of a resident, and David Sheard (2008) explains a training exercise that involves telling participants that they will not be allowed to leave the building to collect their children from school. It is very important that effective de-briefing accompanies any experiential training of this nature. As Judy Arin-Krupp (1982) pointed out, 'Adults do not learn from experience, they learn from processing experience', and this processing needs to take place within a supportive context if empathic insights are to result. Role-play—when undertaken in a safe and trusting environment—can also prompt effective experiential learning, for example, the intensive role-plays used in the Extending Empathy group (Farmer and Bruce, 2010). Short role-plays, too, can be useful as learning tools to assist the development of awareness of the experience of living with dementia. If participants are prepared to briefly set aside their own reality and use their imagination and intuition to enter the world of another, deep learning can result.

Another mistaken belief that contributes to bad practice is that aggressive or otherwise challenging behaviours are 'only to be expected'. 'It's the dementia' (Stokes, 2008) is the erroneous reason too often assumed to explain behaviour that staff have found challenging. Although this explanation is attractive at one level, as it requires virtually no thought, it is completely unhelpful in that it blocks any reflection on what the behaviour may mean and what the person may be trying to communicate. If behaviour is seen simply as a symptom of dementia, then the thoughtless communication, the physical discomfort, or the confusing environment that provoked the individual's distress and led to his or her actions, are never addressed. And so the distress persists, the challenging behaviour continues, and levels of staff stress rise. Stokes (2008) explains that a primary concern in dementia care is to 'wonder why'; to seek the reasons behind any difficult behaviour that has arisen. Training must encourage this quest. Care home staff need to be taught how to look for reasons that lie outside the individual's condition. They need to be supported to become 'dementia care detectives' (Loveday and Murphy, 2009).

Skills development

Although developing knowledge, understanding, and insight will do much to improve the attitudes of care home staff, it is also important that training facilitates the development of the skills through which these improved attitudes can be demonstrated. Summarizing evidence on the effects of training programmes in dementia care, found that particularly positive outcomes were associated with training programmes that teach specific skills (National Collaborating Centre for Mental Health, 2007). The everyday role of a dementia care worker requires many specialist skills. For example, to communicate with someone who has lost almost all of his or her verbal language or to assess the exact help that an individual needs in order to maintain maximum independence in personal care.

Training exercises that focus on real situations can be useful in assisting skills development. Videos, demonstrations, and case studies can promote the development of insight into the potential effect of interactions on the person with dementia, and prompt discussion about useful strategies. Talking about residents and their needs can generate new ideas, and taking part in role-plays offers opportunities to try out new skills. Since the training needs to relate closely to work practices and real-life situations in the home, a key stage in the process of skills development is to encourage participants to implement new interventions with residents. This helps to consolidate learning and flags up potential difficulties or issues for consideration, which can subsequently be brought back to the training and discussed.

Training methods

Hands-on activities and opportunities to immediately put new ideas into practice will particularly benefit learners whose preferred learning style is pragmatic (Honey and Mumford, 1992) or kinaesthetic (Fleming, 2001). The trainer's role with such learners will primarily be to encourage reflection on each new experience. Other learners tend to be more naturally reflective, although they may need encouragement to implement what they have learnt.

The use of a variety of training methods is important in addressing different learning styles: active exercises balanced against thoughtful ones, or experiential processes followed by practical action-planning. Also, more generally, using varied training techniques helps to hold participants' attention and provides multiple opportunities for important concepts to be grasped. New information and guidance will be more easily absorbed if it is delivered in short chunks, interspersed with interactive activities such as brainstorms, quizzes, and games to raise energy levels and prompt other kinds of learning. For care home staff who are particularly motivated and able to study autonomously, it can also be useful to incorporate some independent learning activities in-between training sessions, for example, using an e-learning programme, such as the SCIE Open Dementia Programme (Loveday and Murphy, 2009) to create a blended learning experience.

Addressing needs

In order to ensure that training is meaningful to participants, it is important that the trainer understands their existing level of knowledge and experience, respects and validates this, and builds on it. The trainer must also recognize the range of different learning needs present within any group of staff and strive to be inclusive. For example, many care home staff, particularly in inner cities, have learnt English as a second language and may speak very little of it. So in addition to the challenges of communicating with a person with dementia who may have limited verbal skills, the language barrier presented by a staff member is an additional barrier and one that needs to be acknowledged in any training course.

There is no simple route to overcoming this, but it is very important that the pace of the training is appropriate, that the language used is understandable, and that group discussions are carefully managed to ensure participation by all. Participants should be encouraged to ask questions, and these must always be answered respectfully.

The trainer needs to own the responsibility for enabling all participants to understand and be involved. He or she needs to pitch the course at an appropriate level and provide any necessary support to trainees who are struggling. This may include referring learners to sources of external help or further development, for example functional skills support or English language classes. Similarly, it is important that the trainer identifies and encourages more able learners, pointing them towards opportunities for further development, which could range from short specialist courses—for example in techniques such as validation therapy (see Validation Training Institute Inc.) or Dementia Care Mapping (see University of Bradford)—to formal qualifications such as degrees in dementia studies (available at the universities of Bradford and Stirling).

It is likely that within any group of care home staff, some will have had previously negative experiences in formal learning situations (such as school). In order to engage participants, a trainer must work to counter these experiences. For example, it is essential that the trainer respects all participants as experienced adults, values their contributions, and encourages them to recognize the importance of their own work and feelings. The trainer, therefore, should not present himself or herself as an 'expert', but rather should seek to empower participants to develop their own expertise, through learning about the individuals for whom they are caring and finding the best approaches for each.

Empowerment is a key concept in dementia care training. The trainer, particularly an external one, is only a temporary visitor and is unlikely to become an ongoing source of advice and guidance. Given this, he or she must help to harness and channel participants' strengths and positive motivations and empower them to develop their own capacity for reflective, empathic, creative practice in their work with people with dementia.

Barriers

Sadly, the strengths of staff working in care homes go largely unrecognized. Rates of pay do not value the level of skill required for the work, nor do they provide an incentive to choose a career in dementia care. This area has historically been seen as low status work, best suited to staff of 'low ability, little inspiration, and few qualifications' (Kitwood, 1995). This is a key reason for the training shortfall described earlier in this chapter. Providing quality dementia training has simply not been seen as a priority use of limited resources and the situation has not been helped by the fact that there has been no clear or committed route to obtaining funds.

Some local authorities and primary care trusts (PCTs) have, over recent years, taken steps towards resolving this problem by providing a limited number of free dementia training courses for statutory, voluntary, and private sector care staff. This is done by utilizing monies available through various funding streams from central government and bodies such as the Learning and Skills council, Skills for Care, and regeneration agencies. Inevitably, though, only a small proportion of staff gain places on such training, and it will be down to the care home to work out how to resource the training needs of the rest of the staff group (and how to finance the costs linked to covering the absence of those sent on training courses). Typically, in organizations that do not value staff learning and development, there will only be a minimal budget attached to training, and this will be allocated to areas that relate directly to compliance with the Essential standards of quality and safety (Care Quality Commission 2010). Such topics tend to include moving and handling and health and safety. The result of this is that no dementia training takes place at all, staff are shown a DVD about dementia, and this is thought to meet their training needs, or dementia is included in a short course covering multiple topics, provided by a non-specialist trainer. Clearly, none of these alternatives is going to meaningfully address the need for proper dementia training.

One of the key objectives of the National Dementia Strategy is for 'an informed and effective workforce'. The recommendation made in 'Prepared to Care' (All-Party Parliamentary Group on Dementia, 2009) is that dementia training, in the shape of the Qualifications Credit Framework (QCF) units mentioned earlier, should become a mandatory requirement for care staff working with people with dementia in all care settings. The expectation is that commissioners will have to specify dementia training in contracts with providers and some funding will be made available to increase the likely uptake of training. However, Pitt (2010), writing in 'Community Care', esti-mates the chances of 'an informed and effective workforce' being in place by 2014 as 'weak to moderate'. He puts this down to the 'low status of the social care workforce and lack of clarity about access to training funding'. He also quotes Simon Williams, dementia lead at the Association of Directors of Adult Social Services, who says that 'the key issue is changing assumptions and attitudes among staff'. Therein lies the fundamental challenge for, as has been considered earlier in this chapter, tackling entrenched attitudes and assumptions is no easy task. Sufficient consideration needs to be given to how this can be achieved if improving dementia care is a serious ambi-tion on the part of policy makers and care agencies.

Organizational considerations

When training is provided centrally—for example by local authorities—it is likely that organizations will only be allocated a small number of places on each course. While participants will benefit from the wealth of experience that staff from a range of differ-ent care services bring to the course, the drawbacks are substantial. However inspired they have become, whatever new ideas they are intending to put into practice, it is virtually impossible for one or two individuals to return to their care home and imple-ment new attitudes and approaches when the rest of their team is unchanged. Within any organization, particularly a long-term care setting, behavioural and cultural norms are very powerful and will quickly override the influence of a recently attended train-ing course, particularly if the manager doesn't understand the new way of working and fails to encourage innovative good practices. Thus good intentions quickly wither, new approaches are not sustained, and by the time the next two candidates from the home are sent on the same course, they are in the same position upon their return to work.

For organizations that want dementia training to make a real difference, the most effective practice is when the whole team is able to engage together in the process of learning. This 'team' needs to include everyone who works within the care home, from domestic and kitchen staff to team leaders and managers, as everyone who has contact with residents has the capacity to influence their quality of life. In this way, dementia training can be used as part of a process of team development, recognizing and valuing the input of each team member. Realistically, it is neither possible nor desirable for the whole team to be away from the care home at the same time, but a similar outcome can be achieved by providing two or three 'runs' (depending on the size of the staff team) of the same course in quick succession. Senior staff should be involved from the outset so that they can support the implementation of new learning and the gradual transformation of the culture of care. In large organizations operating a number of care homes, this option is more feasible, as places on each course may be shared between staff from different homes. For smaller care homes, it often proves useful to form a training partnership with another local provider to share places on, and the costs of, training.

Giving serious priority to all staff learning about dementia also means that an organization needs to think about creating its own dementia training pathway. This involves establishing a training 'plan' whereby new staff undertake basic training on dementia as part of their induction, this is subsequently consolidated once they have experience in post, and then further built on by other training opportunities, for example in leadership.

Leadership

It is essential to recognize that training cannot single-handedly transform attitudes and practices. If the training is to make any sustained impact, it needs to be part of a strategy of development within the care home, supported by creative leadership that inspires, guides, and supports the achievement of a vision. 'The importance of good staff management cannot be overestimated' wrote Cantley and Wilson (2002: 93).

At the very least, managers and other senior staff members in care homes need a sound understanding of the nature of dementia and the key principles of person-centred care practice. But more than this, dementia care managers need to develop approaches and techniques for person-centred dementia care leadership, which includes, for example, skills in coaching, promoting reflective practice, and role modelling. Although it is important that staff access formal training on dementia, equally important is the informal on-the-job training and guidance given by effective dementia care leaders. However useful a formal staff training course has been, embedding and implementing new learning is primarily the responsibility of managers (Burgio and Burgio, 1990). Managers can do this, for example, by supporting staff to prioritize their work appropriately (always putting individual needs above tasks), giving clear, constructive feedback on care practice, and making sure that staff have sufficient time to support residents to maximize use of their own abilities (e.g. in personal care tasks).

The National Dementia Strategy calls for 'the development of explicit leadership for dementia care within care homes' (objective 11). However, many managers of dementia care services lack an appreciation of their role in relation to leading the development of person-centred care. Alongside the training needs of care staff is a pressing need for training in the skills of person-centred dementia care management.

Box 24.2 Summary of content of the Dementia Care Leadership Programme

♦ Goals for dementia care: optimizing well-being
♦ Addressing needs and strengths and avoiding secondary losses of ability
♦ Creating guidelines for best practice in dementia care
♦ A partnership approach to care and management
♦ Motivations, strengths, and skills of staff
♦ Key features of person-centred management
♦ The manager as coach: constructive feedback and questions for reflective practice
♦ Evaluating care practice and defining achievable goals
♦ Addressing factors influencing the care approach
♦ Supporting communication and engagement
♦ Being a role model
♦ Getting the most from external professionals
♦ Person-centred risk assessment and management
♦ The use and misuse of medication in dementia care
♦ The dementia care environment
♦ Developing the involvement of relatives and friends as active partners in care
♦ Defining priorities for person-centred care
♦ Team dynamics and communication processes
♦ Assessment and care planning

The Dementia Care Leadership Programme (an accredited training course run by the author) aims to address this deficit with an intensive curriculum of learning and developmental activities (see Box 24.2). Care home managers undertaking the course embark on a series of projects designed to enhance their awareness of the needs of people with dementia and the staff team caring for them, and develop their skills in bringing about the best possible outcomes for both. See Box 24.3 for an example (as described by one of the course students in 2009). It is vital that managers are aware of, and involved with, the everyday lives of residents and staff. Only through having a clear focus on enhancing the well-being of those living in the care home can they guide staff towards achieving this.

Cascade training

A further strategy for maximizing the extent to which staff can be supported to implement new learning, is the use of a 'cascade' training model, whereby managers or team leaders themselves are equipped and resourced to lead dementia training. An example

Box 24.3 Enhancing Tess's well-being*

One of the most upsetting things for Tess is personal care. We have discussed this as a group at a staff meeting as Tess has assaulted three staff this week, all around personal care. I have personally asked three members of staff if they would be prepared to help Tess with her personal care. I explained to each one that the purpose of this assignment was to build a strong relationship based on trust so Tess could be given the opportunity of having someone with whom she could discuss how she felt about personal care.

I have spent 1:1 time with each of these staff members to give them the opportunity to talk through their progress. I have asked them specifics about what is working and what isn't. I have made sure there is time for them to spend with Tess without feeling rushed. The whole staff team have been given all the personal history we have for Tess in order to have a better understanding of her state of mind. We have talked about how Tess could be feeling when the other residents and their families are unkind or disparaging about Tess in her hearing. We also discussed how Tess could be feeling when staff avoid talking to her or avoid eye contact with her (which they have admitted to doing to avoid conflict). We talked about our frustrations and fears and the fact that it is OK to fail sometimes and admit that we don't have all the answers.

......

Three weeks later, we could not have anticipated the improvement to this resident's well-being. Our interventions as a team have transformed Tess from an anxious, unhappy woman spending perhaps 10% of her day in well-being to spending about 75% of her day in well-being. Tess is now continent again taking herself to the toilet both day and night. We have had no assaults on staff for 10 days.

The impact on Tess's well-being is immense. This real team effort has had a positive effect on staff morale as well. We have concluded that the more information we have about an individual the more we can put ourselves in their shoes and have a better understanding on what they may be experiencing. We have also concluded that our resident with the most challenging behaviour was trying to communicate to us how frightened, unhappy, and misunderstood she was feeling.

*Dementia Care Leadership Programme assignment, written by Jacqui Harper, Care Home Manager, Quantum Care.

of this is the Dementia Care Trainers' Programme (see Box 24.4), an accredited course run by the author (for further information see Loveday, 2001). Not only is this a more cost-effective way of providing in-house training, but it also provides a means of ensuring that the training is relevant, grounded, and sustainable. The gap between the classroom and the care home is bridged and the messages delivered in the training seamlessly become the principles guiding the care home's practices.

An excellent example of using the Dementia Care Trainers' Programme as part of a regional strategy was the project spearheaded by Stockport Dementia Care Training (SDCT) in 2010. Sixteen practitioners from local care homes and other social and

Box 24.4 Summary of content of the Dementia Care Trainers' Programme

Module 1—Person-centred dementia care knowledge and practice:

- Facts on dementia
- Person-centred care
- Well-being in dementia
- Focusing on the individual
- Partnership: encouraging independence alongside working with dependency
- Special needs of people with dementia
- Communicating with people who have dementia
- Responding to different realities of people with dementia
- Working with challenging behaviour
- Rights and risk
- Addressing the needs of family carers
- Activities and occupation

Module 2—Person-centred dementia care training skills:

- Adult learning
- Using training equipment
- Practising training skills
- Different training methods
- Analysis of the training process
- Training techniques (e.g. brainstorms, discussions, demonstrations, giving instructions)
- Presentation skills
- Person-centred training
- Preparing and running training sessions
- Managing difficulties and challenges in training
- Possible achievements and limits of training
- Methods for influencing care practice
- Learning to use the Dementia Care Trainers' Resource Pack (a complete set of guidelines and materials for running up to 3 days dementia training)

healthcare settings undertook the course and gained accreditation as dementia care trainers. Using their new skills and resources, and supported by SDCT and their peers, they embarked on a mission to transform dementia care within their care service through training, role modelling, advising, mentoring, and encouraging the implementation of newly learned practices.

Factors influencing care

The quality and type of leadership in a care home has a huge influence on the culture of care. An empowering, cooperative, and supportive management style will play a key part in creating these same qualities in staff interactions with people with dementia (Kitwood, 1997). A number of other factors, too, impact on the potential outcomes of training. These include the organization's policies and procedures, staffing structures and ratios, the physical environment, communication processes (including care planning systems), and relationships with external professionals (including inspectors). Expectations and routines are an important way in which the ethos of an organization is made manifest, and they have a profound influence on the culture of care. Where there is a requirement, for example, that an activities timetable is established and rigidly adhered to, there will inevitably be a reduction in person-centred practice as individuals' choice is compromised and the flexibility to address constantly changing needs is inhibited. If a CQC inspector fails to value the person-centred care plan focused on the promotion of well-being and instead criticizes the written documentation because there are no tick boxes to indicate when each personal care task has been done, then a clear message is conveyed that such tasks are more important than the people themselves. When breakfast is only available in the dining room and within a limited time span, it will unavoidably result in disempowering care practices as staff rush to get residents ready in time and focus on making sure breakfast is consumed rather than enjoyed.

Training alone cannot change the culture of dementia care. At best it can provide a vital component in an organizational strategy; at worst it can be merely a tick-box exercise. In commissioning a training course, it is very important that managers give careful thought to the training needs of their staff, the outcomes they are hoping for, and the role that training can play towards achieving improved care. Too often, the spur for commissioning a training course is an inspector's requirement, but care home managers themselves have to take some responsibility for recognizing the skills gaps and other shortfalls and acknowledging that there is a need for improvement.

Conclusion

Ultimately, the goal of staff attending dementia training is to improve the way they work and enhance the quality of life of residents. Care homes need to give considered thought as to how, once training has been delivered, they will accommodate, support, and sustain changes in practice. Serious questions need to be asked before dementia training takes place: Is the organization open to new ideas and committed to developing person-centred care? Is it prepared to enable and support staff to put their new learning into practice? And how will managers of the care home be equipped to take forward the ideas generated in the training? 'Maintaining person-centred care over time for people with dementia is not an easy or trivial process', writes Dawn Brooker (2007: 41). Although it is clear that training can play a leading role in establishing and maintaining positive attitudes and practices, proper effective training is no casual undertaking and it can only be effective as part of a wider strategy that facilitates a substantial shift in the way that those living with dementia, and those working with people with dementia, are understood and valued.

References

All-Party Parliamentary Group on Dementia (2009). Executive summary. *Prepared to Care: Challenging the Dementia Skills Gap.* London: All-Party Parliamentary Group on Dementia.

Alzheimer's Society (2007). Executive summary, recommendations for action. *Home from Home: Quality of Care for People with Dementia Living in Care Homes.* London: Alzheimer's Society.

Alzheimer's Society and Royal College of Nursing (2001). Staff training and development. *Alzheimer's Society Quality Dementia Care in Care Homes Person-centred Standards.* London: Alzheimer's Society.

Aquilina, C. & Hughes, J. (2006). The return of the living dead: agency lost and found. In: J. Hughes, S. Louw, & S. Sabat (Eds.), *Dementia: Mind, Meaning, and the Person.* Oxford: Oxford University Press pp. 143–161.

Arin-Krupp, J. (1982). *Adult Learner: A Unique Entity.* Manchester: Adult Development and Learning. isbn 096132452X (isbn13: 9780961324520).

Baker, C. (2008). The power of learning through experience. *Journal of Dementia Care, 16,* 27–29.

BBC (2009). *Can Gerry Robinson Fix Dementia Care Homes?* Broadcast on BBC Two at 2100 GMT on Tuesday 8th and Tuesday 15th December.

Brooker, D. (2007). *Person-centred Dementia Care: Making Services Better.* London: Jessica Kingsley Publishers.

Bryan, K., Axelrod, L., Maxim, J., Bell, L., & Jordan, L. (2002). Working with older people with communication difficulties: an evaluation of care worker training. *Aging and Mental Health, 6,* 248–254.

Burgio, L.D. & Burgio, K.L. (1990). Institutional staff training and management: a review of the literature and a model for geriatric, long-term-care facilities. *International Journal of Aging and Human Development, 30,* 287–302.

Cantley, C. & Wilson, R. (2002). *Put Yourself in my Place: Designing and Managing Care Homes for People with Dementia.* Bristol: The Policy Press.

Care Quality Commission (2010). *Guidance about compliance: Essential standards of quality and safety.* Available at: http://www.cqc.org.uk/_db/_documents/Essential_standards_of_ quality_and_safety_March_2010_FINAL.pdf (accessed on 11 February 2011).

Commission for Social Care Inspection (2008). *See Me Not Just the Dementia.* London: Commission for Social Care Inspection.

Davison, T., McCable, M., Visser, S., Hudgson, C., Buchanan, G., & George, K. (2007). Controlled trial of dementia training with a peer support group for aged care staff. *International Journal of Geriatric Psychiatry, 22,* 868–873.

Department of Health (2009). *Living Well With Dementia: A National Dementia Strategy.* London: Department of Health.

Department of Health (2010). *I have Dementia. I Also have a Life.* Awareness raising campaign. Available at: http://www.guardian.co.uk/careandsupportreform/video-dementia (accessed 12 June 2010).

Farmer, J. & Bruce, E. (2010). Role play: refreshing the parts other training can't reach. *Journal of Dementia Care, 18*(2), 28–31.

Feldt, K.S. & Ryden, M.B. (1992). Aggressive behaviour: educating nursing assistants. *Journal of Gerontological Nursing, 18,* 3–12.

Fleming, N.D. (2001). *Teaching and Learning Styles: VARK Strategies.* Honolulu: Community College.

Goffman, E. (1963). *Stigma: Notes on the Management of Spoiled Identity.* London: Prentice-Hall.

Gordon Training International (c. early 1970s). *Conscious Competence Learning Model. Gordon Training International.* Available at: http://www.businessballs.com/consciouscompetence learningmodel.htm (accessed 12 June 2010).

Honey, P. & Mumford, A. (1992). *The Manual of Learning Styles,* 3rd Edition. Maidenhead: Peter Honey.

Kitwood, T. (1995). Cultures of care: tradition and change. In: T. Kitwood & S. Benson (Eds.), *The New Culture of Dementia Care.* (pp. 7–11) London: Hawker.

Kitwood, T. (1997). *Dementia Reconsidered.* Buckingham: Open University Press.

Laing & Buisson (2009). *Care of Elderly People UK Market Survey 2009.* London: Laing & Buisson.

Loveday, B. (2001). 'Cascade training' to develop skills in dementia care. *Journal of Dementia Care, 9*(3), 15–17.

Loveday, B. & Kitwood, T. (1998). *Improving Dementia Care: A Resource for Training and Professional Development.* London: Hawker Publications.

Loveday, B. & Murphy, D. (2009). Section 5: Detective work. In: 'Positive communication', module 7 of *The Open Dementia Programme.* London: Social Care Institute for Excellence.

Luengo-Fernandez, R., Leal, J., & Gray, A. (2010). *Dementia 2010: The Economic Burden of Dementia and Associated Research Funding in the United Kingdom.* Cambridge: Alzheimer's Research Trust.

National Collaborating Centre for Mental Health (2007). *Dementia: NICE-SCIE Guidelines on Supporting People with Dementia and their Carers in Health and Social Care.* The British Psychological Society and Gaskell.

Noel, M.A., Pearce, G.L., & Metcalf, R. (2000). Front line workers in long-term care: the effect of educational interventions and stabilization of staffing ratios on turnover and absenteeism. *Journal of the American Medical Directors Association, 1*(6), 241–247.

Pitt, V. (2010). Things can only get better. *Community Care, 1812,* 26–27.

Schindel-Martin, L., Morden, P., Cetinski, G., et al. (2003). Teaching staff to respond effectively to cognitively impaired residents who display self-protective behaviours. *American Journal of Alzheimer's Disease and Other Dementias, 18,* 273–281.

Schon, D. (1987). *Educating the Reflective Practitioner.* San Francisco: Jossey Bass.

Sheard, D.M. (2008). *Growing: Training that Works in Dementia Care.* London: Alzheimer's Society.

Skills for Care (2006). *Knowledge Set for Dementia.* Available at: http://www.skillsforcare.org. uk/developing_skills/knowledge_sets/dementia.aspx (accessed 12 June 2010).

Stokes, G. (2008). *And Still the Music Plays.* London: Hawker Publications.

Thacker, H. (2007). *Coping with the Influx of Dementia Patients—The Need to Involve the Communities and Church Groups with Medical and Social Program Initiatives.* VDM Verlag Dr. Müeller.

University of Bradford. *Learning to Use Dementia Care Mapping (Basic User Status).* Available at: http://www.brad.ac.uk/health/dementia/DementiaCareMapping/ LearningtoUseDementiaCareMappingBasicUserStatus/ (accessed 11 February 2011).

Validation Training Institute Inc. *Training Program.* Available at: http://www.vfvalidation.org/ web.php?request=Training_Programs (accessed 12 June 2010).

Woods, R.T. (1989). *Alzheimer's Disease: Coping with a Living Death.* London: Souvenir Press.

Chapter 25

My home life: exploring the evidence base for best practice

Julienne Meyer and Tom Owen

Abstract

This chapter summarizes the evidence base underpinning the *My* Home Life (MHL) programme, a UK-wide initiative to promote quality of life in care homes for older people. The work was originally undertaken by members of the National Care Homes Research and Development Forum, who worked collaboratively to update an earlier review of the care needs of older people and family caregivers in continuing care settings. Findings focus on eight relationship-centred themes. The chapter begins by describing the MHL initiative, showing how it has grown from a project into a social movement. The difference between quality of life and quality of care is highlighted and the importance of good relationships between residents, relatives, and staff noted. The evidence base for each of the eight themes is then presented and an argument made for relationship-centred care as the key to best practice in care homes; in particular, for those with dementia.

Introduction

This chapter focuses on the evidence base for best practice in care homes. It draws on the findings from a review of the literature (NCHR&D Forum, 2007); this marked the start of the MHL programme, a UK-wide initiative to promote quality of life for those living, dying, visiting, and working in care homes for older people. This review of the literature updated a previous review by Davies (2001) on the care needs of older people and family caregivers in continuing care settings. The evidence base comprises eight themes, which cluster into three types: transformation, personalization, and navigation (see Table 25.1). Two of the eight themes (transformation) are aimed at managers and are concerned with what they must do to help support their staff put the other six themes into practice: *keeping workforce fit for purpose* and *promoting positive cultures*. Of the six staff themes, three are focused on the approach to care

Table 25.1 MHL: eight evidence-based, relationship-centred themes for promoting quality of life in care homes for older people

MHL themes	
Maintaining identity: (Personalization)	Working creatively with residents to maintain their sense of personal identity and engage in meaningful activity.
Creating community: (Personalization)	Optimizing relationships between and across staff, residents, family, friends, and the wider local community. Encouraging a sense of security, continuity, belonging, purpose, achievement, and significance for all.
Sharing decision-making: (Personalization)	Facilitating informed risk-taking and the involvement of residents, relatives, and staff in shared decision-making in all aspects of home life.
Managing transitions: (Navigation)	Supporting people both to manage the loss and upheaval associated with going into a home and to move forward.
Improving health and healthcare: (Navigation)	Ensuring adequate access to healthcare services and promoting health to optimize resident quality of life.
Supporting good end of life: (Navigation)	Valuing the 'living' and 'dying' in care homes and helping residents to prepare for a 'good death' with the support of their families.
Keeping workforce fit for purpose: (Transformation)	Identifying and meeting ever-changing training needs within the care home workforce.
Promoting a positive culture: (Transformation)	Developing leadership, management, and expertise to deliver a culture of care where care homes are seen as a positive option.

Source: Adapted from NCHR&D Forum (2007). *My Home Life: Quality of Life—Literature Review*. London: Help the Aged.

(personalization): *maintaining identity*, *sharing decision-making*, and *creating community* and the remaining three themes (navigation) are what staff need to do to help support residents and relatives through their journey of care: *managing transitions*, *improving health and healthcare*, and *supporting good end of life*. The mental health of older people in care homes has not been separated out as a particular theme in the MHL vision for best practice; instead mental health issues are integrated throughout the eight themes and are seen to be best addressed by the relational approach that underpins the MHL evidence base. This chapter begins by providing some contextual background on the MHL programme, next it explores what is meant by quality of life for older people in care homes and then goes on to detail the evidence base for best practice, including the relational approach. Finally, it is suggested that while the MHL vision for best practice needs to be continually updated, it nonetheless provides a useful starting point for care homes wishing to improve the mental health of their residents, relatives, and staff.

My home life programme

My Home Life (MHL) is a UK-wide charitable movement promoting quality of life for older people living and dying in care homes, and for those visiting and working with them, through relationship-centred care and evidence-based practice. It is a collaborative scheme bringing together organizations which reflect the interests of care home providers, commissioners, regulators, care home residents, and relatives and those interested in education, research, and practice development. It began in 2006 (phase 1: developing the vision), led by Help the Aged (now merged with Age Concern as Age UK) in partnership with National Care Forum (represents not-for-profit care homes). They commissioned City University London, to pull together the evidence base for best practice in care homes for older people. This work was undertaken in collaboration with the National Care Homes Research and Development Forum (NCHR&D) involving 60 academic researchers from universities across the United Kingdom; they worked together to develop an evidence base for quality of life in care homes. An Appreciative Inquiry approach (Cooperrider et al., 2003) was adopted, so that rather than a focus on research identifying poor practice, the review explored 'what residents want from care homes' and 'what practices work well in care homes'. The findings of this literature review are available on the MHL website (www.myhome.life.org.uk) with a chapter being devoted to each of the eight aforementioned themes. Together these eight themes offer a vision for care homes, a framework from which to deliver good quality of life.

The MHL programme has been very positively received by the sector and is uniquely supported by the Relatives and Residents Association and all the national provider organizations that represent care homes across the United Kingdom.[1] Phase 2 of the MHL programme (disseminating the vision) was funded by BUPA Giving and involved the dissemination of the vision to the 18,000 care homes across the United Kingdom through a number of resources (short report, research briefings, posters, bulletins, and DVD). MHL is now in its third phase of activity (implementing the vision) and, because of the success of the programme, the Joseph Rowntree Foundation has part funded this phase as a formal partner in the programme. MHL began as a project (literature review), developed into a programme of activities (developing resources, creating networks, sustaining change, maintaining the momentum), and is now seen as a social movement for improving quality of life in care homes for older people. Its success is thought to rest on the level of partnership working with the care home sector. To date there are a number of MHL national and regional groups that have organically emerged and are sharing and learning from each other. The largest of these is MHL Wales, which is funded for 3–5 years by the Welsh Assembly to disseminate the MHL vision across the principality. MHL holds the evidence base for the sector and is working to help care homes to professionalize and articulate their expertise. In a recent report 'Residential Care Transformed: Revisiting "The Last Refuge"'

---

[1] National Care Forum, English Community Care Association, National Care Association, Registered Nursing Home Association, Care Forum Wales, Scottish Care, Independent Health and Care Providers for Northern Ireland.

(Johnson et al., 2010), it was suggested that over time there have been some notable improvements in residential care and that there is a need to destigmatize care in this setting. By highlighting the evidence for best practice in care homes, MHL seeks to challenge the commonly held view that residential care is not the preferred choice of some older people in the twenty-first century.

Quality of life

Quality of life is frequently confused or conflated with quality of care. Although the two are often interconnected, they should not be seen as the same (Reed, 2007). Although quality of life may be high, quality of care may be low, that is, people may feel well and satisfied with life even if the care they receive is poor. Conversely, people may have a high quality of care, in that it meets a number of standards, but have a low quality of life.

Quality of life is difficult to define as it is determined by a number of individual dimensions and these may include physical, social, or psychological aspects. Kane (2003) defines the following factors as important aspects of quality of life for older people:

- Physical abilities
- Self-care (autonomy)
- Daily activities
- Social functions
- Sexuality and intimacy
- Psychological well-being and grief
- Cognitive abilities
- Pain/discomfort
- Energy, fatigue
- Self-respect
- Sense of mastery
- Subjective health
- Satisfaction with life.

However, this definition takes a rather reductionist approach. It does not explore how the different dimensions interlink or relate in a conceptual framework that practitioners might find helpful to guide and improve their practice. The MHL evidence-based and relationship-centred themes were identified from the fields of nursing, health, medicine, allied health, social gerontology, social work, and psychology. Synthesis of this diverse literature focused upon the experiences of residents, family caregivers, and staff in order to identify strategies which practitioners could use to enhance the quality of life of residents of care homes, while also supporting caregivers in the most appropriate way. It is important to recognize that there is no evidence that quality of life for care home residents is 'fundamentally different' from anyone else's quality of life (Gerritsen et al., 2004: 612). Nonetheless, it is important that if conceptual frameworks are to be used then they are constructed with the engagement, where possible, of those they are seeking to represent. This is the strength of the MHL vision.

Relationship-centred care

Underpinning the MHL themes is the notion of relationship-centred care (Tresloni and the Pew-Fetzer Task Force, 1994) and the Senses Framework (Nolan et al., 2006). Relationships are thought to be key to quality of life in care homes for older people; not just the relationships between residents, relatives, and staff, but also the relationships between care homes and the wider health and social care community. 'Relationship-centred care', rather than 'Person-centred care', has been selected as the conceptual underpinning for MHL because of its more specific focus on the needs of relatives and staff, as a means of ensuring quality of life for residents. It is also preferred for more semantic reasons. Person-centred care means different things to different people, depending on its historical legacy (Ashburner, 2005) and while those interested in mental health for older people are likely to draw on Kitwood's humanistic theory of person-centred care (Kitwood, 1997), policy makers are using the same words to describe a more consumerist model. For instance, in the National Service Framework for Older People (Department of Health, 2003: 7), the focus has been to 'ensure the provision of **person-centred care**, so that older people are treated as individuals and receive appropriate and timely care tailored to meet their needs'. Although laudable in its aims, the focus is on 'independence' and 'choice' rather than on 'interdependence' and 'reciprocity', which are key elements of ensuring quality of life for those who are frail and living in communal settings. Nonetheless, it is recognized that Kitwood's understanding of 'person-centred care' has had, and continues to have, an important role in care homes (Brooker, 2007).

Currently, the most widely used tool in care homes for assessing the quality of dementia care is Dementia Care Mapping (DCM), which is based upon Tom Kitwood's psychosocial framework about dementia (Surr et al., 2006). A modified shortened version has been created by Professor Dawn Brooker for use by inspectors of care homes (Short Observation Framework for Inspection [SOFI]) and this has clearly had a significant impact on profiling the mental health needs of older people in care homes. DCM does not claim to provide a comprehensive evaluation of care, but to provide the service users' point of view through detailed, skilled, and empathic observation of the person with dementia's activities and interactions with staff. Herein lies one of its main limitations in that it does not consider the experiences of family members or staff. Most accounts of the use of DCM have been enthusiastic about its potential to raise awareness of poor practice (Brooker, 2005), although there have been some suggestions that it can have a negative impact on staff morale, unless feedback is sensitively handled (Davies, 2007). MHL seeks to work with care homes in a more positive way, valuing what staff are trying to do under difficult circumstances and strengthening this activity by sharing the best of what is. Based on empirical evidence from older residents, relatives, and staff in care homes, Nolan et al. (2006) suggest that the fulfilment of six senses (security, belonging, continuity, purpose, achievement, and significance) will assist well-being in care homes and strengthen the relationships between residents, relatives, and staff (see Table 25.2 for a fuller explanation of each of the six senses). MHL sees relationship-centred care and the Senses Framework (Nolan et al., 2006) as key to delivering its evidence-based vision. The next section will explore what is meant by each of the MHL themes, highlighting their particular relevance to mental health in care homes.

Table 25.2 The Senses Framework

A sense of security	
For older people	Attention to essential physiological and psychological needs, to feel safe and free from threat, harm, pain, and discomfort. To receive competent and sensitive care.
For staff	To feel free from physical threat, rebuke, or censure. To have secure conditions of employment. To have the emotional demands of work recognized and to work within a supportive but challenging culture.
For family carers	To feel confident in knowledge and ability to provide good care without detriment to personal well-being. To have access to adequate support networks and timely help when required. To be able to relinquish care when appropriate.

A sense of continuity	
For older people	Recognition and value of personal biography. Skilful use of knowledge of the past to help contextualize the present and future. Seamless, consistent care delivered within an established relationship by known people.
For staff	Positive experience of work with older people from an early stage of career, exposure to good role models and environments of care. Expectations and standards of care communicated clearly and consistently.
For family carers	To maintain shared pleasures/pursuits with the care recipient. To be able to provide competent standards of care, whether delivered by self or others, to ensure that personal standards of care are maintained by others, to maintain involvement in care across care environments as desired/appropriate.

A sense of belonging	
For older people	Opportunities to maintain and/or form meaningful reciprocal relationships, to feel part of a community or group as desired.
For staff	To feel part of a team with a recognized and valued contribution, to belong to a peer group, a community of gerontological practitioners.
For family carers	To be able to maintain/improve valued relationships, to be able to confide in trusted individuals, to feel that you're not 'in this alone'.

A sense of purpose	
For older people	Opportunities to engage in purposeful activity facilitating the constructive passage of time, to be able to identify and pursue goals and challenges, to exercise discretionary choice.

Table 25.2 The Senses Framework *(continued)*

For staff	To have a sense of therapeutic direction, a clear set of goals to which to aspire.
For family carers	To maintain the dignity and integrity, well-being, and 'personhood' of the care recipient, to pursue (re)constructive/reciprocal care.
A sense of achievement	
For older people	Opportunities to meet meaningful and valued goals, to feel satisfied with one's efforts, to make a recognized and valued contribution, to make progress towards therapeutic goals as appropriate.
For staff	To be able to provide good care, to feel satisfied with one's efforts, to contribute towards therapeutic goals as appropriate, to use skills and ability to the full.
For family carers	To feel that you have provided the best possible care, to know you've 'done your best', to meet challenges successfully, to develop new skills and abilities.
A sense of significance	
For older people	To feel recognized and valued as a person of worth, that one's actions and existence are of importance, that you 'matter'.
For staff	To feel that gerontological practice is valued and important, that your work and efforts 'matter'.
For family carers	To feel that one's caring efforts are valued and appreciated, to experience an enhanced sense of self.

Source: Reproduced from Nolan, M., Brown, J., Davies, S., Nolan, J., & Keady, J., *The Senses Framework: Improving Care for Older People through a Relationship-centred Approach*, 2006, University of Sheffield.

Exploring the MHL evidence base

Three of the MHL themes (personalization) are about making care more individualized and person-centred. As such, these themes specify an approach to care that is supportive of the mental health needs of older people in care homes. The themes include *maintaining identity, sharing decision-making*, and *creating community*. Interestingly, a recent review of the literature on older people's experience of acute care (Bridges et al., 2010) has also highlighted these three themes as important, suggesting their wider relevance.

Personalization: maintaining identity

According to Bridges (2007), maintenance of identity (including a sense of gender, occupation, ethnicity, and sexuality) is closely linked to quality of life in old age (McKee et al., 2005). Living in a care home can undermine one's identity in a number of ways (Peace et al., 1997)—firstly, the losses commensurate with moving into a care home (Forte et al., 2006); secondly, the physical and cognitive impairment that most residents experience and impact upon their sense of self; and thirdly, the nature of the collective living environment that can present particular challenges to staff being able to offer individualized care (Coleman and O'Hanlon, 2004).

A number of strategies have been identified in the literature to overcome threats to identity associated with living in a care home including the person-centred approach to care (McCormack, 2004), biographical work (Davies, 2001), and the need to involve the wider community (Lewin, 2002). Much of the literature is anecdotal, reporting on the success of various initiatives to improve care in this area, without the support of formal evaluation. However, the lack of evidence is, to some extent, outweighed by the detail given on these clearly thoughtful and creative person-centred initiatives. The biographical approach to care (reminiscence, life story, autobiography, oral history, life review) is the commonest person-centred approach identified in literature (Goldsmith, 1996). Other issues which enhance a sense of self relate to how individuals dress, personal items they choose to bring into the home, and control over personal space (Tester et al., 2003). Also important are: recognition that belongings, places, animals, and ideas can be sources of security and self-identity for older people (Cookman, 1996); supporting residents to make new friendships and sustain current ones (Cook et al., 2006); and ensuring that meaningful activities are available (McKee et al., 2005). Involving key people and groups from the local community is another route to maintaining a person-centred approach (Lewin, 2002). Also of benefit can be visiting pets (Baun and McCabe, 2000), holding regular cocktail hours (Klein and Jess, 2002), and providing music tailored to individual tastes through providing personal/portable music players and headphones (Burack et al., 2002). Some commentators argue that the spiritual needs of older people with dementia merit a particular focus. Killick (2004) notes how involvement in the creative arts can enable communication, expressiveness, and the continuance of personhood. Forte et al. (2006) note the many challenges and opportunities in care homes for residents to maintain intimate and sexual relationships, another key component of a person's identity.

However, the MHL approach to person-centredness is that it is not just for residents alone. We also need to approach relatives and staff as individuals for care to be offered in a relational way. Ashburner (2005) tried to introduce biographical approaches in a long-term care setting and found that she had started in the wrong place. It was not until the staff had had the chance to tell their own story of care home life that they felt ready to engage with biography work with residents and relatives.

Personalization: sharing decision-making

Sharing decision-making is seen as an important aspect of quality of life in care homes (Davies and Brown-Wilson, 2007a,b). It is thought that a resident's perceived choice over aspects of their daily lives has the potential to prevent depression in long-term care settings (Boyle, 2005). In Boyle's study comparing quality of life, autonomy and mental health in residential and nursing homes in England and Northern Ireland, residents expressed a sense of powerlessness over their everyday lives in homes. They experienced a reduced sense of control through the imposition of regimented routines, restricted scope for decision-making, and diminished sense of freedom.

This resulted in feelings of hopelessness and the development of depression. Based on an ethnographic study of care homes, High and Rowles (1995) describe four broad types of decision-making within this environment: authoritative, given, negotiated, and reflexive and argue the need for more family involvement in decision-making. Davies and Brown-Wilson (2007a,b) suggest little research has been done on decision-making processes in care homes; with the exception of some work on decision-making at the end of life (e.g. Pasman et al., 2004). Most studies have examined the impact of involvement in decision-making at the macro level, for example, making the decision to move into long-term care and choosing a care home. However, the continuing importance of maintaining personal control in day-to-day activities as far as possible has also been demonstrated (Tester et al., 2003).

Good communication is key to sharing decision-making. Murphy et al. (2005) describe the use of 'talking mats', a low technology communication resource to help frail older people, including those with dementia, to express their views and feelings. Patterns of interaction between staff and residents also encourage or inhibit resident involvement in decision-making. For example, Williams et al. (2003) caution against the use of 'elderspeak', a style of speech often indistinguishable from baby talk and felt to be demeaning by residents.

Davies and Brown-Wilson (2007a,b) suggest that enabling residents to make active choices is likely to involve some degree of risk-taking on the part of staff and family. For some family members, a safe environment for their relative is one without risk (Nay and Koch, 2006) and regular communication between all parties is essential to ensure that risk-taking becomes an accepted aspect of good caregiving. Furthermore, staff must feel supported by their managers to adopt some elements of a risk-taking ethos. Managing risk is seen to be key to quality of life in care homes. Owen et al. (2010) suggest that, while there is evidence of a broad range of challenges and dilemmas involved in providing care to an increasingly frail resident population, some care home staff have developed highly individualized (often informal) strategies for supporting residents to manage risk. These staff have demonstrated a range of highly sophisticated communication, negotiation, counselling, reflection, and assessment skills in order to implement good practice.

Recent legislative changes have implications for the involvement of older people with cognitive impairment in decisions that affect them. In England, the Mental Capacity Act (Department for Constitutional Affairs, 2005) is aimed at increasing involvement in decision-making for people with impaired mental capacity and assumes that everyone has capacity until established otherwise. The Act raises questions about the use of proxies to make decisions on behalf of an older person and introduces the idea of a mental capacity advocate—an independent consultant who has responsibility for representing the older person's views and is not a paid member of staff.

Decision-making goes beyond individual care planning—those living, dying, visiting, and working in care homes need to be able to contribute their ideas as to how care home practice might be improved to make life better for all (Aveyard and Davies, 2006). The fact that a resident has severe cognitive impairment does not mean that his or her views should not be sought, although it can be challenging to know how to do so.

This group of residents is particularly at risk if care routines become inflexible and task focused as this makes it more likely that staff will fail to respond to individual needs and preferences (Graneheim et al., 2001).

Personalization: creating communities

For many years, the 'ideal model' for residential care settings has been that of 'home' (Peace and Holland, 2001). However, it may not be realistic to view care homes as 'homelike', given the nature of communal living and the level of dependency of some residents. Instead, creating a sense of community might be a more realistic and desirable aim (Davies and Brown-Wilson, 2007a,b). 'Community' means different things to different people but shared notions include membership, influence, integration, need fulfilment, emotional connection, and commitment to the collective good (Roberts, 1993). Community life is not always easy and becoming part of a community involves effort (Reed et al., 1998). Davies and Brown-Wilson (2007a,b) suggest there are six key areas that need to be recognized as promoting community within care homes. These are:

♦ understanding and respecting the significance of relationships;
♦ recognizing roles, rights, and responsibilities;
♦ creating opportunities for giving and receiving;
♦ creating opportunities for meaningful activity;
♦ building an environment that supports community; and
♦ committing to shared decision-making.

There is now a wealth of research identifying interpersonal relationships as key determinants of experiences within care homes, for residents, their families, and staff (McGilton et al., 2003). Recurrent themes within interview studies involving care home residents highlight the importance of continuity of staff, adequate communication, staff responsiveness, dependability and trust, and a degree of personal control to the development and maintenance of relationships (Edwards et al., 2003). Residents are living with an increased risk of dependency and vulnerability and therefore require dependability, reliability, and continuity from care providers alongside empathy and responsiveness to need (McGilton et al., 2003). There is also evidence that relationships with residents and their families are key factors in shaping the work experiences of staff within care homes (Moyle et al., 2003). For example, nursing assistants have identified their relationships with residents as the most important aspect of their job and the primary reason for staying in the job (Parsons et al., 2003). One study of relationships in care homes also suggested that lack of attachment was a strong predictor of staff burnout and high staff turnover (Sumaya-Smith, 1995).

The built environment can also influence a sense of community. McKee et al. (2005) identified more than 300 features of buildings that have been found to affect quality of life for care home residents. The features can be grouped around 10 resident domains—privacy, personalization, choice/control, community, safety/health, physical comfort, cognitive, awareness, and normality—and 1 staff domain—provisions for staff.

Relationship-centred care and the Senses Framework (see section 'Relationship-centred care') underpins the three *personalization themes* mentioned above, which mainly draw on social care research findings. The following three themes draw more on evidence from healthcare and health services research, focusing on what staff need to do to help residents and relatives navigate their way through the journey of care. These *navigation themes* include *managing transitions, improving health and healthcare*, and *supporting good end of life.*

Navigation: managing transitions

According to O'May (2007), the move into a care home may not always be permanent and, increasingly, homes are offering respite care and/or rehabilitation (e.g. Hart et al., 2005). However, for most it is likely to be where they end their lives. Having a mental health problem, primarily dementia, is a key trigger: this has been identified in 43% of admissions (Office of Fair Trading, 2005). The literature also shows that the majority of admissions are made following a hospitalization, or at a time of acute illness (Stilwell and Kerslake, 2003). In these stressful and time pressured contexts it is unlikely that either the older person or his or her relatives feel included in the decision-making process around admission, which can be very traumatic.

Moving into a care home—with or without mental health problems—is a major life event, involving many potential losses. These include: one's own home and familiar surroundings, control over daily life, social relationships, and, for many, the losses associated with deteriorating health and increasing frailty (Forte et al., 2006). Managing transitions is not just about managing the move into a care home, but also adapting and adjusting to these multiple losses.

Nolan et al. (1996) have suggested that there are (potentially) four types of place-ment: the positive choice, the rationalized alternative, the discredited option, and the fait accompli. The preferred option is positive choice and planning is crucial in all transitions, even if it is wholly unexpected.

Numerous studies have demonstrated the importance of relationships to the experi-ences of family members following an older person's admission to a care home (e.g. Davies and Nolan, 2004). Most family members want to maintain strong links with the cared-for person and seek to work in partnership with care home staff in order to achieve this (Sandberg et al., 2001). Staying involved means establishing new relationships with staff, and with other residents and their families (Davies, 2003).

Although there is some research that focuses on the residents' perspective (Reed et al., 1998) and a growing body of research that focuses on the relatives' perspective (Davies and Nolan, 2003, 2004), little research takes into account the impact on staff of working with continuous loss and bereavement (with the notable exception of Holman et al., 2006). As already noted, for relationships to be good in care homes, consideration needs to be given to the emotional needs of staff, as well as, those of residents and relatives.

Navigation: improving health and healthcare

As recent surveys demonstrate (Continuing Care Conference, 2006), the mental health needs of older people living in care homes are complex (Heath, 2007). A broad range of therapeutic interventions are now available to older people with mental health needs but the extent to which these can be accessed by care home residents varies hugely. Interventions available in better quality homes include activity-based therapy (such as music, art, or exercise), reminiscence, reality orientation, validation, and multisensory stimulation (Snoezelen). There are, however, a much broader range of therapies which appear rarely to be available to those living in care homes. These include psychotherapy, psychodynamic therapy, cognitive behavioural therapy, and counselling (Minardi and Hayes, 2003a,b).

Although two-thirds of care home residents have some form of dementia, only 60% of these individuals are in dementia-registered beds (Alzheimer's Society, 2007). A report by the Alzheimer's Society 'Home from Home' suggests that many homes are still not providing the level of person-centred care people with dementia need. Key challenges include: provision of activities and occupation; treating residents with dementia with dignity and respect; and the relationship between care home and relatives/friends. They also found that the support from external specialist services, for example older people's community mental health teams, was unacceptably variable and often limited.

In a study to identify the unmet needs of people with dementia in care and the characteristics associated with high levels of need, Hancock et al. (2006) assessed 238 people in residential homes using the Camberwell Assessment of Needs for the Elderly (CANE) tool. They found that the environmental and physical health needs of residents with dementia were usually met. Unmet needs included sensory or physical disability needs (including mobility problems and incontinence), mental health, and social needs such as company and daytime activities. These unmet needs were associated with psychological problems, such as anxiety and depression.

Approximately 40% of older people in residential care have significant symptoms of depression (Schneider et al., 1997) and it is suggested that personalized care planning, conducted by suitably trained and supported care staff, might be an effective intervention for detecting and reducing depression in residential care for older people (Lyne et al., 2006).

The research highlights how many older people in care homes do not receive the healthcare services they need (Jacobs and Rummary, 2002). This issue is explored in depth in Chapter 22.

Navigation: supporting good end of life

Nicholson (2007) highlighted that 21% of all deaths in people over 65 years in the United Kingdom occur in care homes (Froggatt, 2004). Since 2000, there has been a burgeoning of research into death and dying in care homes, both within and outside the United Kingdom with researchers exploring the quality and nature of dying (notably Katz and Peace, 2003) and/or identifying and describing possible 'interventions' (Hockley et al., 2005). Hockley et al.'s (2005) work notes that most of the literature on interventions addresses the development of service provision rather than direct resident-focused work.

The very nature of multiple, often chronic, health problems experienced by many care home residents can make it difficult to define with accuracy when someone is actually dying (Froggatt, 2001). In particular, dementia is often not recognized as a 'progressive life-limiting' disease, therefore constraining the potential for open communication and awareness of dying (Henderson, 2006). This uncertainty can sometimes lead to impersonal, reactive, and inadequate care (Kristjanson et al., 2005). Five areas for consideration are proposed that address important aspects of care towards the end of life (Page and Komoramy, 2005): developing a culture of openness, facilitation of the dying process, support for residents in their last days, leadership and support, and respecting and remembering. The Gold Standards Framework (Thomas, 2003) and the preferred-place-of-care initiative (Storey et al., 2003) are UK-wide initiatives to help promote good end of life in care homes for older people. However, as above, these initiatives tend to focus on the needs of residents and relatives, with very limited attention being paid to the needs of staff who are, after all, being asked to introduce the proposed changes.

The six MHL themes mentioned above addressing issues of personalization and navigation are important for all staff working in care homes. The remaining two themes (*transformation around workforce and around culture*) are aimed at care home managers to help them support their staff to deliver the MHL evidence-based, relationship-centred vision.

Transformation: keeping workforce fit for purpose

There is a serious shortage of specialist services for those with mental health problems, including depression and dementia, especially in London (Henwood, 2001), so any approach to improvement needs to be far reaching and support the education of the wider health and social care community (Meyer, 2007). Fitzpatrick and Roberts (2004) identify managing mental health issues as core knowledge and skills required by all care home staff whether they work in a specialist care home or not.

The Royal College of Physicians, Royal College of Nursing, and British Geriatrics Society (2000) emphasized the importance of access to relevant health professionals, in developing positive care for people with dementia and depression in care homes. In its collaborative report, it called for more robust professional input, skill-mix, and a more research-based approach to improving health outcomes for older people in care homes. Training can have a major influence on quality of care (Vaughan, 2002); insufficient training and experience in working with older people with mental health problems can leave staff feeling unsupported and inadequately prepared (Pritchard and Dewing, 1999). A system of supervision for care and ancillary staff is recognized as being particularly important for quality dementia practice (Kitwood, 1997).

In Sweden, Skog et al. (2000) support the concept of teaching nursing homes. The results of a 3-year participant observation study of learning dementia care in three contexts (day care, group dwelling, and nursing home) demonstrated the importance of context, showing that the closer the relationship between trainee and patient, the more the patient seems to be the focus of learning, and the greater the value of practical training. This study revisits an important issue, namely, should practical learning reflect contemporary care or be an 'instrument of reform'? (Gerdman, 1989). The trainees' positive attitude towards the day care setting (teaching ward) led the authors to suggest that the teaching nursing home 'could offer a supreme example of teamwork, minimizing negative image, while strengthening the patient's position as a source of knowledge' (Gerdman, 1989: 156).

Transformation: promoting positive culture

Davies et al. (2003) conducted an action research study in a nursing home that aimed to promote a positive culture of care in a care home for people with dementia. Central to this work is recognition of the interdependence of staff, residents, and their families and the need to consider *all* their perspectives in developing priorities to improve care. The partnership project employed the Senses Framework (see Table 25.2), which helped to identify the nature and aims of good quality care. Using the framework, staff and relatives worked together to identify areas of change in the care home. Activities included a relatives' support group, successful fundraising activities, writing a proposal for funding a part-time occupational therapist, and development of an activities programme. Outcomes included: relatives finding it easier to approach staff, a reduction in episodes of challenging behaviour among residents, and an increase in visits by relatives to the home.

Studies also suggest that we need to change the way we think about older people (Dewar, 2007). The prevalent model in care emphasizes the negative effects of old age where staff 'do things to' residents (Ronch, 2004). This devalues staff as much as residents. A more positive model of care is one that emphasizes personal growth for residents and staff with a shared commitment to ideas, values, goals, and practices by residents, staff, and relatives. This model places a strong focus on the importance of relationships, valuing different perspectives, and fostering creativity, learning, and innovation (Anderson et al., 2003). It is based on a different level and type of learning within organizations, one that challenges beliefs and encourages empathy, as opposed to imparting 'facts' or 'rules'.

Research suggests that a culture strongly based on relationships leads to positive resident outcomes. For instance, being able to say what you mean without fear or retribution has been linked to lower use of restraints, and increased participation in decision-making by registered nurses has been linked to lowered prevalence of aggressive behaviour among residents (Anderson et al., 2003). Conversely, privileging work procedures and rules in combination with surveillance has been linked to higher prevalence of challenging behaviours.

Conclusion

Creating a positive culture for the future requires recognition of the complex and multidimensional nature of life and work in care homes. Person-centred, biographical, and developmental approaches are essential. Homes should work to develop cultures that support relationship-centred care and to disseminate existing initiatives that support its development. A strong message is recognition of the interdependence of staff, residents, and family members: attempts to promote a positive culture need to nurture these important relationships. The MHL vision for best practice was written in 2007 and although it needs continual updating to remain alive to new developments, it nonetheless provides a useful starting point for care homes wishing to improve both the general and mental health of their residents, relatives, and staff. Researchers always identify the need for more research; in this case, it is the action that is required. MHL will continue to exist for as long as it is supported to do so by the care home sector. The messages of MHL are not new, but the engagement of the sector in the initiative is unique and offers a positive and collaborative way forward for developing evidence-based high-quality practice in care homes for older people.

Acknowledgements

This chapter was written in collaboration with Jackie Bridges, Christine Brown-Wilson, Sue Davies, Belinda Dewar, Jennifer Dudman, Hazel Heath, Caroline Nicholson, Fiona O'May, and Jan Reed (drawing on findings from the NCHR&D Forum, 2007).[2]

References

Alzheimer's Society (2007). *Home from Home, Quality of Care for People with Dementia Living in Care Homes*. London: Alzheimer's Society.

Anderson, R., Issel, L.M., & McDaniel, R.R. (2003). Nursing homes as complex adaptive systems: relationship between management practice and resident outcomes. *Nursing Research, 52*, 12–21.

Ashburner, C. (2005). *Person-centred Care: Change through Action Research*, Unpublished PhD thesis. London: City University.

Aveyard, B. & Davies, S. (2006). Moving forward together: evaluation of an action group involving staff and relatives within a nursing home for older people with dementia. *International Journal of Older People Nursing, 1*(2), 95–104.

Baun, M.M. & McCabe, B.W. (2000). The role animals play in enhancing quality of life for the elderly. In: A.H. Fine (Ed.), *Handbook on Animal-assisted Therapy: Theoretical Foundations and Guidelines for Practice* (pp. 237–250). San Diego: Academic Press.

Boyle, G. (2005). The role of autonomy in explaining mental ill-health and depression among older people in long-term care settings. *Ageing and Society, 25*, 741–748.

Bridges, J. (2007). Working to help residents maintain their identity. In NCHR&D Forum. *My Home Life: Quality of Life—Literature Review*. London: Help the Aged.

Bridges, J., Flatley, M., & Meyer, J. (2010). Older people's and relatives' experiences in acute care settings: systematic review and synthesis of qualitative studies. *International Journal of Nursing Studies, 47*, 89–107.

Brooker, D. (2005). Dementia care mapping: a review of the research literature. *Gerontologist, 45*, 11–18.

Brooker, D. (2007). *Person-centred Dementia Care, Making Services Better*. London: Jessica Kingsley Publishers.

Burack, O.R., Jefferson, P., & Libow, L.S. (2002). Individualized music: a route to improving the quality of life for long-term care residents. *Activities, Adaptation and Aging, 27*, 63–76.

Coleman, P. & O'Hanlon, A. (2004). *Ageing and Development*. London: Hodder Arnold.

---

2 Contributions were as follows: Dudman, J. (context), Reed, J. (quality of life), Davies, S. and Heath, H. (quality of care); Bridges, J. (working to help residents maintain their identity); Davies, S. and Brown-Wilson, C. (shared decision-making in care homes and creating community within care homes); O'May, F. (transitions into a care home); Heath, H. (health and healthcare services); Nicholson, C. (end-of-life care); Meyer, J. (keeping the workforce fit for purpose); Belinda, D. (promoting positive culture in care homes).

Continuing Care Conference (2006). *Census of BUPA Care Home Residents.* London: BUPA Care Homes.

Cook, G., Brown-Wilson, C., & Forte, D. (2006). The impact of sensory impairment on relationships between residents in care homes. *International Journal of Older People's Nursing, 1,* 216–224.

Cookman, C.A. (1996). Older people and attachment to things, places, pets, and ideas. *Image: Journal of Nursing Scholarship, 28*(3), 227–231.

Cooperrider, D.L., Whitney, D.L., & Stavros, J. (2003). *Appreciative Inquiry Handbook: The First in a Series of AI Workbooks for Leaders of Change.* Bedford Heights: Lakeshore Communications.

Davies, S. (2001). The care needs of older people and family caregivers in continuing care settings, chapter 5. In: M. Nolan, S. Davies, & G. Grant (Eds.), *Working with Older People and their Families.* (pp. 75–98). Buckingham: Open University Press.

Davies, S. (2003). Creating community: the basis for caring partnerships in nursing homes. In: M. Nolan, G. Grant, J. Keady, & U. Lundh (Eds.), *Partnerships in Family Care* (pp. 218–237). Maidenhead: Open University Press.

Davies, S. & Nolan, M. (2003). 'Making the best of things': relatives' experiences of decision about care-home entry. *Ageing and Society, 23,* 429–450.

Davies, S. & Nolan, M. (2004). 'Making the move': relatives' experiences of the transition to a care home. *Health and Social Care in the Community, 12*(6), 517–526.

Davies, S., Darlington, E., Powell, A., & Aveyard, B. (2003). Developing partnerships at 67 Birch Avenue Nursing Home: the support 67 Action Group Quality in Ageing. *Policy Practice and Research, 4*(4), 32–37.

Davies, S. (2007). Quality of care. In NCHR&D Forum. *My Home Life: Quality of Life—Literature Review.* London: Help the Aged.

Davies, S. & Brown-Wilson, C. (2007a). Creating community within care homes. In NCHR&D Forum. *My Home Life: Quality of Life—Literature Review.* London: Help the Aged.

Davies, S. & Brown-Wilson, C. (2007b). Shared decision-making in care homes. In NCHR&D Forum. *My Home Life: Quality of Life—Literature Review.* London: Help the Aged.

Department for Constitutional Affairs (2005). The Mental Capacity Act. Available at: http://www.opsi.gov.uk/acts/acts2005/20050009.htm (accessed 28 April 2006).

Department of Health (2003). *National Service Framework for Older People.* A report of progress and future challenges. London: Department of Health.

Dewar, B. (2007). Promoting positive culture in care homes. In NCHR&D Forum. *My Home Life: Quality of Life—Literature Review.* London: Help the Aged.

Edwards, H., Courtney, M., & Spencer, L. (2003). Consumer expectations of residential aged care: reflections on the literature. *International Journal of Nursing Practice, 9*(2), 70–77.

Fitzpatrick, J.M. & Roberts, J.D. (2004). Challenges for care homes: education and training of healthcare assistants. *British Journal of Nursing, 13*(21), 1258–1261.

Forte, D., Cotter, A., & Wells, D. (2006). Sexuality and relationships in later life. In: S.G. Redfern & F.M. Ross (Eds.), *Nursing Care of Older People* (pp. 437–455). Edinburgh: Elsevier/Churchill Livingstone.

Froggatt, K. (2001). Palliative care and nursing homes: where next? *Palliative Medicine, 15,* 42–48.

Froggatt, K. (2004). *Palliative Care in Care Homes for Older People.* London: National Council for Palliative Care.

Gerdman, A. (1989). *Klient Praktikant Handledare—Om att Utveckla en Egen Yrkesteori* (Client, Practitioner, Supervisor—How to Develop an Individual Professional Theory). Stockholm: Wahlstrom & Widstrand.

Gerritsen, D.L., Steverink, N., Ooms, M.E., & Ribbe, M.W. (2004). Finding a useful conceptual basis for enhancing the quality of life of nursing home residents. *Quality of Life Research*, *13*, 611–624.

Goldsmith, M. (1996). *Hearing the Voices of People with Dementia: Opportunities and Obstacles*. London: Jessica Kingsley Publishers.

Graneheim, U.H., Norberg, A., & Jansson, L. (2001). Interaction relating to privacy, identity, autonomy and security. An observational study focusing on a woman with dementia and 'behavioural disturbances', and on her care providers. *Journal of Advanced Nursing, 36*(2), 256–265.

Hancock, G., Woods, B., Challis, D., & Orrell, M. (2006). The needs of older people with dementia in residential care. *International Journal of Geriatric Psychiatry, 21*, 43–49.

Hart, E., Lymbery, M., & Gladman, J.R.F. (2005). Away from home: an ethnographic study of a transitional rehabilitation scheme for older people in the UK. *Social Science and Medicine*, *60*, 1241–1250.

Heath, H. (2007). Health and healthcare services, Chapter 8. In: NCHR&D *My Home Life: Quality of life in care homes - Literature Review* (pp. 96–117). London: Help the Aged (available http://www.myhomelife.org.uk).

Henderson, J. (2006). *Lighting Up Lives: A Report on the Palliative Care Needs of People with End-stage Dementia Living in Dumfries and Galloway 2004/2006*. Edinburgh: Alzheimer Scotland.

Henwood, M. (2001). *Future Imperfect: Report of the King's Fund Care and Support Worker Inquiry*. London: King's Fund.

High, D.M. & Rowles, D.G. (1995). Nursing home residents, families and decision-making: towards an understanding of progressive surrogacy. *Journal of Aging Studies, 9*(2), 101–117.

Hockley, J., Dewar, B., & Watson, J. (2005). Promoting end-of-life-care in nursing homes using an 'integrated care pathway for the last days of life'. *Journal of Research in Nursing*, *10*(2), 135–152.

Holman, C., Meyer, J., & Davenhill, R. (2006). Psychoanalytical informed research in an NHS continuing care unit for older people: exploring and developing staff's work with complex loss and grief. *Journal of Social Work and Practice, 20*(3), 315–328.

Jacobs, S. & Rummary, K. (2002). Nursing homes in England and their capacity to provide rehabilitation and intermediate care services. *Social Policy and Administration, 36*(7), 735–752.

Johnson, J., Rolph, S., & Smith, R. (2010). *Residential Care Transformed, Revisiting 'The Last Refuge'*. Basingstoke: Palgrave Macmillan.

Kane, R.A. (2003). Definition, measurement, and correlates of quality of life in nursing homes: toward a reasonable practise, research, and policy agenda. *The Gerontologist, 43*(special issue II), 28–36.

Katz, J.S. & Peace, S.M. (2003). *End of Life in Care Homes: A Palliative Care Approach*. Oxford: Oxford University Press.

Killick, J. (2004). Magic mirrors: what people with dementia show us about ourselves. In: A. Jewell (Ed.), *Ageing, Spirituality and Well-being* (pp. 143–152). London: Jessica Kingsley Publishers.

Kitwood, T. (1997). *Dementia Reconsidered: The Person Comes First*. Buckingham: Open University Press.

Klein, W.C. & Jess, C. (2002). One last pleasure? Alcohol use among elderly people in nursing homes. *Health and Social Work*, *27*(3), 193–203.

Kristjanson, L., Walton, J., & Toye, C. (2005). End of life challenges in residential aged care facilities. *International Journal of Palliative Nursing*, *11*(3), 127–129.

Lewin, M. (2002). *'What I want is a Double Bed': Person-centred Planning and the Development of Community Links in a Residential Home for Older People.* Edinburgh: The City of Edinburgh Council.

Lyne, K.J., Moxon, S., Sinclair, I., Young, P., Kirk, C., & Ellison, S. (2006). Analysis of a care planning intervention for reducing depression in older people in residential care. *Aging and Mental Health*, *10*(4), 394–403.

McCormack, B. (2004). Person-centredness in gerontological nursing: an overview of the literature. *International Journal of Older People Nursing*, *13*(s1), 31–38.

McGilton, K., O'Brien-Pallas, L., Darlington, G., Evans, M., Wynn, F., & Pringle, D. (2003). Effects of a relationship-enhancing programme of care on outcomes. *Journal of Nursing Scholarship*, *35*(2), 151–156.

McKee, K., Downs, M., Gilhooly, M., Gilhooly, K., Tester, S., & Wilson, F. (2005). Frailty, identity and the quality of later life. In: A. Walker (Ed.), *Understanding Quality of Life in Older Age* (pp. 117–129). Maidenhead: Open University Press.

Meyer, J. (2007). Keeping the workforce fit for purpose. In NCHR&D Forum. *My Home Life: Quality of Life—Literature Review.* London: Help the Aged.

Minardi, H. & Hayes, N. (2003a). Nursing older adults with mental health problems: therapeutic interventions, Part 1. *Nursing Older People*, *15*(6), 22–26.

Minardi, H. & Hayes, N. (2003b). Nursing older adults with mental health problems: therapeutic interventions, Part 2. *Nursing Older People*, *15*(7), 20–24.

Moyle, W., Skinner, J., Rowe, G., & Gork, C. (2003). Views of job satisfaction and dis-satisfaction in Australian long-term care. *Journal of Clinical Nursing*, *12*(2), 168–176.

Murphy, J., Tester, S., Hubbard, G., Downs, M., & MacDonald, C. (2005). Enabling frail older people with a communication difficulty to express their views: the use of Talking Mats™ as an interview tool. *Health & Social Care in the Community*, *13*(2), 95–107.

Nay, R. & Koch, S. (2006). Overcoming restraint use: examining barriers in Australian aged care facilities. *Journal of Gerontological Nursing*, *32*, 33–38.

NCHR&D Forum (2007). *My Home Life: Quality of Life—Literature Review.* London: Help the Aged.

Nicholson, C. (2007). End-of-life care. In NCHR&D Forum. *My Home Life: Quality of Life—Literature Review.* London: Help the Aged.

Nolan, M., Brown, J., Davies, S., Nolan, J., & Keady, J. (2006). *The Senses Framework: Improving Care for Older People through a Relationship-centred Approach.* Sheffield: University of Sheffield. ISBN 1-902411-44-7.

Nolan, M.R., Grant, G., & Keady, J. (1996). *Understanding Family Care.* Buckingham: Open University Press.

O'May, F. (2007). Transitions into a care home. In NCHR&D Forum. *My Home Life: Quality of Life—Literature Review.* London: Help the Aged.

Office of Fair Trading (2005). *Survey of Older People in Care Homes.* Annexe F. London: Office of Fair Trading.

Owen, T., Meyer, J., Meehan, L., & Cornell, M. (2010). *Minimising the Use of 'Restraint' in Care Homes: Challenges, Dilemmas and Positive Approaches*, Adults' Services Report 25. London: Social Care Institute for Excellence.

Page, S. & Komaromy, C. (2005). Professional performances: the case of unexpected and expected deaths. *Mortality, 10*(4), 294–307.

Parsons, S., Simmons, W., Penn, K., & Furlough, M. (2003). Determinants of satisfaction and turnover among nursing assistants: the results of a statewide survey. *Journal of Gerontological Nursing, 29*(3), 51–58.

Pasman, H.R.W., Onwuteaka-Philipsen, B.D., Ooms, M.E., Van Wigcheren, P.T., van der Wal, G., Ribbe, M.W. (2004). Forgoing artificial nutrition and hydration in nursing home patients with dementia: Patients, decision making, and participants. *Alzheimer disease and associated disorders, 18*, 154–162.

Peace, S. & Holland, C. (2001). Homely residential care: a contradiction in terms? *Journal of Social Policy, 30*(3), 393–410.

Peace, S., Kellaher, L., & Willcocks, D. (1997). *Re-evaluating Residential Care.* Buckingham: Open University Press.

Pritchard, E. & Dewing, J. (1999). Screening for dementia and depression in older people. *Nursing Standard, 14*(5), 45–52.

Reed, J. (2007). Quality of life. In NCHR&D Forum. *My Home Life: Quality of Life—Literature Review.* London: Help the Aged.

Reed, J., Payton, V.R., & Bond, S. (1998). The importance of place for older people moving into care homes. *Social Science and Medicine, 46*(7), 859–867.

Roberts, D. (1993). Community: the value of social synergy. In: R. Young (Ed.), *Identifying and Implementing the Essential Value of the Profession* (pp. 35–45). San Francisco: Jossey Bass.

Ronch, J.L. (2004). Changing institutional culture: can we re-value the nursing home? *Journal of Gerontological Social Work, 43*, 61–82.

Royal College of Physicians, Royal College of Nursing, and British Geriatrics Society (2000). *The Health and Care of Older People in Care Homes. A Comprehensive Interdisciplinary Approach.* A report of a joint working party. London: Royal College of Physicians.

Sandberg, J., Lundh, U., & Nolan, M.R. (2001). Placing a spouse in a care home: the importance of keeping. *Journal of Clinical Nursing, 10*(3), 406–416.

Schneider, J., Mann, A.H., Levin, E., Mozley, C., & Abbey, A. (1997). *Quality of Care: Testing Some Measures in Homes for Elderly People.* PSSRU Discussion Paper 1245. Canterbury: University of Kent.

Skog, M., Negussie, B., & Grafstrom, M. (2000). Learning dementia care in three contexts: practical training in day-care, group dwelling and nursing home. *Journal of Advanced Nursing, 32*, 148–157.

Stilwell, P. & Kerslake, A. (2003). *What makes Older People Choose Residential Care, and are there Alternatives?* Report for Department of Health: Housing Learning and Improvement Network, South Gloucestershire. Available at: http://ipc.brookes.ac.uk/ChoosingResidential Care SGlos.pdf (accessed 16 January 2006).

Storey, L., Pemberton, C., & O'Donnell, L. (2003). Place of death: Hobson's choice or patient choice? *Cancer Nursing Practice, 2*(4), 33–38.

Sumaya-Smith, I. (1995). Caregiver/resident relationships: surrogate family bonds and surrogate grieving in a skilled nursing facility. *Journal of Advanced Nursing, 21*(3), 447–451.

Surr, C., Brooker, D., & Edwards, P. (2006). Care practice: dementia care mapping update: DCM 8 is ready for action. *Journal of Dementia Care, 14*, 17–19.

Tester, S., Hubbard, G., Downs, M., MacDonald, C., & Murphy, J. (2003). Exploring perceptions of quality of life of frail older people during and after their transition to institutional care. *Research Findings, 24*, 1–4.

Thomas, K. (2003). *Caring for the Dying at Home.* Abingdon: Radcliffe Medical Press.

Tresloni, C.P. & the Pew-Fetzer Task Force (1994). *Health Professions Education and Relationship Centered Care: A Report of the Pew-Fetzer Taskforce on Advancing Psychosocial Education.* San Francisco: Health Professions Commission.

Vaughan, J. (2002). Drive to raise standards of dementia care in care homes. *Professional Nurse, 27*(5), 316.

Williams, K., Kemper, S., & Hummert, M.L. (2003). Practice concepts. Improving nursing home communication: an intervention to reduce elderspeak. *Gerontologist, 43*(2), 242–247.

Chapter 26

Conclusion: key themes and future directions

Tom Dening and Alisoun Milne

Abstract

This final chapter summarizes the current state of care home provision, drawing from the preceding chapters of this book. Several general themes are discussed: (1) the ageing population and the changing profile of care home residents; (2) the changing nature of the care home market; (3) the vulnerability of care home residents and the challenges in hearing an authentic voice especially for older people with dementia; (4) policy and funding issues; (5) the care home workforce and the skills that are required; and (6) how outside agencies, including regulators and other health providers, work with care homes. The authors take a cautiously optimistic view of the future, anticipating that, despite many challenges, improvements in quality will be maintained and a skilled workforce will be able to provide care that promotes mental health, hope, and dignity for older people.

The aim of this concluding chapter is to bring together key themes that have arisen throughout the book and to take a look at what the future may hold for mental health in care homes.

The first overarching theme is that of the ageing population and the profile of care home residents. That the population of most countries is getting older, bringing with it a number of health-related challenges, is widely acknowledged. As an example, by 2050 there will be over 1 million people with dementia in the United Kingdom. As older people are increasingly supported to remain in their own homes—a trend we should celebrate—it is to be expected that the care home population will have higher levels of dependency and frailty. Care home residents often have complex combinations of physical and mental health problems and an increasing proportion have dementia. Most residents are very elderly women. We have also noted in earlier chapters that society is becoming increasingly diverse and heterogeneous and this will be so for care home residents too, though at a slower rate of change. One of the central observations of several authors is that dementia has become the main business of the care home sector; it is also the primary health-related cause of admission.

A second theme relates to the changing nature of the care home market. There have been changes both in the nature of providers and funding. Compared with 20 years ago, care homes are likely to be larger and to be run either by profit or not-for-profit agencies rather than being individual homes run by a single proprietor or homes run by local authorities. The stimulus for the wave of smaller homes was probably the downsizing of long-stay hospital provision, releasing large numbers of older patients in need of care into the care home market. Many were either funded by the National Health Service (NHS) or by social security benefits at this time which also acted as a stimulus to the sector. Small was regarded as beautiful in the 1970s and 1980s, at least in relation to care homes—thus replacing a nineteenth century model of care with one more reminiscent of the eighteenth century (see Parry-Jones, 1972). Centralized funding, including social security, was withdrawn thus shifting responsibility for paying for long-term care to local authorities or the individual themselves. As the main purchasers of care home places, local authorities have driven down profit margins, squeezing many smaller providers out of the sector. During the same period, the nature of the care home environment also changed, from conversions of large Victorian or Edwardian houses to purpose built facilities for larger numbers of residents. The introduction of minimum care home standards and the current inspection regimes have also contributed to the decline of the 'converted mansion', as they often found it difficult to install the necessary en suite bathroom arrangements or to guarantee minimum bedroom dimensions. The growth of the self-funder is also a notable trend.

Our third theme is the invisibility and vulnerability of care home residents. In fact, they would have a legitimate claim to being the most socially excluded group in society. In part, this is a reflection of the continuing or perhaps re-emerging institutional nature of care homes. They tend to exist on the very edge of our communities and to be hidden from public view. The boundaries of care homes are impermeable: they are rarely visited by those from the outside and those on the inside rarely go out (Goffman, 1963). Their marginal status is deepened, hugely, by the fact that the voices and perspectives of care home residents are unheard and unrecorded. This is especially the case for people with dementia who often have serious communication difficulties. This fact amplifies residents' vulnerability to being ignored or worse, being abused or neglected. In homes that have more permeable boundaries and are open to public scrutiny—relatives visiting, local religious leaders popping in, etc.—abuse is less likely. In homes where efforts are made to communicate with residents including those with severe dementia, that adopt a person-centred or relationship-centred approach to care, and that appreciate that care home work is a skilled job beyond the simple performance of a set of tasks, residents tend to be at lower risk of abuse, display lower levels of challenging behaviour, and have enhanced levels of well-being. This shift dovetails with efforts being made in research to capture the subjective experiences of residents. Although many people living in a care home have to manage a host of losses and struggle to retain a sense of self, residents can and do live full lives, interacting with other residents and staff and experiencing a range of normal emotions.

It is clear that we have much to learn from residents, especially those with dementia, about both the negative and positive aspects of living in a care home.

A fourth theme is the significance and influence of policy and funding. Care homes do not operate in isolation from the rest of the economy or the rest of the health and social care sector. As noted above, huge efforts have been made in recent decades to support as many people as possible in their own homes. There is still more that can be done in this regard but it may be that, for dementia, at least, there is a limit to the degree to which it is both cost-effective and actually of benefit to the individual to remain in their own home, especially if they live on their own. There may be a point beyond which a lonely and disorientated person with dementia derives little benefit from being in his or her own home. The drive to promote care in the community as the 'best option' has inevitably positioned care homes as an inferior alternative or even a failure of family and community care; this has of course been amplified by concerns about poor care. This has been recognized in recent policy which has prioritized improvements to the quality of care in residential and nursing homes; care homes are one of the key areas identified in the outcomes framework for the National Dementia Strategy (Banerjee, 2010; Department of Health, 2009). But the big (current) debate is about who should pay for the cost of care. The last UK Government consulted about the funding of long-term care and the present administration has embarked upon a review of the issue. This is just a decade after the last Royal Commission, which published a minority report whose authors supported the Scottish administration's model of free care at the point of delivery. This is certainly not likely to be an alternative on the table of the upcoming review and in fact there appears to be a consensus that some form of additional social insurance may be required in order to share the costs of care between the individual citizen and the state. This is certainly the case in other European countries (Rodrigues and Schmidt, 2010).

Intimately related to funding and quality of care is the role and nature of the care home workforce. This is a large, disparate, predominantly female, often part-time group. Care home workers may well be from a different ethnic background to the older people they care for, and they are often relatively poorly qualified in terms of formal education and qualifications. In certain, often urban, areas they are highly transient and in other areas they may be almost static. Both situations may present problems for maintaining or improving care quality. There is a clear need for care staff to learn more about mental health issues and how to work effectively and positively with residents with dementia in particular. There is also a definite need for the training that is offered to be meaningful and relevant to their work. However, more is required than simply training frontline staff—care home providers have to demonstrate leadership and relentless commitment to high standards. They need to create an open culture where poor practice and untoward events are reported and where there is the opportunity for the whole team to learn from both bad and good practices. This may be one of the areas where large multiple providers have the edge over individual care homes, in that they can instil corporate vision and quality standards supported by leadership that is up to the task. It is now officially sanctioned that people working in residential care that makes specific provision for people with dementia will require specialist knowledge and skills (Department of Health, Skills for Care and Skills for Health, 2010).

A final theme to pick out is about how outside agencies—health and social services and regulators—work with care homes and what help they provide both to individual residents and the care home sector. Despite the existence of a range of innovative models of support by primary and secondary care providers, universal access for care home residents to healthcare services commensurate with those provided to community dwellers remains elusive. Much depends on cultural norms in a given area and on—often informal—relationships between, for example, a committed and respectful community nurse and the care home staff. Although commentators agree that 'the best' needs to be rolled out across the sector there is limited agreement, or funding, about how this can be achieved. The sector has a habit, reflective of its fragmented and fluid nature, of reinventing initiatives which tend not to be sustained as they are often vulnerable to financial cuts and reorganizations. Their impact is also difficult to evaluate. What we do know however is that due to the high level of healthcare need in the resident population, health services are an essential resource for care homes and will continue to be so. Inspection and quality regulation has a distinctive role to play in helping to uphold care standards. In the past, homes were inspected regularly (including unannounced visits); now only those homes that fail to perform to a significant degree will be the focus of 'targeted attention' by the Care Quality Commission. There may be some concerns that this change of focus may be less effective in maintaining the push towards higher standards.

Where are we going?

We hope that the chapters of this book offer a detailed and contemporary commentary on the state of care homes in relation to mental health in older residents. Although it is evident that the sector still has many challenges ahead if it is to achieve a high standard of care, clear improvements have been made over the last decade (see Chapter 7).

Why should this have happened? There is probably no simple answer to this question. Undoubtedly, the specification of clear standards for care homes has meant that they can be measured and those homes that are not fit for purpose have been either refurbished, rebuilt, or eliminated. Other regulatory measures, including inspections and safeguarding have also led to improvements. They have also increased bureaucracy, but arguably this is acceptable if it reduces variation between the worst and the best, in the direction of the best. However, regulation alone is insufficient to drive up standards. There have been important shifts in the approach to caring for older people. These may be summarized as a move towards a more person-centred approach, for example dementia care mapping as it arose from the work of Tom Kitwood and colleagues observing the social psychology around people with dementia in care homes. There are now lots of examples of good practice, some of which have been discussed in this volume. The most imaginative work involves care home residents in producing their own world, be this in performing domestic tasks such as cooking or else in artistic creations ranging from pottery to poetry. A third influence that has contributed to better standards has been an opening up of a public debate about residential care, about how it is funded but also how it is provided. Media exposure, for example the 2009 BBC TV series 'Can Gerry Robinson Fix Dementia Care Homes?'

together with various exposés of poor care, has undoubtedly contributed to greater awareness and openness.

None of this should lead to complacency. There is still much to be done, and there are some difficult questions to be answered in the next few years.

Perhaps the biggest question is how society will cope with growing numbers of older people with dementia over the decades in the middle of this century. Either there will be a gradual increase in the threshold at which people are admitted to care homes or else there will have to be an increased provision of beds. If more people with dementia are going to be cared for in their own homes, then there will need to be improvements in community care to support them or other models of care (such as supported accommodation or 'housing with extra care') will have to become more widespread, fundable, and effective. There are tough questions about what is affordable, how much of the cost should be borne by individuals and/or by the state, and how quality of care can be maintained in difficult times. We certainly do not have the answers to these questions but we are confident that we will see a vigorous debate, occupying not just the rest of our working lives but our retirement years as well.

One approach might be to try to look 10 years into the future. What might the care home sector look like then? In the United Kingdom, as the number of people with dementia approaches the 1 million mark by mid-century, and if a third of this population is likely to require residential care (as at present), that could require up to an extra 80,000 care home places. It would also require a similar additional number of care home staff. The resources required in caring for older people and those with dementia are huge. A simulation model produced by Skills for Care on behalf of the Department of Health projected that a paid social care workforce of between 2 million and 2.5 million would be required by 2025. This figure includes not only community care but also large numbers of care home staff. This scoping study recommended that: 'While all of the workforce will need an enhanced level of awareness and understanding of dementia specific roles will require a range of detailed skills and knowledge to be able to provide an effective service to people with dementia and their carers' (Department of Health, Skills for Care and Skills for Health, 2010: 4). The National Dementia Strategy (Department of Health, 2009) has highlighted living well with dementia in care homes and workforce development as two of its main objectives (objectives 11 and 13, respectively).

However one looks at it, it is difficult to see the number of care home places continuing to fall in the next decade. We would also confidently expect that the number of care homes run by large providers will increase. Probably, the current big providers will continue to grow by acquisitions, but there are also likely to be other entrants to the market too. Given the current political will to widen health service provision and to create more of a market for NHS care, it is likely that the larger homes may start to take on more of a hospital function, for example running rehabilitation services. We may see more specialist physicians working in care homes, as is already the case in Holland, for example. However, given the strength of primary care in the United Kingdom, and the fact its central role has recently been affirmed by the Government, the chances are that most healthcare in care homes will remain with general practitioners and primary care teams. There may be units for people with dementia and challenging behaviour which are run solely or jointly by specialist mental health services. This may even prove attractive for NHS mental health providers as the estate and accommodation costs would be a matter for the care home provider who, in turn, would be able to use the presence of specialist services as a selling point for the home.

Managers of care homes and especially those with responsibility for several homes within a large organization are likely to be increasingly skilled in issues of training and quality care. Their staff will include a larger proportion of people with care qualifications. It is possible, if there is a prolonged downturn in the economy, that staff will stay longer in post and that the status of the work will be enhanced by the fact that at least some care home providers are proving to be very good employers who value their staff. Work that provides personal care for older people is gaining more recognition (e.g. http://www.guardian.co.uk/society/2010/sep/08/heinz-wolff-care-elderly-science) so that the status of care home work is likely to improve, which would be a welcome development. The distinction between nursing and residential care will be further eroded into just 'care' and the costs of care will be calculated much more on an individual needs-led basis than at the current uniform rates. There will be much more emphasis on the potential of residents than on their shortcomings and there will also be more emphasis on creative and artistic pursuits and other enjoyable forms of daytime activity. Work to understand the lived experience of care home residents is also likely to make a greater contribution to the nature of care practice as will an enhanced focus on relationship-centred care.

As a final consideration, what about mental health? The point has been made in earlier chapters that there exists something of a paradox in the interaction between care homes and health services. A greater degree of health input, and perhaps especially from mental health services, is likely to make a care home more like a clinical institution and less 'homely'. What is the appropriate degree of support that health services can, or should, provide? And also, is there not a risk that by emphasizing such problems as dementia and depression, we distract attention from the main issue, which is how to support people in care homes to live fulfilling lives? What is the appropriate balance between autonomy and personal choice on the one hand, and risk and safeguarding on the other? What can we learn about how these tensions can be resolved?

By now, the reader will realize that our stance is in general a cautiously optimistic one; we believe that a resolution is possible. In the same way that psychiatry cannot deny any of its biological, social, or psychological roots, so consideration of mental health in care homes cannot deny the reality of the prevalence of dementia, depression, and other disorders but we also have to bear in mind that we are talking about people, their lives, and the places where they live. This must be prioritized alongside clinical considerations.

Perhaps the best way to approach this compromise position is analogous to the argument made in support of safeguarding (see Chapter 10), where the framework of safeguarding is applied to provide *space* for the vulnerable individual to live a good life. In a similar way, due consideration of the diagnostic and treatment issues, together with regulation and specialist support as required, can provide space within which care home residents have the opportunity to enjoy good mental health and live full lives to the best of their potential. The framework is not sufficient for good quality life in a care home—it is certainly no guarantee—but it can support it. The tone and direction of our book suggests that there is a careful balance to be struck between looking in from outside and offering support from external agencies and developing high quality care from the inside with the shared goal of improving both quality of care and quality of life for all those who live and work in care homes.

References

Banerjee, S. (2010). Living well with dementia—development of the national dementia strategy for England. *International Journal of Geriatric Psychiatry, 25*, 917–922.

Department of Health (2009). *Living Well With Dementia: A National Dementia Strategy.* London: Department of Health.

Department of Health, Skills for Care and Skills for Health (2010). *Working to Support the Implementation of the National Dementia Strategy Project: Scoping Study Report.* London: Department of Health.

Goffman, E. (1963). *Stigma: Notes on the Management of Spoiled Identity.* London: Prentice-Hall.

Parry-Jones, W.L.L. (1972). *The Trade in Lunacy: A Study of Private Madhouses in England in the Eighteenth and Nineteenth Centuries.* London: Routledge & Kegan Paul.

Rodrigues, R. & Schmidt, A. (2010). *Paying for Long Term Care: Policy Brief.* Vienna: European Centre for Social Welfare Policy and Research.

Index

Note: 'vs' indicates differential diagnosis.

AAC (Alternative and Augmentative
    Communication) Research Unit 47
Abbeyfield Society 21, 22, 27
Abbreviated Mental Test Score 165
ABC (Antecedent-Behaviour-Consequence)
    analysis 165, 207, 322
abuse 79, 113–30
  diagnosing cause/source 123, 124
  management 122–8
  preventing 120–2
  range and patterns of 117–18
  vulnerability 116–17, 120
accommodation see home; housing
acetylcholinesterase inhibitors
  Alzheimer's disease 171
  cognitive stimulation therapy enhancing
      effect of 211
  non-Alzheimer's dementia 171–2
  for non-cognitive and behavioural
      problems 172
achievement, sense of (in Senses
    Framework) 351
activities (social and recreational) 209–10
  creative work 29–39
  in dementia 170, 209–10
  female-dominated 239
  manager's account 25–6
  in VIPS framework 287, 288
acute illness 257–8
Addenbrooke's Cognitive Examination-Revised
    (ACE-R) 165
Admiral Nursing 273
admission to care home 151–4, 299
  assessment before see pre-admission
      procedure/assessment
  care plan on 255, 320
  decision 151–2
  in dementia 164–5
  in functional mental illness, routes to 194–5
  impact on mental health 153–4
  psychological adjustment on 214–16
  triggers and predictors for 151, 314
    dementia 139, 152
  weight gain on 259
  see also transition
advanced care planning (ACP) 270
advanced directives (often referred to as
    living wills) 103, 107–8, 109
  resident's view 12

advocacy 42, 321
  in VIPS framework 289
affective disorders see mood disorders
age
  of residents
    and Deprivation of Liberty
        Safeguards 109
    European comparisons of
        distribution 135–9
  of schizophrenia onset 192
ageing population 365
  people with intellectual difficulties 154
  society's need to cope with 369
ageism 3, 317
agency staff, manager's preferring not
    to use 22
aggressive patients
  abuse of 122
  training regarding 334
Alternative and Augmentative Communication
    Research Unit 47
Alzheimer's disease 162
  case study 49–50
  clinical presentation 162
  Down syndrome and 154–5
  therapy
    drugs for cognitive symptoms 171
    psychosocial 212
Alzheimer's Society
  'Home from Home' 356
  study of dementia care in care homes 57
animals, pet 25
Antecedent-Behaviour-Consequence (ABC)
    analysis 165, 207, 322
antibiotics 261
  end-of-life 268
antidepressants 184, 185
  in dementia 172
antihypertensive (hypotensive) drugs 257
antipsychotic drugs (prescribing of) 71, 150,
    172, 199, 200, 260
  atypical 199, 200
  in the media 19
  side-effects 199, 200
appetite loss, dementia 167
appetizing food 258
APPROACH survey 301–2
appropriate care for people with intellectual
    difficulties, lack of 156

aromatherapy 209–10
art therapy 26, 196
assessment
  on admission 320
  of experience of living in case home 45–62
  of health status 253–6
  mental capacity 103–4
  pre-admission *see* pre-admission
  of risk 314–15, 317–19, 321, 323
assets (incl. capital) and eligibility for
    funding 92–3, 94
  spending down 93–5
attitudes, negative *see* negative beliefs and
    attitudes
Austria
  balance of care (home vs care home) 134
  private vs public providers in 140, 141
autonomy 313, 315–16, 323

bedfast patient examination
  fractures 255
  pressure sores 256
behavioural management in dementia 170
behavioural problems/symptoms
  in dementia *see* neuropsychiatric symptoms
  in VIPS framework, discovering reasons
    for 289, 290
  see also challenging behaviour
Belgium, private vs public providers in 141
beliefs, negative *see* negative beliefs and attitudes
belonging, sense of (in Senses Framework) 350
Bennett, David (Rocky), death of 126
best interests 104–7
  deprivation of liberty in 109
bipolar affective disorder 193
bisexual residents 243–5, 246
black and ethnic minority groups 240–3
blood pressure, high 257
Bolam test for negligence 105
boredom 288
Brighton and Hove care homes support
    team 231
Bristol Activities of Daily Living (BADLS) 165
Brown, Molly (patient with dementia), on
    creative writing project 37
Brown Field House, manager's view 21–7
built environment 169
  creating a sense of community 354
  see also physical environment
burnout
  primary carer 195
  staff 215, 285, 354
Burwell village (Cambridgeshire)
  initiatives 45–6, 48–9
'butterfly moments' 210

Camberwell Assessment of Need for the Elderly
    (CANE) 54, 356
Cambridge, Brown Field House,
  manager's view 21–7

Cambridgeshire
  Burwell village initiatives 45–6, 48–9
  libraries creative work projects 29–39
Cambridgeshire Celebrates Age 48
capacity *see* mental capacity; Mental Capacity
    Act
capital assets *see* assets
cardiopulmonary resuscitation in dementia 174
care home (institutional/residential/nursing
    care)
  admission *see* admission
  definition 1
  in Europe
    blurring of boundaries between
      community-based care and 139–40
    comparisons between countries of care at
      home vs 132–5
  good practice inside *see* good practice
  good practice outside of 297–311
  living in *see* living in a care home
  market *see* market
  moving into *see* admission
  numbers in 1
  responsibility for ensuring good care 225–6
Care Home Use of Medicines Study
    (CHUMS) 226
Care Homes for Older People National
    Minimum Standards and Regulations 337
Care Quality Commission (CQC) 22, 27, 75,
    79, 81, 315, 316, 342
Care Standards Act 2000 73, 74, 75, 79
carers (informal - incl. family/relatives)
  abuse by 117
  in end-of-life, supporting 273–4
  experiences of
    daughter's personal account 41–2, 43–4
    discrepancy from residents' experiences 61
    partner's personal account 13–20
  inclusion in dementia care 173–4
  people with intellectual difficulties 154
  risk of losing contact with 293
  transition to residential care and role of 152
  visits by *see* visits
caring (feeling concern and empathy for
    others) 50
  presenting oneself as 58
cascade training 339–41
Celebration Event (Cambridge Central
    Library) 35, 38
centres of learning 228
cerebrovascular disease, dementia *see* vascular
    dementia
challenging behaviours 290
  labelling of 317, 318
  male residents 239
  management 322
    Newcastle care home support team
      and 231
    psychosocial 206–7
    training example 340

training regarding 334
understanding causes 322
Charging for Residential Accommodation Guide (CRAG) 90
children, treating residents as 292
chiropodists 10, 301
choice (preferences), individual (residents) 287, 288, 313, 316
in end-of-life issues 272
inquiring at admission about 320
positive choice of care home placement 355
risk weighed against at 321–2, 323
see also decisions
chronic disease 256–7, 299
Clare, L 59
closure of home due to poor performance 83
clozapine 200
cognitive behavioural therapy (CBT) 214
schizophrenia 200
cognitive stimulation therapy (CST) 170, 210–11
cognitive symptoms (incl. deficits)
decision-making with 353
dementia 162–3
drug therapy 171–2
functional mental illness 198
in mood disorders 198–9
see also mental capacity
Commission for Social Care Inspection 74, 226, 283, 315
sexual orientation and 245
using SOFI 56
commissioners and GPs, local enhanced service agreement (for individual care homes) between 224–5
communication and interaction
residents developing/enhancing skills in 46–7, 57
staff–resident (and their carers)
in admission to care home 254–5
in *My* Home Life themes 353
quality impacting on well-being 56
in VIPS framework 284–5, 289–90, 292
staff–staff, with infrequent GP visits 223
community
admission in functional mental illness from the 195
creating a sense of, in care homes 346, 351, 354–5
resources/facilities 298
and improving quality of life 48–9
in VIPS framework 291
community setting
of abuse 117
care in, in Europe
blurring of boundaries between institutional care and 139–40
payments to dementia patients in Germany for 139

comorbid psychiatric problems
in dementia 168
in functional mental illness 198–9
compulsion (staff) to hurt others 118
confidentiality
medical records 255
sexual orientation 244
continence problems *see* incontinence
continuity, sense of (in Senses Framework) 350
coping styles and depression 181
core temperature measurement 255
Cornell Scale for Depression in Dementia (CSDD) 182, 182–3
costs (incl. fees) of caring 89, 93–4
in dementia, annual 161
high, reasons for 95
see also funding; payment
court-appointed deputies 107
creative work 29–39
culture (of care/care home)
abuse relating to 118, 119
leadership and training influencing 342
positive, promotion in *My home life* themes 345, 346, 358
Czech Republic
balance of care (home vs care home) 134
private vs public providers in 141

daily living routines 25
dangers *see* risk; safety; vulnerability
death (mortality) 262
abuse-related 126
on being told of another resident's (view of a resident) 12
carer's account of partner's 19–20
depression and 186
schizophrenia and 199
staff fear of being blamed for 269
see also end-of-life; suicide
decisions and decision-making
in best interests *see* best interest
on end-of-life care, carers/family 273
to move into care home 151–2
by residents 313
capacity to make *see* mental capacity
sharing, in *My* Home Life themes 346, 351, 352–4
see also choice
dedicated primary care service 225, 230–3
deferred payment agreements 93
dehydration in dementia 167
delirium 257–8
dementia vs 166
delusions, schizophrenia 192
dementia 41–65, 150, 161–77, 327–44, 356
as admission trigger 139, 152
advanced/severe
advance care planning for 270
end-of-life care 174, 222, 266
symptoms 266

dementia (*cont.*)
  assessment/diagnosis/investigations 164–6
  black and ethnic minority groups 241
  clinical features 162–3
  creative work 29–39
  depression comorbid with 168, 182, 187
  differential diagnosis 166
  empathic support 328, 331, 333, 334, 336, 349
  epidemiology/prevalence among
      residents 161
    in Europe 139
  fear of 42–3
  functional mental illness comorbid with 198
  hearing the voice of people with 41–51
  intellectual difficulties and 154–5
    better care 157
  interventions/management/care 168–72
    antipsychotic drugs *see* antipsychotic drugs
    assessing quality (with Dementia Care
        Mapping) 54, 55, 61, 121, 165, 215,
        228, 333–4, 349, 368
    Malignant Social Psychology (MSP)
        of care 292–3
    psychosocial 170–1, 205–14
    specialist care 173, 260, 273, 320
    training *see* training
  living in a care home with *see* living in a
      care home
  manager's account of her education in caring
      for people with 24
  mental capacity in *see* mental capacity
  mental health and 168
  needs in *see* needs
  proportion of residents with 150
  rating scales 165
  risk assessment and management in 316–21
  syndrome of 162
  types 162
    see also specific types
Dementia Care Leadership Programme 339, 340
Dementia Care Mapping (DCM) 54, 55, 61,
    121, 165, 215, 228, 333–4, 349, 368
Dementia Care Trainers' Programme 340, 341
Dementia Champions 289
Dementia UK 272
denial of dementia 49
Denmark
  age distribution of residents 136
  balance of care (home vs care home) 133, 134
depression 150–1, 179–90
  black and ethnic minority
      groups 241, 242, 243
  causes 180–2
  comorbid
    in dementia patients 168, 182, 187
    in schizophrenia 198
  dementia vs 166
  diagnosis 179–80, 182–3
  impact of admission 153–4
  outcome and prognosis 186–7

physical health and 166–8, 181
prevalence and incidence 180
treatment and management 184–6
  in *My* Home Life themes 356
Deprivation of Liberty Safeguards
    (DoLS) 71, 101, 102, 108–12, 114
deputies, court-appointed 107
deputy manager, manager's view 23
Diagnostic and Statistical Manual of Mental
    Disorders (DSM-IV), depression 180, 182
diet *see* food; nutrition and diet
digital recording, assessment using 56
Dignity in Care initiative 31–2, 34
disability 299
disclosure of sexual preference 243–4, 246
discomfort (physical) 291
discussion, stimulating participation and 46–7
disease *see* physical health problems
disempowerment 317
district nurse 10, 125, 165, 222,
    301, 302, 303, 304, 368
doctors/physicians
  family *see* general practitioners
  specialist 233–4
donepezil 171, 172
Down syndrome and Alzheimer's-type
    dementia 154–5
Downes, Jim (carer of patient with dementia),
    on creative writing project 37
drop-in centre, Burwell 48
drugs and medicines 226–7, 259–60, 299
  dementia patients 171–2
  depression 184
  in functional mental illness 199–200
    adverse effects 199, 200
  management issues 78, 226–7, 259–60
  see also specific (types of) drugs
DSM-IV, depression 180, 182
duration of long-term care and depression 182
Durham care homes team 231
Durrant, Kate, on creative writing project 38
dying *see* end-of-life; terminal illness

eating difficulties at end-of-life 267
  see also feeding; food; nutrition
education
  professionals *see* training and education
  residents 25–6
elderly *see* older people
electroconvulsive therapy (ECT) 184
emotional needs in VIPS framework 292
empathy
  in dementia care 328, 331, 333, 334, 336, 349
  in VIPS framework 289, 290
empowerment *see* power
enabling in VIPS framework 291
end-of-life
  care at 24, 262, 265–76
    dementia 174, 222, 266
    improving 269–74

in *My* Home Life themes 346, 356–7
  patient choice 271, 272
  providing good care 268–9
identifying residents approaching 268
moving through dementia pathway to 43–4
symptoms 266–9
End of Life Strategy 222
enforcement powers (of regulatory bodies) 72
  changes (in 2008) from old (2000) regime 80
  closure of home 83
  examples 73
engagement (principle to work by) 307
England
  age distribution of residents 136
  balance of care (home vs care home) 133, 134
English as second language, staff with 335
Enriched Opportunities Programme 288–9
enteral feeding 259
  end-of-life 267
environment (care home)
  depression and the 181–2
  importance (beneficial) 284
    in creating a sense of community 354
    dementia 169
    manager's view 24–5
  staff controlling (in risk management) 318
  in VIPS framework
    physical 289
    social (=S) 283, 291–3
equity (principle to work by) 307
equity release 93
essential oils (aromatherapy) 210
Estonia
  age distribution of residents 136
  balance of care (home vs care home) 134
  gender distribution of residents 137
ethical issues 313–25
  closure of care home due to poor
    performance 83
ethnic minority groups
  residents 240–3
  staff, with English as second language 335
Europe, comparisons of long-term care 131–45
European Court of Human Rights
  (ECtHR) 108, 110
Everett, Debbie (hospital chaplain in
  Canada) 30
evidence-based best practice 345–64
examination of resident 255–6
exercise, physical 209
experience
  of living in a care home *see* living in a care home
  past *see* life history work
Extending Empathy group 334
extra care housing 44–6, 96, 196, 318

faecal incontinence, dementia patients 167
Fair Access to Care Services 90, 314
Fairview Court 125–6
falling, preventing risk 318, 318–19

family
  as carers *see* carers
  having a role in 58
fear of dementia 42–3
feeding, help with 259
  see also eating difficulties; food; nutrition
feelings (individuals)
  best interests and weight given to wishes
    and 105–6
  in VIPS framework 292
fees and costs *see* costs
females *see* women
finances, managing one's 11–12
  see also assets; cost; funding; payment
Finland
  age distribution of residents 136
  balance of care (home vs care home) 134
  private vs public providers in 141
focus groups in assessment 56–7
food
  appetizing 258
  help with feeding 259
  a resident's opinion 11
  see also appetite; eating; nutrition
football memorabilia 47
fractures, examination of bedfast patients for 255
France
  age distribution of residents 136
  balance of care (home vs care home) 134
  gender distribution of residents 138
  private vs public providers in 141
free care 92, 93, 96
  Scotland 367
freedom *see* liberty
frontotemporal dementia 162
  clinical features 163
functional displacement 209
functional impact of dementia 165
functional mental illness 191–204
  definitions 191–2
  epidemiology 192
  meeting residents' needs 197
  models of care 201
  physical health problems 199
  providing long-term care 195–6
  routes to care home admission 194–5
  social exclusion 194
  support services 197–201
  treatment 199–201
  types 192–3
funding of care/services 89–99, 367
  dementia 45
  impact of downward trend 84
  policy 90–1, 367
  see also self-funding

galantamine 171
gender of residents, European
  comparisons 137–9
  see also men; women

general medical service (GMS) contract 222–3
    with having a special interest 224
general practitioners (GP; doctor) and
        primary care 222–6, 300–1
    access to 222–6, 300–1
        dementia care 173
        manager's view 26
        resident's view 10–11
    joint reviews with specialists 229–30
    medicines management 226–7
    retainer fees 224, 300–1
    see also dedicated primary care service
Geriatric Depression Scale (GDS) 180, 182
geriatricians 222, 227, 228, 298, 300
Germany
    age distribution of residents 136
    balance of care (home vs
        care home) 134, 135
    community-based dementia services,
        payments for 139
    gender distribution of residents 138
    inspections in 142
    private vs public providers in 140, 141
Glasgow Caledonian University and football
        memorabilia 47
Gloucestershire, Partnership for Older People
        Project 231
Gold Standards Framework 222, 269, 271–2
good practice/care 279–311, 368
    inside care homes 279–95
        in dementia 319, 328
    outside care homes 297–311
    see also evidence-based best practice; quality
government policies see policies
group (treatment in)
    depression 185
    reality orientation 211
group homes, long-term mental illness 195

hairdresser 10
hallucinations, schizophrenia 192
health
    improving, in My Home Life
        themes 346, 355–6
    mental and physical see mental health;
        physical health
    promotion see promoting health and
        well-being
Health and Social Care Act (2001) 93
Health and Social Care Act (2008a,b) 79, 80, 83
health needs
    as indicator of external support 298–9
    meeting
        mental health 149–60
        physical health see physical health
health professionals 298–305
    see also specific posts
Health Research Service Delivery and
        Organisation (NIHR-SDO)-funded
        APPROACH study 301–2

healthcare services 297–311
    future needs 306–8, 368
    how older people define needs 299
    initiatives supporting and improving 302–3
        My Home Life themes 346, 355–6
    resident's view of access to 10–11
hearing the voice of people with
        dementia 41–51
heterosexism, assumption of 245
Hollingsworth, Peter, poem written by 30
home (lived in)
    care at, vs care homes, European
        comparisons 132–5
    ownership, and eligibility for
        funding 92–3, 95–6
    see also assets; housing
'home' (sense of care home as) 24–5,
        29–30, 354
homosexual men and women 243–5, 246
honesty (principle to work by) 307
hospitals
    discharge in functional mental illness 194–5
    health service viewing care homes
        much like 308
hostel accommodation, long-term
        mental illness 195
housing/accommodation 44–5, 95–6
    extra care 44–6, 96, 196, 318
    housing with care model (older people) 45
    long-term mental illness 195–6
    see also home
human resource management (in VIPS
        framework) 283
100 care homes study 283, 284–5, 286–7, 288,
        289, 291–2, 293
Hungary
    age distribution of residents 136
    balance of care (home vs care home) 134
    gender distribution of residents 138
hydration 258–9
    maintaining 259
    status, assessment 255, 258
    see also dehydration
hyperactive patients, nutrition 258
hypertension 257
hypnotics 168
hypotensive drugs 257

ICD-10, depression 179–80
Iceland
    age distribution of residents 136, 137
    balance of care (home vs care
        home) 133, 134
    gender distribution of residents 138
    private vs public providers in 141
identity, retaining sense of 56
    men 238, 240
    in My Home Life themes 346, 351, 351–2
    in VIPS framework 288, 292, 293
Improving Dementia Services in England 228

inappropriate care for people with intellectual difficulties 156
incontinence
  abuse in patients with 122
  dementia patients 167
independence 313, 316
independent safeguarding system with abuse 126–8
individualized approach (I in VIPS framework) 283, 287–9
  see also person-centred care
infections 261
  control 261
  dementia and 166–7
  end-of-life 268
in-reach teams, nursing 303
insomnia, dementia 168
inspections (of services) 11, 72, 80–1, 142
  thematic (in 100 care homes study) 283
  see also Commission for Social Care Inspection
institutional abuse 117, 118–20
  see also staff
institutional care see care home
integrated approach
  in community to improving quality of life 48–9
  healthcare services working with care homes 301–2, 303–5
    barriers 304–5
    models 303–5
intellectual difficulties 154–7
interaction see communication and interaction
interdisciplinary team see multidisciplinary team
International Classification of Diseases (ICD-10), depression 179–80
international comparisons of long-term care 131–45
interview, assessment by 56–7
  on admission 320
'invisibility' of residents 2, 366
Ireland
  age distribution of residents 136
  balance of care (home vs care home) 133, 134
  gender distribution of residents 138
Israel
  balance of care (home vs care home) 134
  gender distribution of residents 138
Italy
  age distribution of residents 136, 137
  balance of care (home vs care home) 134
  gender distribution of residents 138

joint reviews with GPs and specialists 229–30
Joseph Rowntree Foundation
  My Home Life programme funding 347
  Older People's Vision for Long-term Care 152

regulatory framework for care homes 72–4
social well-being in extra care housing 45, 48
workforce development 306

Killick, John, and the creative writing project 31, 32, 33–4, 34, 35, 37, 38
Kingman, Bryan (patient with dementia), on creative writing project 37
knowledge and understanding (and possible lack)
  in dementia training 331–3, 333
  of experience of living in a care home (incl. residents with dementia), experience 60–2

labelling of challenging behaviours 317, 318
laboratory tests, dementia 165–6
language barriers in dementia training 335
lasting power of attorney 107, 270
Latvia, balance of care (home vs care home) 134
law see legislation
leadership 367
  culture of care and the influence of 342
  in dementia training 338–9, 339–40
  in VIPS framework for person-centred care 284
learning disabilities (intellectual difficulties) 154–7
legislation 43, 101–12
  cognitive impairment-related 353
  post-2000 74, 75, 101–12
  sexual orientation-related 244–5
length of time in care and depression 182
lesbian, gay, bisexual, transgender residents 243–5, 246
'Let Me Decide' programme (Australia) 270
Lewy bodies, dementia with 162
  clinical features 163
liberty (freedom) 313, 316
  in advancing dementia, maintaining 49–50
  balance between safety and 24, 114–16, 314, 316, 320, 321
  Deprivation of Liberty Safeguards (DoLS) 71, 101, 102, 108–12, 114
libraries, creative work projects 29–39
life history (past experience) work 24, 46–7, 50, 58, 213–14
  lack of understanding about 333
  in VIPS framework 287, 288, 290
limb fractures, examination of bedfast patients for 255
listening to people with dementia 41–51
Lithuania
  age distribution of residents 136
  balance of care (home vs care home) 134
  gender distribution of residents 137, 138
  private vs public providers in 141
Liverpool Care Pathway 262, 269, 272

living in a care home (incl. residents with
    dementia), experience 53–65
  relationships determining 254
  research evidence 55–65
  staff training simulating 334
  subjective *see* subjective experience
  in transition phase *see* transition
  understanding 60–2
living wills *see* advanced directives
local authority
  funding of dementia training 336
  funding of residents 91
    disqualification from 92, 93
  negotiate with homes on fees in their area 94
  serious case review 126
local enhanced services 224–5, 227
long-term (chronic) conditions/health
    problems 256–7, 299
loving care 50
Luxembourg
  age distribution of residents 136
  balance of care (home vs care home) 134
  gender distribution of residents 138

males *see* men
Malignant Social Psychology (MSP) of
    dementia care 292–3
malnutrition 258, 259, 342
managers
  in dementia training 339–40
    enhancing their own skills and
        understanding 339
    responsibilities 338
  personal account 21–7
  staff-related abuse (with inadequate
      levels) and 127–8
  survey asking about working with healthcare
      services 301–2
  in VIPS framework, importance 285–6
  see also leadership
Many Happy Returns 1940s 47
market, care home
  changing nature 366
  a decade ahead (from 2010) 369–70
  Europe 140–1
Martin, Linda, and the creative writing
    project 31, 32, 34–6
meaningful relationships 216, 313, 317
means testing 90, 91, 94, 95, 97, 253
media 368
  antipsychotic drugs in 19
  dementia awareness 42
medical conditions *see* physical
    health problems
medicines *see* drugs and medicines
meeting, residents' 11
memantine 171
men
  gay 243–5, 246
  as minority group in care home 238–40

mental capacity 101
  assessment 103–4
  impaired/lack 353
    assumption of, in risk management 318
    end-of-life care and 270
    required for deprivation of liberty 108, 109
  see also cognitive symptoms
Mental Capacity Act 2005 43, 71, 102–8, 114,
    270, 321, 351
  Deprivation of Liberty Safeguards
      (DoLS) 71, 101, 102, 108–12, 114
mental health
  book's focus on (and not just problems) 3
  a decade ahead (from 2010) 370
  dementia and 168
  impact of admission on 153–4
  meeting needs in 149–60
  see also health; well-being
Mental Health Act 1983 90, 101, 109, 111–12
  Deprivation of Liberty and Safeguards
      and 111–12
mental health problems/illness 161–219
  comorbid *see* comorbid psychiatric problems
  functional *see* functional mental illness
  high levels 150
  intellectual difficulties and 154–5
  manager's perspectives 26–7
  see also specific problems
mentoring 32, 234
methicillin-resistant *Staphylococcus aureus*
    (MRSA) 261
Miller, Daisy (patient with dementia), on
    creative writing project 37
Mini Mental State Examination (MMSE) 165, 183
Minimum Data Set (MDS)-based depression
    rating scale 182, 183
minorities 237–49
  ethnic *see* ethnic minority groups
monetary issues *see* assets; cost; finances;
    funding; payment
money *see* finances; funding
mood (affective) disorders
  comorbid in functional
      mental illness 198, 198–9
  in dementia 164
  see also bipolar affective disorder
mortality *see* death
moving into nursing home *see* admission;
    transition
MRSA (methicillin-resistant *Staphylococcus
    aureus*) 261
multidisciplinary (interdisciplinary)
    team 167, 225, 230–3, 303, 305
  dementia 169
  reviewing medication 227
  see also staff
multisensory stimulation 171, 210
music therapy 171, 209–10
mutual learning (principle to work by) 307
My Home Life programme 152, 285, 308, 345–64

nasogastric tube feeding 267
National Care Standards Commission 74, 226
National Council for Palliative care
  (NCPC) 272
National Dementia Strategy 1, 2, 43, 49, 222,
  228, 237, 328
  individualized care 289
  key themes and future directions 367, 369
  leadership for dementia care 338
  quality of life 172
  workforce/staff 337
  training 234, 338
National Development Team for Inclusion 61
National Framework for NHS Continuing
  Healthcare and NHS-funded
  Nursing Care 92
National Institute for Health and Clinical
  Excellence see NICE
National Minimum Standards (NMS) 75–6, 77,
  226, 337
navigation in *My* Home Life
  themes 345, 346, 355–7
needs
  meeting/supporting
    in dementia training 335–6
    health see health needs
    in long-term functional
      mental illness 197
    National Minimum Standards (NMS)
      and 76–7
    of staff in end-of-life care 273–4
  unmet
    challenging behaviours relating to 209
    in dementia 356
negative beliefs and attitudes 120, 318
  of residents, depression associated with 181
  of staff and healthcare persons 197, 318, 333–4
    chronic mental illness 199
    dementia 333–4
    need to address 358
negative symptoms, schizophrenia 192
neglect 94, 113, 115, 117, 118, 119, 121, 123,
  128, 129, 133
negligence, *Bolam* test 105
Netherlands
  age distribution of residents 136, 137
  balance of care (home vs care home) 134
  gender distribution of residents 138
  quality of care rankings 142
  small institutional units dementia
    patients 139
neuropsychiatric (behavioural and
  psychological/non-cognitive) symptoms in
  dementia 163, 164, 168, 267
  treatment 170, 172
  end-of-life 267
Neuropsychiatric Inventory (NPI) 165
Nevill, Connie (patient with dementia), on
  creative writing project 37
Newcastle challenging behaviour service 231

NHS (National Health Service)
  funding (incl. NHS continuing healthcare
    scheme) 91, 91–3
  inequitable access to services 298
NICE/NIHCE (National Institute for Health
  and Clinical Excellence) guidelines in
  dementia
  assessment and diagnosis 164–5
  end-of-life care 174
  investigations 165–6
  pressure sores 261–2
  training 328
  treatment of dementia 170, 171, 173
night 290
  routine and indiscriminate checking at 318
  sedation at 252, 260
No Secrets 70, 113–14, 117
nominated point of contact 229
non-cognitive symptoms in dementia see
  neuropsychiatric symptoms
Norway
  age distribution of residents 136
  balance of care (home vs care home) 133, 134
nurse
  district 10, 125, 165, 222, 301, 302,
    303, 304, 368
  in risk management 318–19
nurse specialists (specialist nurses) 298, 301,
  302, 303, 305
  dementia care 273
  South East London CHST 232
nursing home see care home
nursing in-reach teams 303
nutrition and diet 73, 258–9
  dementia and 167, 168
  depression and 168
  see also appetite; eating; food

objective assessment of quality of life and
  care 54–5, 61
observational methods of assessment 55–6
occupation (in care home), having an 58
  in VIPS framework 287
O'Driscoll, Richard, on creative writing
  project 38
older people/elderly
  dementia in see dementia
  how they define health and healthcare
    needs 299
  with intellectual difficulties,
    better care 156–7
  negative beliefs about see negative beliefs
  see also geriatricians
Older People's Vision for Long-term Care 152
100 care homes study 283, 284–5, 286–7,
  288, 289, 291–2, 293
organizational issues in dementia
  training 337–8
out-of-area placement of people with
  intellectual difficulties 155–6

outcomes
  for depression 186–7
  safeguarding from abuse 127
  for service users (in regulatory
    frameworks) 76, 77, 78–9, 80, 81
  improving 83
outreach services 229

pain management
  dementia 167–8
  end-of-life 267
  neglecting 291
palliative care 265–76
Parkinsonism and Parkinson's disease 181, 256
  and dementias 162, 168
participation
  of resident, stimulating discussion and 46–7
  in working relationships 307–8
partners (in care home), carers
  account of 13–20
Partnership for Older People Project
  (Gloucestershire) 231
past experience see life history work
Patient Health Questionnaire (PHQ-2) 183
Patient Outcomes Research Team (PORT)
  study 199
payment (for care) 89–99
  GP retainer fee 224, 300–1
percutaneous endoscopic gastrostomy 267
performance
  improving 72
  poor, closure of home due to 83
Perrin, Tessa 30
person-centred (individualized) care 45, 56,
  206, 279, 280, 283–94, 368
  current bias towards 303
  dementia 173, 332–3
  end-of-life 269
  My Home Life programme and 349, 351, 352
  role of staff 173
  training in 329, 330, 332–3, 338, 341
  VIPS framework 283–94
personal care, abuse in management of 122
personal possessions in VIPS framework 287
personalization (and its
  encouragement) 49–50, 113–14
  in My Home Life themes 345, 346, 351, 351–4
perspectives (P in VIPS
  framework) 283, 284, 289–91
pet animals 25
Pettit, Sally Jane, poem by 33–4
pharmacy 226–7
physical abuse see abuse
physical contact (touch) 17, 18
physical environment in VIPS
  framework 289
  see also built environment
physical examination 255–6
physical exercise 209

physical health (residents)
  assessment 253–6
  maintaining 251–63
    dementia 171
    in VIPS framework 289
  see also health; well-being
physical health problems (medical conditions/
    disease) 256–9, 299
  acute 257–8
  chronic/long-term 256–7, 299
  in dementia 166–7, 181
  depression related to 181
  in functional mental illness 199
  high levels 150
  intellectual difficulties and 154–5
  see also terminal illness
physical restraint 126, 168, 319, 321
physician see doctor
planning of care
  on admission to care home 255, 320
  advanced (for end-of-life) 269–70
  in dementia 168–9
  review see review
  in VIPS framework 287, 288
poet, resident, and creative writing
  projects 29–39
Poland
  age distribution of residents 136
  balance of care (home vs care home) 133, 134
  gender distribution of residents 137, 138
policies (government) 367
  extra care housing 96
  funding 90–1, 367
  regulating quality of care 70
polypharmacy 168, 299
Portugal, balance of care (home vs care
  home) 133, 134
power and empowerment
  staff 230, 233, 284
    regulation facilitating 84
    in training 330, 331, 336
  user/resident 140, 170, 313, 317
power of attorney, lasting 107, 270
powerlessness, resident 317
Pratchett, Sir Terry 42
pre-admission procedure/assessment 273
  health status 253
  manager's view 23–4
preferences see choice
pressure sores (bed sores) 261–2
  abuse and 125
  examination of bedfast patients for 256
prevention
  of abuse 120–2
  of accidents see safety
primary care trusts, funding of dementia
  training 336
  see also general practitioners
primary prevention of abuse 121

Prioritising Need in the Context of Putting People First 90
private care
  in Europe, public vs 140–2
  paying for *see* self-funding
private contracts between care home
    and GP 224
PRN (prescription as required) 260
promoting health and well-being 277–371
  black and ethnic minority groups 242–3
  men 239–40
protection *see* safety
provision of long-term care
  functional mental illness 195–6
  manager's view 23–4
  market in Europe 140–1
  see also services
psychiatric illness *see* mental
    health problems
psychological adjustment on admission to care
    home 214–16
psychological interventions *see* psychosocial
psychological symptoms in dementia *see*
    neuropsychiatric symptoms
psychosocial (psychological)
    interventions 150, 205–19
  dementia 170–1, 205–14
  depression 184–5
  functional mental illness 200–1
psychotic symptoms in dementia 164, 168
public (the)
  informing them of service
      performance/quality 72, 81
  media informing the *see* media
public funding
  charges lower than self-funding 94
  disqualification/ineligibility for 92–3
  in Europe, vs private funding 140–2
  qualification/eligibility for 90–1, 92, 95
public inquiries 315
  into abuse 126
purpose, sense of (in Senses
    Framework) 350–1

Qualifications and Credit Framework (QCF)
    units 331, 337
quality (of care)
  assurance (in VIPS framework) 284
  care home's responsibility 225–6
  in dementia, assessment tool
      (Dementia Care Mapping) 54, 55, 61,
      121, 165, 215, 228, 333–4, 349, 368
  improving 81
    Europe 140
  ratings system 77
  regulating *see* regulation
  standards for 75–9
  see also good practice
Quality and Risk Profile (QRP) 80, 81

quality of life (QoL) 348–9
  assessment 50–1, 54–5, 61
    community resources 48–9
  defining 348–9
  improving/enhancing
    dementia 172–3, 328–9
    principles underpinning and 313
quasi-market in care 140–1

rapid eye movement (REM) sleep
    behaviour disorder 168
reality-based training 329–30, 334–5
reality orientation therapy 170, 211
recreational activities *see* activities
Reed, Sarah, and Many Happy
    Returns 1940s 47
regime (care home), abuse
    relating to 118, 119
regulation 69–87
  defining 71–2
  European countries 142
  future of 83–4, 368
  impact on care home quality 81–3
  pre-1985 to present 72–5
  sexual orientation-related 244–5
relationships (residents'
    interpersonal) 58, 354–5
  care centred on 349–50
  culture based on 358
  experienced determined by 354
  meaningful 216, 313, 317
relatives as carers *see* carers
REM sleep behaviour disorder 168
reminiscence therapy 123–4, 170
research evidence, living in care home
    with dementia 55–65
resident(s)
  activities *see* activities
  communication *see*
      communication
  European comparisons of
      profile of 135–9
  inclusion in dementia 173–4
  'invisibility' 2, 366
  needs *see* needs
  profile, future directions 365–6
  views/experiences
    discrepancy from carers' views 61
    personal account 9–12
  vulnerability *see* vulnerability
residential care *see* care home
Residential Care Transformed: Revisiting
    "The Last Refuge" 347
respect in VIPS framework 291
respiratory rate assessment 255
restraint 79, 319, 321–2
  physical 126, 168, 319, 321
resuscitation in dementia 174
retainer fee, GP 224, 300–1

review
  of care plan
    resident's account 11
    in VIPS framework 287
  of health status 253
rewards for staff 285, 286
risk 313–25
  assessment and
    perceptions of 314–15, 317–19, 321, 323
  defining 314–15
  management 317–19, 321–2
  managing (protection and
    overprotection) 24, 114–16, 314, 319–22
  reframing 322–3
  see also safety; vulnerability
rivastigmine 171, 171–2
Robinson, Gerry 329, 368
role play in dementia training 334
room (resident's own), carer's view 19
routines in daily living 25
Royal Commission on Long
  Term Care 91, 94, 96, 367
Russian Federation, balance of care (home vs
  care home) 134

safeguarding 42–3, 113–14
  from abuse 123–6
    independent system 126–8
  definition 113–14
safety (protection and overprotection) and
  security 313–25
  improving 81
  liberty and, balance between 24, 114–16,
    314, 316, 320, 321
  sense of
    false 323
    in Senses Framework 350
  standards 75–9
  see also risk; vulnerability
schizoaffective disorder 193, 198
schizophrenia 192–3
  cognitive impairment 198
  physical health problems 199
  psychiatric comorbidity 198
  social exclusion 194
  treatment 199, 200
schizophrenia and, death 199
Scotland
  free care 367
  study of staff controlling environment 318
screening
  dementia 165
  depression 182–3, 184, 188
  malnutrition 258
secondary care see specialist care
secondary prevention of abuse 121
security see safety and security
sedation 260
  night 252, 260

self-funding (private paying) 92–3
  charges higher than publically-funded
    residents 94
selfhood (sense of self)
  factors influencing 58
  preservation of 56
Semashko model 135
Senses Framework 62, 285, 349,
  350–1, 354, 358
serious adverse event 315
serious case review by local authority 126
services (support) 221–36, 297–311
  assessing what really matters to
    users of 80
  care and welfare of users of 78
  external/outside, access to 221–36, 297–311
    future perspectives 368
    manager's view 26–7
    resident's view 10–11, 11
  functional mental illness 197–201
  inspection 11, 72, 80–1, 142
  outcomes for users of see outcomes
  regulation see regulation
  safety of users see safety
  see also provision
sex see gender; men; women
sexism 317
sexual orientation of residents 243–5, 246
Shaping the Future of Care Together 2, 91, 96
Sheffield care homes support team 231
Short Observation Framework for Inspection
  (SOFI) 55–6, 78, 228, 349
  in 100 care homes study 283
significance, sense of (in Senses
  Framework) 351
simulated presence therapy 209
singing 48
skills development
  residents, communication 46–7, 57
  staff
    in dementia 334–5
    future needs 367
skin care 261–2
sleep disorders, dementia 168
Slovak Republic
  balance of care (home vs
    care home) 133, 134
  gender distribution of residents 137, 138
Slovenia
  age distribution of residents 136
  balance of care (home vs
    care home) 133, 134
  gender distribution of residents 138
Snoezelen therapy 171, 210
Snow, Iris (patient with dementia), on creative
  writing project 37
social activities see activities
Social Care Institute for Clinical Excellence on
  dementia training 328

social environment and social psychology
  (S in VIPS framework) 283, 291–3
social exclusion 48
  account of 58–9
  functional mental illness 194
social history, depression 181
social inclusion 48–9, 291
social interventions, depression 185
social role, having a 58
social services, future needs 368
South East London Care Homes
  Support Team 227, 232
South West Yorkshire continuing
  care team 231, 232
Spain
  age distribution of residents 136
  balance of care (home vs care home) 134
  gender distribution of residents 138
  private vs public providers in 140, 141
SPECAL (Specialized Early Care for
  Alzheimer's) 212
specialist (secondary) care 227–34
  dementia 173, 260, 273, 320
  innovations 229–33
  see also nurse specialists
spending down of assets 93–5
sports memorabilia 47
spouse (in care home)
  carers account of 13–20
  negative beliefs see negative beliefs
staff/workers/workforce 327–44, 367
  abuse by 118–20
    causes/contributing factors 118, 120
    challenged by new members 119
    with inadequate staffing levels 127–8
    management 124–8
  carer's observations 18
  communication with residents see
    communication
  controlling environment (in risk
    management) 318
  dementia care 173, 327–44
    Malignant Social Psychology (MSP) 292–3
  depression detected by 183
  fear of blame for death 269
  future perspectives 367, 370
  GP relationship with, with
    infrequent visits 223
  keeping them fit for purpose (in My Home
    Life themes) 345, 346, 357–8
  male residents and 239
  manager's account 22–3
  regulatory requirements relating to 79
  resident's view 11
  role and nature of workforce 367
  stress or burnout 215, 285, 354
  support of 305
    in end-of-life care 273–4
  training see training

in VIPS framework 285–6
  valuing 284, 285–6
  see also multidisciplinary team
stakeholders, informing them of service
  performance 72
standards for quality and safety 75–9
statin drugs 259
stigmatization 31
  countering 32, 348
  dementia 42, 58
  gay men and women 244
  male residents 239
  tardive dyskinesia 200
Stockport Dementia Care Training 340–1
stress, staff 215, 285
subjective experience of living in a care home
  (incl. people with dementia) 57–80
  assessing 57–60
  personal accounts
    carers see carers
    manager 21–7
    resident 9–12
suicide
  depression and 187
  male residents 240
support services see services
Surr, CA 58–9
swallowing difficulties at end-of-life 267
Sweden
  age distribution of residents 136, 137
  balance of care (home vs
    care home) 133, 134
  gender distribution of residents 138
  private vs public providers in 140, 141
  small institutional units dementia
    patients 139
  teaching care homes 357
Switzerland
  age distribution of residents 136
  balance of care (home vs care home) 134
  gender distribution of residents 138
  private vs public providers in 141
Szczepura review 230–1, 303, 304, 305

Talking Mats 47, 57, 353
tardive dyskinesia 200
teaching care homes 228, 357
team
  dementia training 337–9
  multidisciplinary see
    multidisciplinary team
temperature measurement, core 255
terminal illness 266
  see also end-of-life
tertiary prevention of abuse 121
thematic inspection (in 100 care
  homes study) 283
time in care and depression 182
touch (physical contact) 17, 18

training and education 228, 234,
    305–6, 327–44, 367
  dementia care 150, 173, 327–44
    addressing needs 335–6
    barriers 336–7
    importance 328–9
    knowledge and its lack 331–3
    manager's own experiences 24
    methods 335
    organizational issues 337–8
    readiness to learn 330–1
    reality-based 329–30, 334–5
    skills development 334–5
  depression detection and treatment 184
  future needs 367
  manager's view of 23
  in *My* Home Life themes 357
  in VIPS framework 284
  see also teaching care homes
transformation in *My* Home Life
    themes 345, 346, 357–8
transgender residents 243–5, 246
transition to living in a care home
  managing 152
    in *My* Home Life 346, 355
    role of informal carers 152
  psychological adjustment 214–16
treats for staff 286

Ukraine, balance of care (home vs care home) 134
understanding *see* knowledge and
    understanding
United Kingdom
  age distribution of residents 136
  balance of care (home vs care home) 133, 134
  private vs public providers in 141
  see also England; Scotland
urinary incontinence, dementia patients 167
urinary tract infections 261

validation, in VIPS framework 291
validation therapy 170, 211–12, 336

valuing (V in VIPS framework) 283, 284
  staff 284, 285–6
Van Spyk, Peter, poem by 35–6
vascular dementia (in cerebrovascular
    disease) 162
  account of being diagnosed with 42–3
video recording, assessment using 56
VIPS framework, person-centred care 283–94
'virus', abuse as a 119
vision, care home (in VIPS framework) 283
visits by carers to care home
  carer's account 16, 17
    looking for a home 14, 15
    seeing other residents with no visitors 18
  resident's view 10
vital signs assessment 255
vulnerability 366–7
  to abuse 116–17, 120
  see also risk; safety

Wallace, Dr Daphne, diagnosed with vascular
    dementia 42–3
Wanless Social Care Review 93
warmth (towards residents) in VIPS
    framework 291
weight
  gain on admission 259
  loss, causes 258
well-being (physical and mental)
  factors impacting on sense of 56, 58
  promoting *see* promoting health and well-being
Wieczorek, Jacqueline (librarian), on creative
    writing project 38
Williams, May (resident) 280–3
wishes and feelings (individual's), best interests
    and weight given to 105–6
women
  gay 243–5, 246
  as majority in care homes 238
  men socializing with 240
workforce *see* staff
writing, creative 29–39